IARC Handbooks of Cancer Prevention

Volume 2

Carotenoids

Erratum

Please replace the legend following Figure 7 on page 234 by the following:

Figure 7. The antimutagenicity profile displays the performance of β-carotene to modulate mutagen-induced genetic and related effects. The profile contains quantitative results from the data in Tables 53-55 and is organized using chemical abbreviations and test codes to identify each item on the profile. The abbreviations mark the initial occurrence of each mutagen and all tests as labeled across the x-axis. In the upper panel doses are plotted in molar units for both the mutagens and β-carotene. In the lower panel positive values are the maximum percent inhibition of the mutagen-induced effects, negative values are the maximum percent enhancement of the effects, and values equal to zero indicate that no significant differences were observed relative to the mutagen-induced effects. A brief description of the anti-mutagenicity profile methodology and test code definitions are given in the appendices. Chemicals abbreviated here are: ADR, adriamycin; AfB_1, aflatoxin B_1; BP, benzo[*a*]pyrene; BLM, bleomycin; CPA, cyclophosphamide; DENA, diethyl-nitrosamine; DMBA, 7,12-dimethylbenz[*a*]anthracene; ENU, *N*-ethyl-*N*-nitrosourea; GA, gallic acid; HP, hydrogen peroxide; MCA, 3-methylcholanthrene; MMC mitomycin C; MMS, methylmethane sulfonate; MNNG, *N*-methyl-*N'*-nitro-*N*-nitrosoguanidine; MNU, *N*-methyl-*N*-nitrosourea; MOP, 8-methoxypsoralen + UV–A; MYL, myleran; 2NF, 2-nitrofluorene; 3NFA, 3-nitrofluoranthene; NO, nitric oxide; 1NP, 1-nitropyrene; NQO, 4-nitroquinoline 1-oxide; TA, tannic acid; Trp-P-1, 3-Amino-3,4-dimethyl-5H-pyrido[4,3-b]indole.

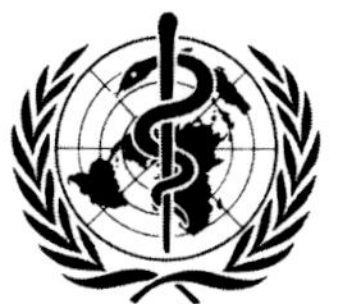

WORLD HEALTH ORGANIZATION

INTERNATIONAL AGENCY FOR RESEARCH ON CANCER

IARC Handbooks of Cancer Prevention

Volume 3

Vitamin A

This publication represents the views and expert opinions
of an IARC Working Group on the
Evaluation of Cancer-preventive Agents,
which met in Lyon,

13 – 19 May 1998

1998

Published by the International Agency for Research on Cancer,
150 cours Albert Thomas, F-69372 Lyon cedex 08, France

Distributed by Oxford University Press, Walton Street, Oxford, OX2 6DP, UK (Fax: +44 1865 267782) and in the USA by Oxford University Press, 2001 Evans Road, Carey, NC 27513, USA (Fax: +1 919 677 1303).
All IARC publications can also be ordered directly from IARC*Press*
(Fax: +33 4 72 73 83 02; E-mail: press@iarc.fr).

IARC Library Cataloguing in Publication Data

Vitamin A/
IARC Working Group on the Evaluation of
Cancer Preventive Agents (1998 : Lyon, France)

(IARC handbooks of cancer prevention ; 3)

1. Vitamin A – congresses. I. IARC Working Group on the Evaluation of Cancer Preventive Agents II Series

ISBN 92 832 3003 5 (NLM Classification: W1)
ISSN 1027-5622

Printed in France

International Agency For Research On Cancer

The International Agency for Research on Cancer (IARC) was established in 1965 by the World Health Assembly, as an independently financed organization within the framework of the World Health Organization. The headquarters of the Agency are in Lyon, France.

The Agency conducts a programme of research concentrating particularly on the epidemiology of cancer and the study of potential carcinogens in the human environment. Its field studies are supplemented by biological and chemical research carried out in the Agency's laboratories in Lyon and, through collaborative research agreements, in national research institutions in many countries. The Agency also conducts a programme for the education and training of personnel for cancer research.

The publications of the Agency contribute to the dissemination of authoritative information on different aspects of cancer research. A complete list is printed at the back of this book. Information about IARC publications, and how to order them, is also available via the Internet at: **http://www.iarc.fr/**

Note to the Reader

Anyone who is aware of published data that may influence any consideration in these *Handbooks* is encouraged to make the information available to the Unit of Chemoprevention, International Agency for Research on Cancer, 150 Cours Albert Thomas, 69372 Lyon Cedex 08, France

Although all efforts are made to prepare the *Handbooks* as accurately as possible, mistakes may occur. Readers are requested to communicate any errors to the Unit of Chemoprevention, so that corrections can be reported in future volumes.

Acknowledgements

The Foundation for Promotion of Cancer Research, Japan, is gratefully acknowledged for its generous support to the meeting of the Working Group and the production of this volume of the *IARC Handbooks of Cancer Prevention.*

Contents

List of participants

Volume 3. Vitamin A

Lyon, 13–19 May 1998

W. S. Blaner
Hammer Health Sciences Building
Department of Medicine
Columbia University
701 West 168th Street
New York, NY 10032
USA

T. Byers *(Chairman)*
Department of Preventive Medicine & Biometrics
University of Colorado
School of Medicine
Box C245
4200 East Ninth Avenue
Denver, CO 80262
USA

J.A. Crowell
Chemoprevention Branch
Division of Cancer Prevention and Control
National Institutes of Health
National Cancer Institute
Bethesda, MD 20892
USA

M.I. Dawson
SRI International
333 Ravenswood Avenue
Menlo Park,CA 94025
USA

S. De Flora
Institute of Hygiene and Preventive Medicine
University of Genoa
Via A. Pastore 1
I-16132 Genoa
Italy

N. De Vries
Department of Otolaryngology
Saint Lucas - Andreas Hospital
Jan Tooropstraat 164
1016 AE Amsterdam
The Netherlands

L.O. Dragsted
Institute of Food Safety and Toxicology
Morhoj Bygade 19
DK 2860 Soborg
Denmark

S. Franceschi
Epidemiology Unit
Aviano Cancer Centre
Via Pedemontana Occidentale 12
33081 Aviano PN
Italy

D.J. Hunter
Harvard School of Public Health and Channing Laboratory
Boston, MA 02115
USA

C. IJsselmuiden
Department of Community Health
University of Pretoria
PO Box 667
Pretoria 0001
South Africa

R. Lotan
Department of Tumor Biology
University of Texas
M.D. Anderson Cancer Center
1515 Holcombe Boulevard
Houston, TX 77030
USA

R. Mehta
The University of Illinois at Chicago
Department of Surgical Oncology
Clinical Sciences Building
840 South Wood Street (m/c 820)
Chicago, IL 60912-7322
USA

J.O. Moskaug
Institute for Nutrition Research
University of Oslo
PO Box 1046
Blindern
N 0316 Oslo

H. Nau
Department of Food Toxicology
Centre of Food Sciences
School of Veterinary Medicine Hannover
Bischofsholer Damm15
D-30173 Hannover
Germany

P. Nettesheim
National Institute of Environmental Health Sciences
Research Triangle Park, NC 27709
USA

J.A. Olson
Iowa State University
Biochemistry and Biophysics Department
Ames, IA 50011
USA

D.I. Thurnham *(Vice-Chairman)*
Northern Ireland Centre for Diet and Health
University of Ulster
Coleraine, County Londonderry
BT52 1SA
Northern Ireland

H. Tsuda
National Cancer Center Research Institute
Experimental Pathology and Chemotherapy Division
5-1-1 Tsukiji
Chuo-ku
Tokyo 104-0045
Japan

A. Woodward
Wellington School of Medicine
University of Otago
PO Box 7343
Wellington South
New Zealand

R.A. Woutersen
TNO-Nutrition and Food Research Institute
Toxicology Division
PO Box 360
3700 AJ Zeist
The Netherlands

Observers:

U. Wiegand
Hoffmann-La Roche Ltd
CH-4070 Basel
Switzerland

Secretariat:

J. Cheney *(Editor)*
V. Krutovskikh
C. Malaveille
H. Ohshima
B. Pignatelli
M. Rautalahti
R. Sankaranarayanan
P. Toniolo
H. Vainio *(Responsible Officer)*
A.L. Van Kappel-Dufour
J. Wilbourn

Technical Assistance:

M. Lézère
A. Meneghel
D. Mietton
J. Mitchell
S. Reynaud
S. Ruiz
J. Thévenoux

Abbreviations

ALAT	Alanine aminotransferase
apoB48	Apolipoprotein B-48
apo-RBP	Unbound retinol-binding protein
apoE	Apolipoprotein E
ARAT	Acyl-coenzyme A:retinol acyltransferase
AUC	Area under the concentration-time curve
BBN	*N*-Butyl-*N*-(4-hydroxybutyl)-nitrosamine
BCC	Basal cell carcinoma
bFGF	Basic fibroblast growth factor
BP	Benzo[*a*]pyrene
BPV	Bovine papillomavirus
CARET	Beta-Carotene and Retinol Efficacy Trial
CETP	Cholesteryl ester transfer protein
CHD	Coronary heart disease
CHEL	Chinese hamster epithelial liver
CHO	Chinese hamster ovary
CI	95% Confidence interval
CIN	Cervical intraepithelial neoplasia
CRABP	Cellular retinoic acid-binding protein
CralBP	Cellular retinal-binding protein
CRBP	Cellular retinol-binding proteins
CSF	Colony-stimulating factor
CYP	Cytochrome P450
DEN	*N*-Nitrosodiethylamine
DMBA	7,12-Dimethylbenz[*a*]anthracene*
DPT	Diphtheria/pertussis/tetanus
EGF	Epidermal growth factor
FANFT	*N*-[4-(5-Nitro-2-furyl)-2-thiazolyl]-formamide
αFGF	α-Fibroblast growth factor
GGT	γ-Glutamyltranspeptidase
HDL	High-density lipoprotein
HGPRT	Hypoxanthine phosphoribosyl transferase
HIV	Human immunodeficiency virus
Holo-RBP	Retinol–RBP complex
4-HP	*N*-(4-Hydroxyphenyl)retinamide
HPLC	High-performance liquid chromatography
14-HRR	14-Hydroxy-4,14-retro-retinol
HSPG	Heparin sulfate proteoglycans
IR	Infrared
IRBP	Interphotoreceptor retinol-binding protein
IU	International unit
LD_{50}	Dose that is lethal to 50% of individuals
LDL	Low-density lipoprotein
LDL-R	Low-density lipoprotein receptor
LPL	Lipoprotein lipase
LRAT	Lecithin:retinol acyltransferase
LRP	LDL receptor-related protein
LSR	Lipolysis-stimulated receptor
MCA	3-Methylcholanthrene
MNNG	*N*-Methyl-*N′*-nitro-*N*-nitroso-guanidine
MNU	*N*-Methyl-*N*-nitrosourea
MRDR	Modified relative dose response
NK	Natural killer
NMR	Nuclear magnetic resonance
ODC	Ornithine decarboxylase
PASI	Psoriasis Area and Severity Index
PDGF	Platelet-derived growth factor
RAP	Receptor-associated protein
RAR	Retinoic acid receptor
RARE	Retinoic acid response element
RBP	Retinol-binding protein
RDA	Recommended dietary allowance
RDR	Relative dose response
RE	Retinol equivalents
RPE	Retinal pigment epithelium
RR	Relative risk
RXR	Retinoid X receptor
SCC	Squamous cell carcinoma
SCE	Sister chromatid exchanges
SCID	Severe combined immunodeficient
TGF	Transforming growth factor
TNF	Tumour necrosis factor
TPA	12-*O*-Tetradecanoylphorbol 13-acetate
TTR	Transthyretin
UDS	Unscheduled DNA synthesis
UNICEF	United Nations Children's Fund
UV	Ultraviolet
VLDL	Very low-density lipoprotein

*Alternative nomenclature: 9,12-dimethyl-1,2-benzanthracene

Preamble to the *IARC Handbooks of Cancer Prevention*

The prevention of cancer is one of the key objectives of the International Agency for Research on Cancer (IARC). This may be achieved by avoiding exposures to known cancer-causing agents, by increasing host defences through immunization or chemoprevention or by modifying lifestyle. The aim of the *IARC Monographs* programme is to evaluate carcinogenic risks of human exposure to chemical, physical and biological agents, providing a scientific basis for national or international decisions on avoidance of exposures. The aim of the series of *IARC Handbooks of Cancer Prevention* is to evaluate scientific information on agents and interventions that may reduce the incidence of or mortality from cancer. This preamble is divided into two parts. The first addresses the general scope, objectives and structure of the *Handbooks*. The second describes the procedures for evaluating cancer-preventive agents.

Part One

Scope

Cancer-preventive strategies embrace chemical, immunological, dietary and behavioural interventions that may retard, block or reverse carcinogenic processes or reduce underlying risk factors. The term 'chemoprevention' is used to refer to interventions with pharmaceuticals, vitamins, minerals and other chemicals to reduce cancer incidence. The *IARC Handbooks* address the efficacy, safety and mechanisms of cancer-preventive strategies and the adequacy of the available data, including those on timing, dose, duration and indications for use.

Preventive strategies can be applied across a continuum of: (1) the general population; (2) subgroups with particular predisposing host or environmental risk factors, including genetic susceptibility to cancer; (3) persons with precancerous lesions; and (4) cancer patients at risk for second primary tumours. Use of the same strategies or agents in the treatment of cancer patients to control the growth, metastasis and recurrence of tumours is considered to be patient management, not prevention, although data from clinical trials may be relevant when making a *Handbooks* evaluation.

Objective

The objective of the *Handbooks* programme is the preparation of critical reviews and evaluations of evidence for cancer-prevention and other relevant properties of a wide range of potential cancer-preventive agents and strategies by international working groups of experts. The resulting *Handbooks* may also indicate where additional research is needed.

The *Handbooks* may assist national and international authorities in devising programmes of health promotion and cancer prevention and in making benefit–risk assessments. The evaluations of IARC working groups are scientific judgements about the available evidence for cancer-preventive efficacy and safety. No recommendation is given with regard to national and international regulation or legislation, which are the responsibility of individual governments and/or other international authorities. No recommendations for specific research trials are made.

IARC Working Groups

Reviews and evaluations are formulated by international working groups of experts convened by the IARC. The tasks of each group are: (1) to ascertain that all appropriate data have been collected; (2) to select the data relevant for the evaluation on the basis of scientific merit; (3) to prepare accurate summaries of the data to enable the reader to follow the reasoning of the Working Group; (4) to evaluate the significance of the available data from human studies and experimental models on cancer-preventive activity, carcinogenicity and other beneficial and adverse effects; and (5) to evaluate data relevant to the understanding of mechanisms of action.

Working Group participants who contributed to the considerations and evaluations within a particular *Handbook* are listed, with their addresses, at the beginning of each publication. Each participant serves as an individual scientist and not as a representative of any organization, government or industry. In addition, scientists nominated by national and international agencies, industrial associations and consumer and/or environmental organizations may be invited as observers. IARC staff involved in the preparation of the *Handbooks* are listed.

Working procedures

Approximately 13 months before a working group meets, the topics of the *Handbook* are announced, and participants are selected by IARC staff in consultation with other experts. Subsequently, relevant clinical, experimental and human data are collected by the IARC from all available sources of published information. Representatives of producer or consumer associations may assist in the preparation of sections on production and use, as appropriate.

About eight months before the meeting, the material collected is sent to meeting participants to prepare sections for the first drafts of the *Handbooks*. These are then compiled by IARC staff and sent, before the meeting, to all participants of the Working Group for review. There is an opportunity to return the compiled specialized sections of the draft to the experts, inviting preliminary comments, before the complete first-draft document is distributed to all members of the Working Group.

Data for *Handbooks*

The *Handbooks* do not necessarily cite all of the literature on the agent or strategy being evaluated. Only those data considered by the Working Group to be relevant to making the evaluation are included. In principle, meeting abstracts and other reports that do not provide sufficient detail upon which to base an assessment of their quality are not considered.

With regard to data from toxicological, epidemiological and experimental studies and from clinical trials, only reports that have been published or accepted for publication in the openly available scientific literature are reviewed by the Working Group. In certain instances, government agency reports that have undergone peer review and are widely available are considered. Exceptions may be made on an ad-hoc basis to include unpublished reports that are in their final form and publicly available, if their inclusion is considered pertinent to making a final evaluation. In the sections on chemical and physical properties, on production, on use, on analysis and on human exposure, unpublished sources of information may be used.

The available studies are summarized by the Working Group, with particular regard to the qualitative aspects discussed below. In general, numerical findings are indicated as they appear in the original report; units are converted when necessary for easier comparison. The Working Goup may conduct additional analyses of the published data and use them in their assesment of the evidence; the results of such supplementary analyses are given in square brackets. When an important aspect of a study, directly impinging on its interpretation, should be brought to the attention of the reader, a comment is given in square brackets.

Criteria for selection of topics for evaluation

Agents, classes of agents and interventions to be evaluated in the *Handbooks* are selected on the basis of one or more of the following criteria.

- The available evidence suggests potential for significantly reducing the incidence of cancers.
- There is a substantial body of human, experimental, clinical and/or mechanistic data suitable for evaluation.
- The agent is in widespread use and of putative protective value, but of uncertain efficacy and safety.
- The agent shows exceptional promise in experimental studies but has not been used in humans.
- The agent is available for further studies of human use.

Outline of data presentation scheme for evaluating cancer-preventive agents

1. Chemical and physical characteristics

2. Occurrence, production, use, analysis and human exposure

- 2.1 Occurrence
- 2.2 Production
- 2.3 Use
- 2.4 Analysis
- 2.5 Human exposure

3. Metabolism, kinetics and genetic variation

- 3.1 Human studies
- 3.2 Experimental models

4. Cancer-preventive effects

- 4.1 Human studies
  - 4.1.1 Epidemiology studies
  - 4.1.2 Intervention trials
  - 4.1.3 Intermediate end-points
- 4.2 Experimental models
  - 4.2.1 Tumour induction
  - 4.2.2 Intermediate biomarkers
  - 4.2.3 *In-vitro* models
- 4.3 Mechanisms of cancer-prevention

5. Other beneficial effects

6. Carcinogenicity

- 6.1 Human studies
- 6.2 Experimental models

7. Other toxic effects

- 7.1 Adverse effects
  - 7.1.1 Human studies
  - 7.1.2 Experimental studies
- 7.2 Reproductive and developmental effects
  - 7.2.1 Human studies
  - 7.2.2 Experimental studies
- 7.3 Genetic and related effects
  - 7.3.1 Human studies
  - 7.3.2 Experimental studies

8. Summary of data

- 8.1 Chemistry, occurrence and human exposure
- 8.2 Metabolism and kinetic properties
- 8.3 Cancer-preventive effects
  - 8.3.1 Human studies
  - 8.3.2 Experimental studies
  - 8.3.3 Mechanisms of cancer-prevention
- 8.4 Other beneficial effects
- 8.5 Carcinogenic effects
  - 8.5.1 Human studies
  - 8.5.2 Experimental animals
- 8.6 Toxic effects
  - 8.6.1 Human studies
  - 8.6.2 Experimental studies

9. Recommendations for research

10. Evaluation

- 10.1 Cancer-preventive activity
  - 10.1.1 Humans
  - 10.1.2 Experimental animals
- 10.2 Overall evaluation

11. References

Part Two

Evaluation of cancer-preventive agents

A wide range of findings must be taken into account before a particular agent can be recognized as preventing cancer. On the basis of experience from the *IARC Monographs* programme, a systematized approach to data presentation is adopted for *Handbooks* evaluations.

1. Chemical and physical characteristics of the agent

The Chemical Abstracts Services Registry Number, the latest Chemical Abstracts Primary Name, the IUPAC Systematic Name and other definitive information (such as genus and species of plants) are given as appropriate. Information on chemical and physical properties and, in particular, data relevant to identification, occurrence and biological activity are included. A description of technical products of chemicals includes trade names, relevant specifications and available information on composition and impurities. Some of the trade names given may be those of mixtures in which the agent being evaluated is only one of the ingredients.

2. Occurrence, production, use, analysis and human exposure

2.1 Occurrence

Information on the occurrence of an agent or mixture in the environment is obtained from data derived from the monitoring and surveillance of levels in occupational environments, air, water, soil, foods and animal and human tissues. When available, data on the generation, persistence and bioaccumulation of the agent are included. For mixtures, information is given about all agents present.

2.2 Production

The dates of first synthesis and of first commercial production of a chemical or mixture are provided; for agents that do not occur naturally, this information may allow a reasonable estimate to be made of the date before which no human use of, or exposure to, the agent could have occurred. The dates of first reported occurrence of an exposure are also provided. In addition, methods of synthesis used in past and present commercial production and methods of production that may give rise to different impurities are described.

2.3 Use

Data on production, international trade and uses and applications are obtained for representative regions. Some identified uses may not be current or major applications, and the coverage is not necessarily comprehensive. In the case of drugs, mention of their therapeutic applications does not necessarily represent current practice, nor does it imply judgement as to their therapeutic efficacy.

2.4 Analysis

An overview of current methods of analysis or detection is presented. Methods for monitoring human exposure are also given, when available.

2.5 Human exposure

Human uses of, or exposure to, the agent are described. If an agent is used as a prescribed or over-the-counter pharmaceutical product, then the type of person receiving the product in terms of health status, age, sex and medical condition being treated are described. For nonpharmaceutical agents, particularly those taken because of cultural traditions, the characteristics of use or exposure and the relevant populations are described. In all cases, quantitative data, such as dose–response relationships, are considered to be of special importance.

3. Metabolism, kinetics and genetic variation

In evaluating the potential utility of a suspected cancer-preventive agent or strategy, a number of different properties, in addition to direct effects upon cancer incidence, are described and weighed. Furthermore, as many of the data leading to an evaluation are expected to come from studies in experimental animals, information that facilitates interspecies extrapolation is particularly important; this includes metabolic, kinetic and genetic data. Whenever possible, quantitative data, including information on dose, duration and potency, are considered.

Information is given on absorption, distribution (including placental transfer), metabolism and excretion in humans and experimental animals. Kinetic properties within the target species may affect the interpretation and extrapolation of dose–response relationships, such as blood concentrations, protein binding, tissue concentrations, plasma half-lives and elimination rates. Comparative information on the relationship between use or exposure and the dose that reaches the target site may be of particular importance for extrapolation between species. Studies that indicate the metabolic pathways and fate of the agent in humans and experimental animals are summarized, and data on humans and experimental animals are compared when possible. Observations are made on inter-individual variations and relevant metabolic polymorphisms. Data indicating long-term accumulation in human tissues are included. Physiologically based pharmacokinetic models and their parameter values are relevant and are included whenever they are available. Information on the fate of the compound within tissues and cells (transport, role of cellular receptors, compartmentalization, binding to macromolecules) is given.

Genotyping will be used increasingly, not only to identify subpopulations at increased or decreased risk for cancers but also to characterize variation in the biotransformation of, and responses to, cancer-preventive agents.

This subsection can include effects of the compound on gene expression, enzyme induction or inhibition, or pro-oxidant status, when such data are not described elsewhere. It covers data obtained in humans and experimental animals, with particular attention to effects of long-term use and exposure.

4. Cancer-preventive effects

4.1 Human studies

Types of study considered. Human data are derived from experimental and non-experimental study designs and are focused on cancer, precancer or intermediate biological end-points. The experimental designs include randomized controlled trials and short-term experimental studies; non-experimental designs include cohort, case–control and cross-sectional studies.

Cohort and case–control studies relate individual use of, or exposure to, the agents under study to the occurrence of cancer in individuals and provide an estimate of relative risk (ratio of incidence or mortality in those exposed to incidence or mortality in those not exposed) as the main measure of association. Cohort and case–control studies follow an observational approach, in which the use of, or exposure to, the agent is not controlled by the investigator.

Intervention studies are experimental in design — that is, the use of, or exposure to, the agent is assigned by the investigator. The intervention study or clinical trial is the design that can provide the strongest and most direct evidence of a protective or preventive effect; however, for practical and ethical reasons, such studies are limited to observation of the effects among specifically defined study subjects of interventions of 10 years or fewer, which is relatively short when compared with the overall lifespan.

Intervention studies may be undertaken in individuals or communities and may or may not involve randomization to use or exposure. The differences between these designs is important in relation to analytical methods and interpretation of findings.

In addition, information can be obtained from reports of correlation (ecological) studies and case series; however, limitations inherent in these approaches usually mean that such studies carry limited weight in the evaluation of a preventive effect.

Quality of studies considered. The *Handbooks* are not intended to summarize all published studies. It is important that the Working Group consider the following aspects: (1) the relevance of the study; (2) the appropriateness of the design and analysis to the question being asked; (3) the adequacy and completeness of the presentation of the data; and (4) the degree to which chance, bias and confounding may have affected the results.

Studies that are judged to be inadequate or irrelevant to the evaluation are generally omitted. They may be mentioned briefly, particularly when the information is considered to be a useful supplement to that in other reports or when it provides the only data available. Their inclusion does not imply acceptance of the adequacy of the study design, nor of the analysis and interpretation of the results, and their limitations are outlined.

Assessment of the cancer-preventive effect at different doses and durations. The Working Group gives special attention to quantitative assessment of the preventive effect of the agent under study, by assessing data from studies at different doses. The Working Group also addresses issues of timing and duration of use or exposure. Such quantitative assessment is important to clarify the circumstances under which a preventive effect can be achieved, as well as the dose at which a toxic effect has been shown.

Criteria for a cancer-preventive effect. After summarizing and assessing the individual studies, the Working Group makes a judgement concerning the evidence that the agent in question prevents cancer in humans. In making their judgement, the Working Group considers several criteria for each relevant cancer site.

Evidence of protection derived from intervention studies of good quality is particularly informative. Evidence of a substantial and significant reduction in risk, including a dose–response relationship, is more likely to indicate a real effect. Nevertheless, a small effect, or an effect without a dose–response relationship, does not imply lack of real benefit and may be important for public health if the cancer is common.

Evidence is frequently available from different types of study and is evaluated as a whole. Findings that are replicated in several studies of the same design or using different approaches are more likely to provide evidence of a true protective effect than isolated observations from single studies.

The Working Group evaluates possible explanations for inconsistencies across studies, including differences in use of, or exposure to, the agent, differences in the underlying risk of cancer and metabolism and genetic differences in the population.

The results of studies judged to be of high quality are given more weight. Note is taken of both the applicability of preventive action to several cancers and of possible differences in activity, including contradictory findings, across cancer sites.

Data from human studies (as well as from experimental models) that suggest plausible mechanisms for a cancer-preventive effect are important in assessing the overall evidence.

The Working Group may also determine whether, on aggregate, the evidence from human studies is consistent with a lack of preventive effect.

4.2 Experimental models

4.2.1 Experimental animals

Animal models are an important component of research into cancer prevention. They provide a means of identifying effective compounds, of carrying out fundamental investigations into their mechanisms of action, of determining how they can be used optimally, of evaluating toxicity and, ultimately, of providing an information base for developing intervention trials in humans. Models that permit evaluation of the effects of cancer-preventive agents on the occurrence of cancer in most major organ sites are available. Major groups of animal models include: those in which cancer is produced by the administration of chemical or physical carcinogens; those involving genetically engineered animals; and those in which tumours develop spontaneously. Most cancer-preventive agents investigated in such studies can be placed into one of three categories: compounds that prevent molecules from reaching or reacting with critical target sites (blocking agents); compounds that decrease the sensitivity of target tissues to carcinogenic stimuli; and compounds that prevent evolution of the neoplastic process (suppressing agents). There is increasing interest in the use of combinations of agents as a means of improving efficacy and minimizing toxicity. Animal models are useful in evaluating such combinations. The development of optimal strategies for human intervention trials can be facilitated by the use of animal models that mimic the neoplastic process in humans.

Specific factors to be considered in such experiments are: (1) the temporal requirements of administration of the cancer-preventive agents; (2) dose–response effects; (3) the site-specificity of cancer-preventive activity; and (4) the number and structural diversity of carcinogens whose activity can be reduced by the agent being evaluated.

An important variable in the evaluation of the cancer-preventive response is the time and the duration of administration of the agent in relation to any carcinogenic treatment, or in transgenic or other experimental models in which no carcinogen is administered. Furthermore, concurrent administration of a cancer-preventive agent may result in a decreased incidence of tumours in a given organ and an increase in another organ of the same animal. Thus, in these experiments it is important that multiple organs be examined.

For all these studies, the nature and extent of impurities or contaminants present in the cancer-preventive agent or agents being evaluated are given when available. For experimental studies of mixtures, consideration is given to the possibility of changes in the physicochemical properties of the test substance during collection, storage, extraction, concentration and delivery. Chemical and toxicological interactions of the components of mixtures may result in nonlinear dose–response relationships.

As certain components of commonly used diets of experimental animals are themselves known to have cancer-preventive activity, particular consideration should be given to the interaction between the diet and the apparent effect of the agent being studied. Likewise, restriction of diet may be important. The appropriateness of the diet given relative to the composition of human diets may be commented on by the Working Group.

Qualitative aspects. An assessment of the experimental prevention of cancer involves several considerations of qualitative importance, including: (1) the experimental conditions under which the test was performed (route and schedule of exposure, species, strain, sex and age of animals studied, duration of the exposure, and duration of the study); (2) the consistency of the results, for example across species and target organ(s); (3) the stage or stages of the neoplastic process, from preneoplastic lesions and benign tumours to malignant neoplasms, studied and (4) the possible role of modifying factors.

Considerations of importance to the Working Group in the interpretation and evaluation of a particular study include: (1) how clearly the agent was defined and, in the case of mixtures, how adequately the sample composition was reported; (2) the composition of the diet and the stability of the agent in the diet; (3) whether the source, strain and quality of the animals was reported; (4) whether the dose and schedule of treatment with the known carcinogen were appropriate in assays of combined treatment; (5) whether the doses of the cancer-preventive agent were adequately monitored; (6) whether the agent(s) was absorbed, as shown by blood concentrations; (7) whether the survival of treated animals was similar to that of controls; (8) whether the body and organ weights of treated animals were similar to those of controls; (9) whether there were adequate numbers of animals, of appropriate age, per group; (10) whether animals of each sex were used, if appropriate; (11) whether animals were allocated randomly to groups; (12) whether appropriate respective controls were used; (13) whether the duration of the experiment was adequate; (14) whether there was adequate statistical analysis; and (15) whether the data were adequately reported. If available, recent data on the incidence of specific tumours in historical controls, as well as in concurrent controls, are taken into account in the evaluation of tumour response.

Quantitative aspects. The probability that tumours will occur may depend on the species, sex, strain and age of the animals, the dose of carcinogen (if any), the dose of the agent and the route and duration of exposure. A decreased incidence and/or decreased multiplicity of neoplasms in adequately designed studies provides evidence of a cancer-preventive effect. A dose-related decrease in incidence and/or multiplicity further strengthens this association.

Statistical analysis. Major factors considered in the statistical analysis by the Working Group include the adequacy of the data for each treatment group: (1) the initial and final effective numbers of animals studied and the survival rate; (2) body weights; and (3) tumour incidence and multiplicity. The statistical methods used should be clearly stated and should be the generally accepted techniques refined for this purpose. In particular, the statistical methods should be appropriate for the characteristics of the expected data distribution and should account for interactions in multifactorial studies. Consideration is given as to whether the appropriate adjustment was made for differences in survival.

4.2.2 Intermediate biomarkers

Other types of study include experiments in which the end-point is not cancer but a defined preneoplastic lesion or tumour-related, intermediate biomarker.

The observation of effects on the occurrence of lesions presumed to be preneoplastic or the emergence of benign or malignant tumours may aid in assessing the mode of action of the presumed cancer-preventive agent. Particular attention is given to assessing the reversibility of these lesions and their predictive value in relation to cancer development.

4.2.3 In-vitro models

Cell systems *in vitro* contribute to the early identification of potential cancer-preventive agents and to elucidation of mechanisms of cancer prevention. A number of assays in prokaryotic and eukaryotic systems are used for this purpose. Evaluation of the results of such assays includes consideration of: (1) the nature of the cell type used; (2) whether primary cell cultures or cell lines (tumorigenic or nontumorigenic) were studied; (3) the appropriateness of controls; (4) whether toxic effects were considered in the outcome; (5) whether the data were appropriately summated and analysed; (6) whether appropriate quality controls were used; (7) whether appropriate concentration ranges were used; (8) whether adequate numbers of independent measurements were made per group; and (9) the relevance of the end-points, including inhibition of mutagenesis, morphological transformation, anchorage-independent growth, cell–cell communication, calcium tolerance and differentiation.

4.3 Mechanisms of cancer prevention

Data on mechanisms can be derived from both human studies and experimental models. For a rational implementation of cancer-preventive measures, it is essential not only to assess protective end-points but also to understand the mechanisms by which the agents exert their anticarcinogenic action. Information on the mechanisms of cancer-preventive activity can be inferred from relationships between chemical structure and biological activity, from analysis of interactions between agents and specific molecular targets, from studies of specific end-points *in vitro*, from studies of the inhibition of tumorigenesis *in vivo*, from the effects of modulating intermediate biomarkers, and from human studies. Therefore, the Working Group takes account of data on mechanisms in making the final evaluation of cancer prevention.

Several classifications of mechanisms have been proposed, as have several systems for evaluating them. Cancer-preventive agents may act at several distinct levels. Their action may be: (1) extracellular, for example, inhibiting the uptake or endogenous formation of carcinogens, or forming complexes with, diluting and/or deactivating carcinogens; (2) intracellular, for example, trapping carcinogens in non-target cells, modifying transmembrane transport, modulating metabolism, blocking reactive molecules, inhibiting cell replication or modulating gene expression or DNA metabolism; or (3) at the level of the cell, tissue or organism, for example, affecting cell differentiation, intercellular communication, proteases, signal transduction, growth factors, cell adhesion molecules, angiogenesis, interactions with the extracellular matrix, hormonal status and the immune system.

Many cancer-preventive agents are known or suspected to act by several mechanisms, which may operate in a coordinated manner and allow them a broader spectrum of anticarcinogenic activity. Therefore, multiple mechanisms of action are taken into account in the evaluation of cancer-prevention.

Beneficial interactions, generally resulting from exposure to inhibitors that work through complementary mechanisms, are exploited in combined cancer-prevention. Because organisms are naturally exposed not only to mixtures of carcinogenic agents but also to mixtures of protective agents, it is also important to understand the mechanisms of interactions between inhibitors.

5. Other beneficial effects

This section contains mainly background information on preventive activity; use is described in Section 2.3. An expanded description is given, when appropriate, of the efficacy of the agent in the maintenance of a normal healthy state and the treatment of particular diseases. Information on the mechanisms involved in these activities is described. Reviews, rather than individual studies, may be cited as references.

The physiological functions of agents such as vitamins and micronutrients can be described briefly, with reference to reviews. Data on the therapeutic effects of drugs approved for clinical use are summarized.

6. Carcinogenicity

Some agents may have both carcinogenic and anticarcinogenic activities. If the agent has been evaluated within the *IARC Monographs on the Evaluation of Carcinogenic Risks to Humans*, that evaluation is accepted, unless significant new data have appeared that may lead the Working Group to reconsider the evidence. When a re-evaluation is necessary or when no carcinogenic evaluation has been made, the procedures described in the Preamble to the *IARC Monographs on the Evaluation of Carcinogenic Risks to Humans* are adopted as guidelines.

7. Other toxic effects

Toxic effects are of particular importance in the case of agents that may be used widely over long periods in healthy populations. Data are given on acute and chronic toxic effects, such as organ toxicity, increased cell proliferation, immunotoxicity and adverse endocrine effects. If the agent occurs naturally or has been in clinical use previously, the doses and durations used in cancer-prevention trials are compared with intakes from the diet, in the case of vitamins, and previous clinical exposure, in the case of drugs already approved for human use. When extensive data are available, only summaries are presented; if adequate reviews are available, reference may be made to these. If there are no relevant reviews, the evaluation is made on the basis of the same criteria as are applied to epidemiological studies of cancer. Differences in response as a consequence of species, sex, age and genetic variability are presented when the information is available.

Data demonstrating the presence or absence of adverse effects in humans are included; equally, lack of data on specific adverse effects is stated clearly.

Findings in human and experimental studies are presented sequentially under the headings 'Adverse effects', 'Reproductive and developmental effects' and 'Genetic and related effects'.

The section 'Adverse effects' includes information on immunotoxicity, neurotoxicity, cardiotoxicity, haematological effects and toxicity to other target organs. Specific case reports in humans and any previous clinical data are noted. Other biochemical effects thought to be relevant to adverse effects are mentioned.

The section on 'Reproductive and developmental effects' includes effects on fertility, teratogenicity, foetotoxicity and embryotoxicity. Information from nonmammalian systems and *in vitro* are presented only if they have clear mechanistic significance.

The section 'Genetic and related effects' includes results from studies in mammalian and nonmammalian systems *in vivo* and *in vitro*. Information on whether DNA damage occurs via direct interaction with the agent or via indirect mechanisms (e.g. generation of free radicals) is included, as is information on other genetic effects such as mutation, recombination, chromosomal damage, aneuploidy, cell immortalization and transformation, and effects on cell–cell communication. The presence and toxicological significance of cellular receptors for the cancer-preventive agent are described.

The adequacy of epidemiological studies of toxic effects, including reproductive outcomes and genetic and related effects in humans, is evaluated by the same criteria as are applied to epidemiological studies of cancer. For each of these studies, the adequacy of the reporting of sample characterization is considered and, where necessary, commented upon. The available data are interpreted critically according to the end-points used. The doses and concentrations used are given, and, for experiments *in vitro*, mention is made of whether the presence of an exogenous metabolic system affected the observations. For studies *in vivo*, the route of administration and the formulation in which the agent was administered are included. The dosing regimens, including the duration of treatment, are also given. Genetic data are given as listings of test systems, data and references; bar graphs (activity profiles) and corresponding summary tables with detailed information on the preparation of genetic activity profiles are given in appendices. Genetic and other activity in humans and experimental mammals is regarded as being of greater relevance than that in other organisms. The *in-vitro* experiments providing these data must be carefully evaluated, since there are many trivial reasons why a response to one agent may be modified by the addition of another.

Structure–activity relationships that may be relevant to the evaluation of the toxicity of an agent are described.

Studies on the interaction of the suspected cancer-preventive agent with toxic and subtoxic doses of other substances are described, the objective being to determine whether there is inhibition or enhancement, additivity, synergism or potentiation of toxic effects over an extended dose range.

Biochemical investigations that may have a bearing on the mechanisms of toxicity and cancer-prevention are described. These are carefully evaluated for their relevance and the appropriateness of the results.

8. Summary of data

In this section, the relevant human and experimental data are summarized. Inadequate studies are generally not summarized; such studies, if cited, are identified in the preceding text.

8.1 Chemistry, occurrence and human exposure

Human exposure to an agent is summarized on the basis of elements that may include production, use, occurrence in the environment and determinations in human tissues and body fluids. Quantitative data are summarized when available.

8.2 Metabolism and kinetic properties

Data on metabolism and kinetic properties in humans and in experimental animals are given when these are considered relevant to the possible mechanisms of cancer-preventive, carcinogenic and toxic activity.

8.3 Cancer-preventive effects

8.3.1 Human studies

The results of relevant studies are summarized, including case reports and correlation studies when considered important.

8.3.2 Experimental studies

Data relevant to an evaluation of cancer-preventive activity in experimental models are summarized. For each animal species and route of administration, it is stated whether a change in the incidence of neoplasms or preneoplastic lesions was observed, and the tumour sites are indicated. Negative findings are also summarized. Dose– response relationships and other quantitative data may be given when available.

8.3.3 Mechanism of cancer-prevention

Data relevant to the mechanisms of cancer-preventive activity are summarized.

8.4 Other beneficial effects

When beneficial effects other than cancer prevention have been identified, the relevant data are summarized.

8.5 Carcinogenic effects

Normally, the agent will have been reviewed and evaluated within the *IARC Monographs* programme, and that summary is used with the inclusion of more recent data, if appropriate.

8.5.1 Human studies

The results of epidemiological studies that are considered to be pertinent to an assessment of human carcinogenicity are summarized. When relevant, case reports and correlation studies are also summarized.

8.5.2 Experimental animals

Data relevant to an evaluation of carcinogenic effects in animal models are summarized. For each animal species and route of administration, it is stated whether a change in the incidence of neoplasms or preneoplastic lesions was observed, and the tumour sites are indicated. Negative findings are also summarized. Dose–response relationships and other quantitative data may be mentioned when available.

8.6 Toxic effects

Adverse effects in humans are summarized, together with data on general toxicological effects and cytotoxicity, receptor binding and hormonal and immunological effects. The results of investigations on the reproductive, genetic and related effects are summarized. Toxic effects are summarized for whole animals, cultured mammalian cells and non-mammalian systems. When available, data for humans and for animals are compared.

Structure–activity relationships are mentioned when relevant to toxicity.

9. Recommendations for research

During the evaluation process, it is likely that opportunities for further research will be identified. These are clearly stated, with the understanding that the areas are recommended for future investigation. It is made clear that these research opportunities are identified in general terms on the basis of the data currently available.

10. Evaluation

Evaluations of the strength of the evidence for cancer-preventive activity and carcinogenic effects from studies in humans and experimental models are made, using standard terms. These terms may also be applied to other beneficial and adverse effects, when indicated. When appropriate, reference is made to specific organs and populations.

It is recognized that the criteria for these evaluation categories, described below, cannot encompass all factors that may be relevant to an evaluation of cancer-preventive activity. In considering all the relevant scientific data, the Working Group may assign the agent or other intervention to a higher or lower category than a strict interpretation of these criteria would indicate.

10.1 Cancer-preventive activity

The evaluation categories refer to the strength of the evidence that an agent prevents cancer. The evaluations may change as new information becomes available.

Evaluations are inevitably limited to the cancer sites, conditions and levels of exposure and length of observation covered by the available studies. An evaluation of degree of evidence, whether for a single agent or a mixture, is limited to the materials tested, as defined physically, chemically or biologically. When the agents evaluated are considered by the Working Group to be sufficiently closely related, they may be grouped for the purpose of a single evaluation of degree of evidence.

Information on mechanisms of action is taken into account when evaluating the strength of evidence in humans and in experimental animals, as well as in assessing the consistency of results between studies in humans and experimental models.

10.1.1 Cancer-preventive activity in humans

The evidence relevant to cancer prevention in humans is classified into one of the following categories.

- *Sufficient evidence of cancer-preventive activity*
  The Working Group considers that a causal relationship has been established between use of the agent and the prevention of human cancer in studies in which chance, bias and confounding could be ruled out with reasonable confidence.
- *Limited evidence of cancer-preventive activity*
  The data suggest a reduced risk for cancer with use of the agent but are limited for making a definitive evaluation either because chance, bias or confounding could not be ruled out with reasonable confidence or because the data are restricted to intermediary biomarkers of uncertain validity in the putative pathway to cancer.
- *Inadequate evidence of cancer-preventive activity*
  The available studies are of insufficient quality, consistency or statistical power to permit a conclusion regarding a cancer-preventive effect of the agent, or no data on the prevention of cancer in humans are available.
- *Evidence suggesting lack of cancer-preventive activity*
  Several adequate studies of use or exposure are mutually consistent in not showing a preventive effect.

The strength of the evidence for any carcinogenic effect is assessed in parallel.

Both cancer-preventive activity and carcinogenic effects are identified and, when appropriate, tabulated by organ site. The evaluation also cites the population subgroups concerned, specifying age, sex, genetic or environmental predisposing risk factors and the relevance of precancerous lesions.

10.1.2 Cancer-preventive activity in experimental animals

Evidence for cancer prevention in experimental animals is classified into one of the following categories.

- *Sufficient evidence of cancer-preventive activity*
  The Working Group considers that a causal relationship has been established between the agent and a decreased incidence and/or multiplicity of neoplasms.
- *Limited evidence of cancer-preventive activity*
  The data suggest a cancer-preventive effect but are limited for making a definitive evaluation because, for example, the evidence of cancer prevention is restricted to a single experiment, the agent decreases the incidence and/or multiplicity only of benign neoplasms or lesions of uncertain neoplastic potential or there is conflicting evidence.
- *Inadequate evidence of cancer-preventive activity*
  The studies cannot be interpreted as showing either the presence or absence of a preventive effect because of major qualitative or quantitative limitations (unresolved questions regarding the adequacy of the design, conduct or interpretation of the study), or no data on cancer prevention in experimental animals are available.
- *Evidence suggesting lack of cancer-preventive activity*
  Adequate evidence from conclusive studies in several models shows that, within the limits of the tests used, the agent does not prevent cancer.

10.2 Overall evaluation

Finally, the body of evidence is considered as a whole, and summary statements are made that encompass the effects of the agents in humans with regard to cancer-preventive activity, carcinogenic effects and other beneficial and adverse effects, as appropriate.

General Remarks

Introduction and definitions

In much of the scientific literature on nutrition, 'vitamin A' is used as a generic term referring to both preformed vitamin A (largely all-trans-retinol and its esters) and some of the carotenoids. This Handbook, the third in the IARC series of *Handbooks of Cancer Prevention*, focuses on the cancer-preventive effects of the preformed vitamin A compounds, principally retinol and retinyl esters. Volume 2 of the series reviewed the carotenoids (IARC, 1998) and the forthcoming Volume 4 will review in detail retinoic acid, metabolites of retinol and related synthetic retinoid compounds. The full scientific terminology, common abbreviated names and relevant general terms used to describe both individual compounds and broad classes of vitamin A compounds are summarized in Table 1.

Compounds in the vitamin A, or retinol, family, as defined by the International Union of Pure and Applied Chemistry/International Union of Biology (IUPAC-IUB) Joint Commission on Biochemical Nomenclature, belong to a class derived from four isoprenoid units joined in a head-to-tail manner to produce a monocyclic parent having five carbon–carbon double bonds and a functional group at the acyclic terminus. The parent compound in preformed vitamin A, from which retinal and retinyl esters are derived, is all-*trans*-retinol (hereinafter referred to as retinol). The structures, physical properties and sources of retinol, retinyl esters, retinal and retinoic acid are listed in Section 1 of this Handbook.

Many of the significant discoveries in chemistry and biology that have led to our understanding of the critical roles in nutrition played by retinol, retinal, retinoic acid and their analogues, have been thoroughly reviewed (Moore, 1957; Tee, 1992; Blomhoff, 1994; Sporn *et al.*, 1994). In 1913, McCollum and Davies as well as, independently, Osborne and Mendel identified a lipid-soluble dietary factor needed for the growth of rats. It was later termed 'fat-soluble A'. In 1931, Karrer and co-workers determined

Table 1. Nomenclature of vitamin A compounds

Full name	Common abbreviated names	Included in class known as:		
		'Preformed vitamin A'	'Vitamin A precursors'	'Total vitamin A'
All-*trans*-retinol	Retinol	Yes		Yes
All-*trans*-retinol palmitate	Retinyl palmitate	Yes		Yes
All-*trans*-retinol acetate	Retinyl acetate[a]	Yes		Yes
Provitamin A carotenoids [b]			Yes	Yes
All-*trans*-retinal	Retinal, retinaldehyde[c]			
All-*trans*-retinoic acid	Retinoic acid			
9-*cis*-Retinoic acid	9-*cis*-Retinoic acid			
Other natural metabolites				
Retinoid[d]				
Synthetic retinoids[e]				

[a] Retinyl acetate is a usable form of preformed vitamin A, but it is found in only small amounts in the diet.
[b] Carotenoids that are metabolized to retinol in vivo. In the diet, these are largely α- and β-carotene and β-cryptoxanthin.
[c] The term retinaldehyde is used in this volume only if confusion could occur with the adjective 'retinal' relating to the retina of the eye.
[d] A member of the vitamin A family the structure of which is related to those of retinol, retinal or retinoic acid or their derivatives.
[e] A synthetic retinoid having structural modifications not found in natural compounds. Generally, this term is used in reference to analogues of retinoic acid and its double-bond isomers. These compounds will be covered in detail in Volume 4 of the IARC Handbook series.

the structure of retinol, and soon thereafter the structure of β-carotene. In 1937, retinol was first crystallized from fish liver oil, from which the first crystalline esters were also isolated five years later. In 1946, Van Dorp and Arens synthesized retinoic acid and in 1947 the Isler group reported a commercially feasible synthesis of retinol. In 1950, Karrer and Eugster synthesized β-carotene. Synthetic retinol serves as the precursor for the retinyl esters used widely in vitamin A supplements and in food fortificants. These early developments have been summarized by Moore (1957).

Both plants and animals are sources of vitamin A for humans. Plants contain carotenoids, some of which are provitamin A compounds, but they contain no preformed vitamin A. Over 600 naturally occurring carotenoids have been identified, but only about 10 are major sources of vitamin A (Olson, 1994). Animal products contain vitamin A predominantly in the form of retinyl esters, but also as retinol and, in small amounts, as provitamin A carotenoids originating from plants consumed by the animals. Both synthetic and natural vitamin A and carotenoids are also found in pharmaceuticals and cosmetics. Section 2 of this Handbook covers the major sources of vitamin A.

Because of the low water-solubility of retinol, retinal and retinoic acid, the retinoid-binding proteins play an important role in providing a source of stable, solubilized retinoids for target tissues. Specific binding proteins selectively compartmentalize and regulate retinol levels. The nuclear retinoic acid receptor proteins function as transcription factors, permitting the retinoids to act as hormones that modulate the activity of retinoid-responsive genes. The binding proteins are therefore thought both to regulate the metabolic transformations of vitamin A and to prevent toxic effects that could be caused by high levels of unbound retinoids. The distribution of retinoids in tissues and their metabolic transformations, functions and characteristics are further described in Section 3 of this Handbook.

Vitamin A in human nutrition and cancer

In 1922, Mori observed corneal and conjunctival keratinization and interference with tear production in vitamin A-deficient rats. In 1925, Wolbach and Howe observed metaplastic changes in gastrointestinal, genitourinary, ocular and respiratory epithelia (replacement of columnar and transitional cells by squamous, keratinized cells) in animals deprived of vitamin A. These changes were morphologically similar to, but distinct from, certain pre-neoplastic lesions (reviewed by Shapiro, 1986). The observation of inhibitory action of vitamin A on the induction of tumours of the forestomach and cervix (Chu & Malmgren, 1965) and of bronchotracheal tumours (Saffiotti *et al.*, 1967) stimulated much interest in the relationship between vitamin A-dependent cell differentiation and cancer. In the next 15 years, the interactive roles of retinoids in the chemoprevention of carcinogenesis were carefully explored (Sporn & Roberts, 1983). Subsequently, the roles of retinoic acid and its 9-*cis* isomer in controlling cell differentiation, growth and reproduction were established (reviewed in Gudas *et al.*, 1994; Mangelsdorf *et al.*, 1994; Blomhoff, 1994). Several reviews on cancer prevention studies using vitamin A in cell culture, in animals and in man have been published in recent years (Hong & Itri, 1994; Moon *et al.*, 1994; Alberts & Garcia, 1995; Kelloff *et al.*, 1996; Minna & Mangelsdorf, 1997; Sankaranarayanan *et al.*, 1997).

'Chemoprevention' is a term that has been widely used to describe intentional chemical interference with the process of carcinogenesis by inducing a variety of biological mechanisms. Chemoprevention can be achieved by preventing the onset of carcinogenesis by protecting against initiation or by arresting or reversing stages of carcinogenesis at various steps in the processes of promotion and progression. The use of agents to prevent cancer in healthy individuals falls within the framework of 'primary prevention'. Chemoprevention used to arrest or reverse carcinogenesis in individuals who have been identified as having a pre-malignant lesion falls within the framework of 'secondary prevention' (the prevention of disease at a pre-clinical stage). 'Tertiary prevention', defined as the prevention of complications (recurrence, invasion, metastases) among people already diagnosed with symptomatic disease, is best regarded in the context of clinical management of the cancer patient. Tertiary prevention is not considered in this Handbook.

The discoveries that have enhanced our understanding of the various phases in the multi-step process of carcinogenesis have also led to the current understanding that preventive agents may act in different ways at different stages of progression. Hence, potential cancer-preventive agents, such as vitamin A, appear to be useful for either primary or secondary cancer prevention, or for both. Potential chemopreventive agents could be useful among individuals at average cancer risk, or among those at high cancer risk due to other behavioural or genetic factors (e.g., smokers or carriers of cancer-relevant genetic mutations). Section 4 reviews human observational and intervention studies using primary and secondary prevention strategies among subjects at various levels of cancer risk, as well as animal experimental studies.

Vitamin A deficiency is clearly a continuing public health problem in many areas of the world (Sommer & West, 1996). Because vitamin A deficiency can lead to increased risk for many health problems including infection and blindness, programmes to supplement and fortify foods for undernourished populations continue to be an important public health priority. The public health problem of vitamin A deficiency and the potential role of vitamin A in cancer prevention are two important but distinctly different issues. The implications and inferences that can be drawn from epidemiological observational studies and from the limited set of intervention studies using supplements of preformed vitamin A are reviewed in Section 4.

Dietary factors are thought to have a major causative role in cancer induction. Though the contribution of diet to cancer risk probably varies across populations, it has been estimated that in the United States possibly one third of all cancer deaths may be attributable to nutritional factors (Doll & Peto, 1981). A consistent finding for many cancer sites has been that diets with a high proportion of fruits and vegetables, and hence high levels of carotenoids, are associated with lower cancer risk (IARC, 1998). This Handbook focuses more specifically on the evidence for a protective effect of preformed vitamin A.

Issues in research on vitamin A

Knowledge of the effects of vitamin A and its molecular mechanisms of action is continually expanding. Thus, over the past several decades, as methods and understanding have advanced, findings from older studies need to be viewed in their historical context. As in other areas of cancer prevention research, studies of vitamin A have been carried out using a wide variety of methods, including animal experiments *in vitro* and *in vivo*, observational human studies, and, ultimately, intervention trials in humans. Thus, it has been a formidable challenge to compare and contrast findings across different study designs and settings to produce a coherent evaluation of the overall potential of vitamin A as a cancer-preventive agent in human populations. Nonetheless, the Working Group has conducted such an evaluation, first summarizing the convergent and divergent data in support of the general conclusions (Section 8), and finally producing an overall evaluation of the cancer-preventive potential of vitamin A (Section 10). These summaries and conclusions afforded the Working Group the opportunity to identify research areas critical for the advancement of cancer prevention that could lead to implementation of successful prophylactic treatments. Thus, future research should be directed to areas listed in Section 9 that the Working Group considered of high priority.

An important limitation of the use of preformed vitamin A in cancer prevention in humans is the toxicity that is seen at high doses. Toxic effects are seen in various organs, including the skin, circulation (e.g., hypertriglyceridaemia), liver, nervous system and bones (see Section 7). Some aspects of toxicity could be explained by overwhelming of the binding capacity of cellular and extracellular binding proteins by excess vitamin A or retinoids, which would result in the presence of unbound ('free') vitamin A, which might interact differently with receptors or other sites of retinoid action. Of particular concern regarding the widespread ingestion of preformed vitamin A supplements is the apparent sensitivity of the developing embryo to teratogenesis by daily supplemental retinyl palmitate at 25 000 IU per day or possibly less (Nau *et al.*, 1994). Such effects have prompted the development of literally thousands of synthetic retinoids designed to have more specific beneficial properties, but with lower toxic potential. The cancer-preventive potential of these synthetic retinoids will be covered in detail in Volume 4 of the IARC Handbook series. An active retinoid without teratogenic potential is yet to be identified, which suggests that retinoid receptors may play important roles in aspects of both the desired activity and the teratogenicity and reproductive toxicity.

One of the particular challenges in interpreting the effects of vitamin A on cancer is that studies have been performed at widely differing levels of vitamin A nutritive status. Obviously, experimental studies in humans maintained in a vitamin A-deficient state cannot be ethically justified. Therefore, studies have been performed in animals. For instance, several studies have indicated greater effects with supplementation in animals that were first fed vitamin A-deficient diets than in animals on normal diets. In animal studies, it is also possible to test the effects of vitamin A at high doses, where toxicity is often seen, whereas this type of research in human populations is also not justifiable.

A striking feature of vitamin A physiology is the elaborate mechanism of homeostatic control of circulating concentrations of plasma retinol across a broad range of intakes of preformed vitamin A and provitamin A. Therefore, much of the human observational and experimental work, which has been carried out within this homeostatically controlled range, may not be comparable to animal experimental studies with vitamin A at levels of deprivation or excess. Also related to the phenomenon of homeostasis is the limitation of the use of serum retinol levels as a measure of vitamin A status (see Section 2). Circulating retinol concentrations remain fairly constant until liver reserves fall to very low levels (below 0.07 mmol/g) (Olson, 1994), and factors other than intake, especially infection, infestation, malnutrition and acute stress, can affect circulating retinol levels (Section 5.2), thus limiting the value of plasma levels in other than long-term prospective studies. Vitamin A status can now be estimated by the relative dose–response and the modified relative dose–response tests, which have been widely used to assess vitamin A deficiency states. A more precise method of estimating total body stores, namely the isotope dilution method using deuterated retinol (Olson, 1994), has not been widely used, as it is technically demanding.

Purposes of this Handbook

The review and commentary in this Handbook is intended for use by researchers, clinicians, educators, and public health policy makers interested in cancer prevention and nutrition. This handbook is intended to provide a comprehensive review of the relevant information in the published scientific literature available to the Working Group on the role of vitamin A in cancer prevention. The focus of this critical review and commentary is on retinol and the retinyl esters. Some scientific literature in this field overlaps with reports dealing with vitamin A metabolites, vitamin A precursors and total dietary vitamin A (which is a combination of preformed vitamin A and its precursors), so information from this wide range of research is included in the current review when it was deemed relevant to our understanding of the observed effects of retinol or retinyl esters on cancer development. The observed effects of preformed vitamin A in cell and organ culture, in animal models and in human dietary observational epidemiological studies and intervention studies are reviewed. Based on this review, the Working Group offers recommendations for future research on the use of vitamin A in cancer prevention (Section 9) and an overall evaluation of the strength of the evidence for a role of vitamin A for cancer prevention in humans (Section 10).

References

Alberts, D.S. & Garcia, D.J. (1995) An overview of clinical cancer chemoprevention studies with emphasis on positive phase III studies. *J. Nutr.*, **125**, 692S–697S

Blomhoff, R., ed. (1994) *Vitamin A in Health and Disease*, New York, Marcel Dekker

Chu, E.W. & Malmgren, R.A. (1965) An inhibitory effect of vitamin A on the induction of tumors of forestomach and cervix in the Syrian hamster by carcinogenic polycyclic hydrocarbons. *Cancer Res.*, **25**, 884–895

Doll, R. & Peto, R. (1981) The causes of cancer: quantitative estimates of avoidable risks of cancer in the United States today. *J. Natl Cancer Inst.*, **66**, 1191–1308

Gudas, L.J., Sporn, M.B. & Roberts, A.B. (1994). Cellular biology and biochemistry of retinoids. In: Sporn, M.B., Roberts, A.B. & Goodman, D.S., eds, The Retinoids. Biology, Chemistry, and Medicine, 2nd ed., New York, Raven Press, pp. 443–520

Hong, W.K. & Itri, L.M. (1994) Retinoids and human cancer. In: Sporn, M.B., Roberts, A.B. & Goodman, D.S., eds, *The Retinoids. Biology, Chemistry, and Medicine,* 2nd ed., New York, Raven Press, pp. 597–630

IARC (1998) *IARC Handbooks of Cancer Prevention.* Volume 2, *Carotenoids*, Lyon

Kelloff, G.J., Crowell, J.A., Hawk, E.T., Steele, V.E., Lubet, R.A., Boone, C.W., Covey, J.M., Doody, L.A., Omenn, G.S., Greenwald, P., Hong, W.K., Parkinson, D.R., Bagheri, D., Baxter, G.T., Blunden, M., Doeltz, M.K., Eisenhauser, K.M., Johnson, K., Knapp, G.G., Longfellow, D.G., Malone, W.F., Nayfield, S.G., Seifried, H.E., Swall, L.M. & Sigman, C.C. (1996) Clinical development plans for cancer chemopreventive agents: vitamin A. *J. Cell. Biochem.*, **Suppl. 26**, 269–306

Mangelsdorf, D.J., Umesono, K. & Evans, R.M. (1994) The retinoid receptors. In: Sporn, M.B., Roberts, A.B. & Goodman, D.S., eds, *The Retinoids. Biology, Chemistry, and Medicine*, 2nd ed., New York, Raven Press, pp. 319–350

Minna, J.D. & Mangelsdorf, D.J. (1997) Retinoic acid receptor expression abnormalities in lung cancer: important clues or major obstacles? *J. Natl. Cancer Inst.*, **89**, 602–604

Moon, R.C., Mehta, R.G. & Rao, K.V.N. (1994) Retinoids and cancer in experimental animals. In: Sporn, M.B., Roberts, A.B. & Goodman, D.S., eds, *The Retinoids: Biology, Chemistry and Medicine*, 2nd ed., Raven Press, New York, pp. 573–595

Moore, T. (1957) *Vitamin A*, Amsterdam, Elsevier

Nau, K., Chahoud, I., Dencker, L., Lammer, E.J. & Scott, W.J. (1994) Teratogenicity of vitamin A and retinoids. In: Blomhoff, R., ed., *Vitamin A in Health and Disease*, New York, Marcel Dekker, pp. 615–663

Olson, J.A. (1994) Vitamin A, retinoids and carotenoids. In: Shils, M., Olson, J.A., & Shike, M., eds, *Modern Nutrition in Health and Disease,* 8th ed., Philadelphia, Lea & Febiger, pp. 287–307

Saffiotti, U., Montesano, R., Sellakumar, A.R. & Borg, S.A. (1967) Experimental cancer of the lung—inhibition by vitamin A of tracho-bronchial squamous metaplasia and squamous cell tumors. *Cancer*, **20**, 857–864

Sankaranarayanan, R., Mathew, B., Varghese, C., Sudhakaran, P.R., Menon, V., Jayadeep, A., Nair, M.K., Mathews, C., Mahalingam, T.R., Balaram, P. & Nair, P.P. (1997) Chemoprevention of oral leukoplakia with vitamin A and beta-carotene: an assessment. *Eur. J. Cancer, Oral Oncol.*, **33**, 231–236

Shapiro, S.S. (1986) Retinoids and epithelial differentiation. In: Sherman, M.I., ed., *Retinoids and Cell Differentiation*, Boca Raton, CRC Press, pp. 29–59

Sommer, A. & West, K.P., Jr, eds (1996) *Vitamin A Deficiency. Health, Survival and Vision,* Oxford, Oxford University Press

Sporn, M.B. & Roberts, A.B. (1984). Biological methods for analysis and assay of retinoids – relationships between structure and activity. In: Sporn, M.B., Roberts, A.B. & Goodman, D.S., eds, *The Retinoids,* Vol. 1, Orlando, Academic Press, pp. 235–279

Sporn, M.B., Roberts, A.B. & Goodman, D.S., eds (1994) *The Retinoids. Biology, Chemistry, and Medicine*, 2nd ed., New York, Raven Press

Tee, E.-S. (1992) Carotenoids and retinoids in human nutrition. *Crit. Rev. Food Sci. Nutr.*, **31**, 103–156

Vitamin A

1. Chemical and physical characteristics

The general characteristics of retinol, retinyl acetate, retinyl palmitate and β-retinal have been obtained from the following: Beilstein (Boit, 1966); *Directory of Chemical Producers* (MDL Information Systems, 1998); *Kirk-Othmer Encyclopedia of Chemical Technology*, 4th ed. (Kroschwitz, 1998); Kelloff *et al.* (1994a); *Martindale. The Extra Pharmacopoeia* (Reynolds, 1989); *The Merck Index*, 12th ed. (Budavari, 1996); and the *Physicians' Desk Reference* (1997).

1.1 Retinol

1.1.1 Name

Chemical Abstracts Services Registry Number
68-26-8

Chemical Abstracts Primary Name
Retinol

IUPAC Systematic Name
(All-*E*)-3,7-Dimethyl-9-(2,6,6-trimethyl-1-cyclohexen-1-yl)-2,4,6,8-nonatetraen-1-ol

Synonyms
All-*trans*-retinol; anti-infective vitamin; antixerophthalmic vitamin; 15-apo-β-caroten-15-ol; axerol; axerophthol; axerophtholum; biosterol; (*E*)-3,7-dimethyl-9-(2,6,6-trimethylcyclohexenyl)-2,4,6,8-nonatetraenol; (*E*)-3,7-dimethyl-9-(2,6,6-trimethylcyclohexen-1-yl)-2,4,6,8-nonatetraenol; fat-soluble A (obsolete); (*E*)-9-hydroxy-3,7-dimethyl-9-(2,6,6-trimethylcyclohexenyl)-1,3,5,7-nonatetraene; lard factor; oleovitamin A; ophthalamin (obsolete); *trans*-retinol; 2-*trans*,4-*trans*,6-*trans*,8-*trans*-retinol; vitamin A; vitamin A_1; vitamin A_1 alcohol; vitamin A alcohol; vitaminum A.

1.1.2 Structural and molecular formulae and relative molecular mass

CH_2OH

$C_{20}H_{30}O$

Relative molecular mass: 286.46

1.1.3 Physical and chemical properties

Description
Pale yellow prisms

Melting-point
62–64°C (yellow prisms from ethyl formate, petroleum ether, propylene oxide)

Solubility
Soluble in most organic solvents (acetone, chloroform, dimethyl sulfoxide, ether, ethanol, hexane, isopropanol, methanol) and in fats and mineral oils (2.5 mol/L) (Boit, 1966); practically insoluble in water (0.06 μmol/L) (Szuts & Harosi, 1991) and glycerol.

Spectroscopy
Double-bond isomers of retinol do not show differences in their infrared spectra, which are briefly mentioned in the review by Frickel (1984) and more extensively covered in that by Isler *et al.* (1971). The ultraviolet (UV) absorption spectrum in ethanol has λ_{max} at 325 nm; $E^{1\%}_{1\,cm}$ = 1835 (Tee, 1992). Retinol exhibits yellow-green fluorescence at 510 nm after excitation at 327 nm and at 470 nm after excitation at 325 nm. The infrared (IR) and proton magnetic resonance (^{1}H-NMR) spectra of retinol can be found in the relevant Aldrich Library volumes (Pouchert, 1985; Pouchert & Behnke, 1993).

Stability
Photo-induced bond isomerization from *trans* to *cis* gives the other known retinol isomers: 11-*cis* (neo b), 13-*cis* (neo a), 9,13-di-*cis* (iso b), 9-*cis* (iso a), and 11,13-di-*cis* (neo c) (Tee, 1992). Particularly in oil solution, retinol can be protected from isomerization by preventing exposure to UV and sunlight. Bond isomerization can also be caused by heat and iodine. High levels of illumination can induce polymerization. Retinol is sensitive to oxygen and is optimally stored at below 4°C under an inert gas (argon or nitrogen) or in the presence of an antioxidant, such as butylated hydroxytoluene. Heat and trace metals accelerate retinol decomposition by oxygen and light (Kroschwitz, 1998). Retinol is unstable to acids, which cause bond rearrangement to retrovitamin A, isomerization, and dehydration to anhydrovitamin A, sometimes followed by solvent addition; it is also unstable to alkali in the presence of oxygen (Tee, 1992). Unlike the palmitate ester, the alcohol and its acetate can bind strongly to polyvinyl chloride in plastics used for administration.

1.1.4 Technical products

Commercial preparations of retinol may contain antioxidants (low levels of butylated hydroxyanisole and butylated hydroxytoluene, dispersants and antimicrobial agents when diluted with edible oils or solid dispersants (Polysorbate 20). One international unit (IU) of vitamin A is defined as 0.3 μg of pure all-*trans*-retinol.

The major producers of vitamin A are BASF AG (Germany), BASF Corp. (USA), BASF Mexicana (Mexico), Bayer AG (Germany), Gaveteco S.A.I.C.I. e I. (Argentina), Hoffmann-La Roche AG (Germany) and Rhone-Poulenc Animal Nutrition (France).

1.2 Retinyl acetate

1.2.1 Name

Chemical Abstracts Services Registry Number
127-47-9

Chemical Abstracts Primary Name
Retinol acetate

IUPAC Systematic Name
(*E*)-9-Acetoyl-3,7-dimethyl-9-(2,6,6-trimethylcyclohexenyl)-2,4,6,8-nonatetraenol

Synonyms
Acetic acid (*E*)-3,7-dimethyl-9-(2,6,6-trimethylcyclohexenyl)-2,4,6,8-nonatetraenyl ester; acetic acid retinyl ester; all-*trans*-retinyl acetate; all-*trans*-retinol acetate; *O*-acetoxy-all-*trans*-retinol; *O*-acetyl-all-*trans*-retinol; retinyl acetate; 2-*trans*,4-*trans*,6-*trans*,8-*trans*-retinol acetate; 2-*trans*,4-*trans*,6-*trans*,8-*trans*-retinyl acetate; vitamin A acetate.

1.2.2 Structural and molecular formulae and relative molecular mass

CH_2OCOCH_3

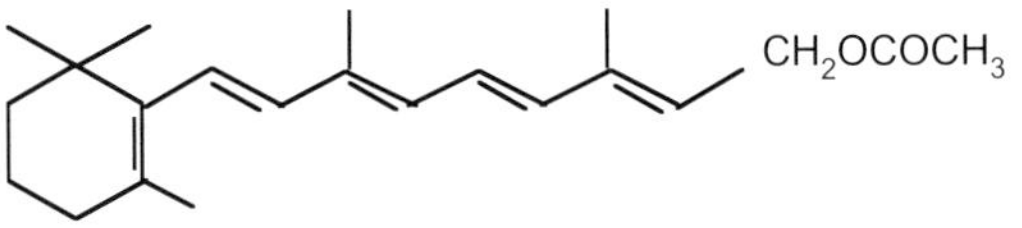

$C_{22}H_{32}O_2$

Relative molecular mass: 328.5

1.2.3 Physical and chemical properties

Description
Pale yellow prisms or yellow supercooled, viscous liquid

Melting point
57–58°C

Solubility
Soluble in most organic solvents (acetone, chloroform, ethanol, isopropanol) and in fats and oils (750 g/100 mL); insoluble in water and glycerol.

Spectroscopy
UV–visible: λ_{max} 326 nm (in ethanol); $E^{1\%}_{1\,cm}$ 1550.

Fluorescence
Emission λ_{max} at 470 nm for excitation at 325 nm

Stability
More stable than retinol. For stability in crystalline form and in solution, see Guerrant

et al. (1948); for stability to hydrolysis in ethanolic sodium hydroxide at 40° and 60°C, see Isler *et al.* (1949). Store at below 4°C.

1.2.4 Technical products

Activity is based on high-performance liquid chromatographic comparison with the international standard. The international unit (IU) was defined by the WHO Expert Committee on Biological Standardization as the activity of 0.344 μg of pure all-*trans*-retinyl acetate. Synthetic material may be sold dispersed in a corn starch–gelatin matrix (Sigma, USA) or in gelatin, sucrose, peanut oil, and calcium phosphate-containing butylated hydroxyanisole and butylated hydroxytoluene (USB, USA), and in pure form (2 800 000 IU/g, Sigma). Major producers are BASF AG (Germany), F. Hoffman-La Roche AG (Germany) and Roche AG (Switzerland). In one pharmaceutical source (Materna prenatal tablets; Lederle, USA), retinyl acetate is combined with β-carotene and vitamins D, E, B_1, B_2, B_6, B_{12}, biotin, pantothenic acid and minerals.

1.3 Retinyl palmitate

1.3.1 Name

Chemical Abstracts Services Registry Number
79-81-2

Chemical Abstracts Primary Name
Retinol hexadecanoate

IUPAC Systematic Name
(*E*)-3,7-Dimethyl-9-*O*-palmitoyl-9-(2,6,6-trimethylcyclohexenyl)-2,4,6,8-nonatetraenol

Synonyms
Palmitic acid (*E*)-3,7-dimethyl-9-(2,6,6-trimethylcyclohexenyl)-2,4,6,8-nonatetraenyl ester; palmitic acid retinyl ester; *O*-palmitoyl-all-*trans*-retinol; *O*-palmitoyl-retinol; *O*-palmitoyl-retinol; retinyl palmitate; 2-*trans*,4-*trans*,6-*trans*,8-*trans*-retinyl palmitate; 2-*trans*,4-*trans*,6-*trans*,8-*trans*-retinol palmitate; *trans*-retinol palmitate; *trans*-retinyl palmitate; vitamin A palmitate.

1.3.2 Structural and molecular formulae and relative molecular mass

$CH_2OC(O)(CH_2)_{14}CH_3$

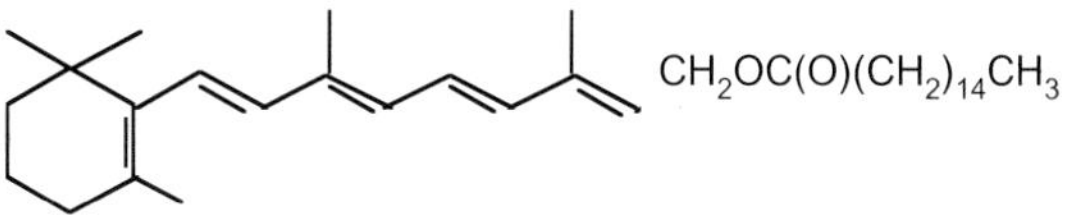

$C_{36}H_{60}O_2$

Relative molecular mass: 524.8

1.3.3 Physical and chemical properties

Description
Yellow, crystalline or amorphous powder, n_D^{20} 1.5558 (Tee, 1992)

Melting-point
27–29°C (Tee, 1992)

Solubility
Soluble in most organic solvents (ethanol, isopropanol, chloroform, acetone) and in fats and oils insoluble in water and glycerol.

Spectroscopy
UV–visible: λ_{max} 325–328 nm (in ethanol); $E_{1\,cm}^{1\%}$ 940–975

Fluorescence
Emission λ_{max} at 470 nm for excitation at 325 nm

Stability
More stable than retinol to oxidation in air; rate of hydrolysis in ethanolic sodium hydroxide was reported by Isler *et al.* (1949). Store at below 4°C.

1.3.4 Technical products

One IU of vitamin A is contained in 0.55 μg of pure all-*trans*-retinyl palmitate. Major producers of retinyl palmitate are BASF AG (Germany), BASF Mexicana, S.A. de C.V. (Mexico), F. Hoffman-La Roche AG (Switzerland) and Piramal Health-care Limited (India). A pharmaceutical source is Aquasol A (capsules or the parental form is water-miscible by solubilization in polysorbate 80; Carlson

Laboratories, USA). Retinyl palmitate is also available in a corn starch–gelatin matrix containing butylated hydroxyanisole and butylated hydroxytoluene, in a water-dispersible starch–gelatin matrix containing butylated hydroxyanisole and butylated hydroxytoluene, in a mixture of acacia, lactose, coconut oil, butylated hydroxytoluene, sodium benzoate, sorbic acid, and silicon dioxide, or in corn oil (USB, USA).

1.4 Retinal

1.4.1 Name

Chemical Abstracts Service Registry Number
116-31-4

Chemical Abstracts Primary Name
Retinal

IUPAC Systematic Name
(All-E)-3,7-Dimethyl-2-(2,6,6-trimethyl-1-cyclohexen-1-yl)2,4,6,8-nonatetraenol

Synonyms
All-*trans*-retinal, axerophthal, retinaldehyde, retinene, vitamin A aldehyde

1.4.2 Structural and molecular formulae and relative molecular mass

CHO

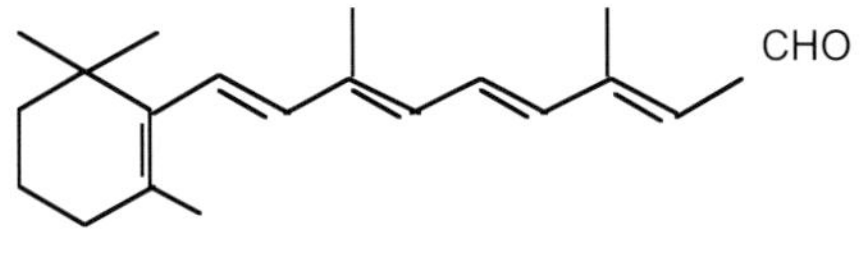

$C_{20}H_{28}O$

Relative molecular mass 284.4

1.4.3 Physical and chemical properties

Description
Orange crystals (from petroleum ether)

Melting point
64–65°C

Solubility
Soluble in ethanol, chloroform, cyclohexane, petroleum ether and oils; virtually insoluble in water.

Spectroscopy
IR (Rockley *et al.*, 1986); NMR (Patel, 1969)

UV–visible
λ_{max} 383 nm (*E* 4.288 x 10^4 in ethanol); λ_{max} 368 nm (*E* 4.88 x 10^4 in hexane) (Hubbard *et al.*, 1971)

Stability
Sensitive to light and oxygen. Store under an inert gas (argon or nitrogen) at < 4°C.

Commercial sources
Retinal can be obtained from the following suppliers: Sigma (USA), Crescent Chemical Co. (USA), Nacalia Tesque, Inc. (Japan) and Kanto Chemicals Co. (Japan).

1.5 Retinoic acid

1.5.1 Name

Chemical Abstracts Services Registry Number
302-79-4

Chemical Abstracts Primary Name
Retinoic acid

IUPAC Systematic Name
All-*trans*-retinoic acid

Synonyms
(All-*E*)-3,7-dimethyl-9-(2,2,6-trimethylcyclohexenyl)nona-2,4,6,8-tetraenoic acid, *trans*-retinoic acid, tretinoin, vitamin A acid, vitamin A_1 acid.

1.5.2 Structural and molecular formulae and relative molecular mass

COOH

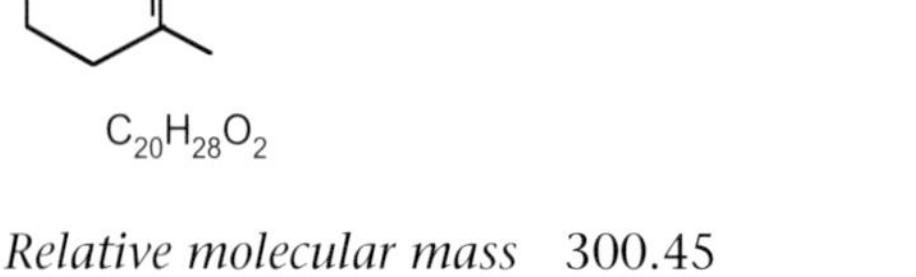

$C_{20}H_{28}O_2$

Relative molecular mass 300.45

1.5.3 Physical and chemical properties

Description
Yellow crystals

Melting-point
180–182°C (Tee, 1992).

Solubility
Soluble in most organic solvents, fats, and oils; low solubility in water (0.21 μmol/L) (Szuts & Harosi, 1991)

Spectroscopy
UV–visible: λ_{max} 350 (ethanol), $E^{1\%}_{1\,cm}$ 1510 (Tee, 1992).

Stability
Unstable to light, oxygen and heat, but less so than retinol. Store under inert gas at below 4°C or in the presence of an antioxidant.

2. Occurrence, Production, Use, Analysis and Human Exposure

2.1 Occurrence

The primary source of vitamin A is the precursor compounds, the carotenoids. There are more than 600 naturally occurring carotenoids, but only 50–60 of them possess vitamin A activity, producing at least one intact molecule of retinol or retinoic acid when metabolized, and only about 10 of them have nutritional relevance (Pfander, 1987).

The second important dietary source of vitamin A is retinyl esters, which are found in foods of animal origin. Retinyl esters are derivatives of retinol with fatty acids. The most important dietary retinyl ester is retinyl palmitate, with smaller amounts of retinyl oleate and retinyl stearate (Ong, 1994).

In several developing countries, synthetic vitamin A, often in the form of palmityl ester, is added to commonly consumed foods. Monosodium glutamate has been used as a vehicle in Indonesia (Muhilal *et al.*, 1988) and the Philippines, while vitamin A is added to sugar in several central American countries (Mejia & Arroyave, 1982), and ghee is used in Pakistan. However, while food fortification may be a short-term measure to cope with inadequacy of dietary intake, more sustainable measures must involve promoting the consumption of locally grown fruit and vegetables and improving social conditions.

In the developed world, synthetic vitamin A and carotenoids are added to a small number of foods such as dairy products and are also found in pharmaceuticals and cosmetics for oncological and dermatological use. β-Carotene and other carotenoids are also used extensively as food colourants (IARC, 1998).

2.2 Production

Retinol can be synthesized chemically. Early developments have been described by Moore (1957) and more recent approaches by Frickel (1984) and by Dawson & Hobbs (1994). Several pharmaceutical companies supply retinol with 99% purity. Provitamin A carotenoids may be converted to vitamin A by central cleavage to yield one or two molecules of retinal. This conversion is catalysed by a 15,15′-dioxygenase enzyme that is found in the intestinal mucosa, liver and other tissues (Devery & Milborrow, 1994; Nagao *et al.*, 1996). Retinal is then reduced by an aldehyde reductase to retinol. Eccentric cleavage of carotenoids yields β-apo-carotenals with different chain lengths, which then may be shortened by β-oxidation to retinol. In addition, there is evidence that retinoic acid may be formed directly from such carotenoids as β-carotene by a still undefined pathway (Wang *et al.*, 1992).

Preformed vitamin A is found in the diet primarily in the form of retinyl esters. Retinol is formed in the intestine by hydrolysis of the long-chain retinyl esters catalysed by a brush border retinyl hydrolase and a non-specific pancreatic hydrolase (Blaner & Olson, 1994) (see Section 3.2.2).

2.3 Use and application

Vitamin A is an essential micronutrient for animals and man. Humans obtain their dietary supply from foods of both animal and plant origin, but the more dependent they are on plant sources, the more difficult it is to meet metabolic needs. Dietary requirements for vitamin A have been investigated by many workers and their findings have been reviewed in various reports and by both national and international bodies (Olson, 1987; FAO/WHO, 1988; National Research Council, 1989). There are some wide differences between countries in the amounts of vitamin A considered essential to meet dietary requirements (McLaren, 1994), but most countries have generally adopted the arguments discussed in the FAO/WHO (1988) handbook. Requirements for infants are generally arrived at from the amount of vitamin A in breast milk (340–400 mg/day) and as children get progressively older, this amount is increased to allow for growth. In adults, requirements are based on the catabolism of total body vitamin A, with allowances for body size and storage. These calculations give figures of 700 mg/day for men and 600 mg/day for women. In addition, about 400 mg/day must be added during lactation. Despite the abundance of carotenoids in vegetables and fruits, more than 200 million children worldwide suffer from various degrees of vitamin A deficiency. Therefore, vitamin A is used as a supplement or in fortification of a large number of processed foods. In terms of the degree of public health importance of vitamin A deficiency, the World Health Organization (WHO) categorizes countries into those that have clinical or subclinical vitamin A deficiency and those that have no vitamin A deficiency-related problems (McLaren & Frigg, 1997). The group with subclinical problems is further subclassified as having severe, moderate or mild vitamin A deficiency, based on prevalence of low serum retinol levels in children (WHO, 1996). Vitamin A- and retinol-deficient states such as xerophthalmia and night-blindness can be reversed by treatment with vitamin A (retinyl acetate or palmitate) from either animal or synthetic sources (Tee, 1992). In subclinically vitamin A-deficient populations, supplementation during measles infection will reduce mortality, morbidity and the length of hospital stay (Barclay *et al.*, 1987; Hussey & Klein, 1990). The WHO, United Nations Children's Fund (UNICEF), the United States Agency for International Development, and many other national and non-governmental organizations aim to eliminate vitamin A deficiency as a public health problem in all countries by the year 2000 through a combination of supplementation, food fortification and nutrition education.

The following dosages are recommended by WHO and UNICEF for alleviating vitamin A-deficiency disorders in children in areas of high risk (McLaren & Frigg, 1997).

Subject	Oral dose (IU)
Children 1–6 years	200 000 every 3–6 months
Infants 6–11 months	100 000 every 3–6 months
Lactating mothers	200 000 once (within 3 months of delivery)

In cases where xerophthalmia has been diagnosed or in children with measles in marginally vitamin A-deficient populations, the supplemention would be as shown below.

Time of administration after diagnosis	Dose (IU) < 1 year old	> 1 year old
Immediately	100 000	200 000
Next day	100 000	200 000
2–4 weeks later	100 000	200 000

The well documented effects of retinoic acid and synthetic retinoids on several dermatological disorders (for review, see Vahlquist, 1994) led to the development of commercial ointments containing retinyl esters. Several prescription drugs containing retinoic acid and its 13-*cis*-isomer are available for treating acne and photo-ageing skin. Vitamin A is also used in topical non-prescription cosmetics for improvement of appearance of wrinkles. The effect of these topical preparations is limited to the skin and does not contribute substantially to the vitamin A status of the body.

2.4 Human exposure

Preformed vitamin A in the diet is obtained from vertebrate animal sources rich in retinyl esters (tissues such as liver, kidney, dairy products and eggs). Liver and fish oils are the richest dietary sources of preformed vitamin A and concern has been expressed by some authorities about potentially teratogenic effects of liver consumption during pregnancy (Eckhoff & Nau, 1990b). However, for many populations worldwide, these foods are used only sparingly. Hence, plant provitamin A carotenoids are usually the major food source of vitamin A. Unfortunately, poor bioavailability of carotenoids in vegetables restricts their usefulness, because the cellulose walls of plant cells are not easily broken down (de Pee & West, 1996). In contrast, carotenoids in fruits are more bioavailable. Fruits such as mangoes and pawpaw are good sources of vitamin A, but their consumption may be restricted to short seasonal periods. Volume 2 of the *IARC Handbooks of Cancer Prevention* treats this subject in depth. The average daily dietary intake of vitamin A in the United States is about 2.25 mg of retinol equivalents, of which 47% is derived from fruits and vegetables; 27% from fats, oils and dairy products and 27% from meat, fish and eggs. Provitamin A carotenoids provide about 50% of this intake (Tee, 1992).

The vitamin A activity of β-carotene and other provitamin A carotenoids has been arbitrarily defined as one-sixth and one-twelfth of that of retinol. Calculation of vitamin A intakes is generally satisfactory if retinol or β-carotene is in the main food constituents, but this is often not the case. Calculations of vitamin A intakes are made more difficult by variability in the way data are presented in food composition tables, some of which combine provitamin A carotenoids and retinol as vitamin A, while others separate them (Tee, 199).

The dietary intake of vitamin A in different populations in the world varies greatly. In addition, intake data outside the industrialized world are incomplete, particularly where vitamin A deficiency is a problem. The incompleteness of food composition tables for carotenoids in foods also makes accurate measurements of total vitamin A intake difficult and complicates the design of supplementation programmes (McLaren & Frigg, 1997). Substantial amounts of vitamin A may also be taken as single or multivitamin supplements. These usually contain vitamin A in the range of 3000 to 10 000 IU. In a study by Willett *et al.* (1983), supplementation of well nourished adults with β-carotene (30 mg daily for 16 weeks) increased the plasma levels of β-carotene but not the plasma retinol levels. Also, a daily retinyl ester supplement (25 000 IU) did not increase the plasma retinol levels, illustrating the fact that plasma retinol concentration is under homeostatic control (see Section 3.1).

2.5 Analysis

Measurement of plasma retinol is probably the most common method used to assess vitamin A status. As mentioned above however, the concentration of plasma retinol is homeostatically controlled over most of the range found in human subjects, so that interpreting status from low plasma values can be difficult.

In many developing countries, plasma retinol levels are lower than those seen in the western world, particularly in environments where viral and bacterial infections and parasite infestations are common (Thurnham, 1997). The WHO (1996) has suggested that serum levels of ≤0.7 mmol/L indicate a high risk of vitamin A deficiency. There is evidence that concurrent infection lowers concentrations of circulating retinol by suppressing the synthesis of retinol-binding protein (RBP) in the liver (Rosales & Ross, 1996). Frequent infections also contribute to poor vitamin A status by reducing intake and increasing the potential excretion of retinol in urine (Stephensen *et al.*, 1994).

The concentration of plasma carotenoids also gives information on vitamin A status. The concentration of plasma β-carotene depends on dietary intake and availability of preformed vitamin A in the diet. Based on currently available data, the higher the vitamin A intake, the lower the conversion of provitamin A carotenoids to retinol. Levels of non-provitamin A carotenoids like lutein also provide information on vegetable intake. The presence of lutein in the plasma indicates that green vegetables are consumed, implying that β-carotene, even if undetectable in the plasma (Thurnham *et al.*, 1997), is present in the diet. It is therefore advisable to measure several markers of vitamin A status and some of the more useful methods currently being used are described below. In the following descriptions, the terms plasma and serum are used interchangeably.

2.5.1 Functional methods

2.5.1.1 Night-blindness

This method of assessment involves an ophthalmological instrument, the dark adaptometer, which measures the speed of adaptation of the eye to low light conditions. However, the method is not suitable for field conditions and night-blindness is usually assessed by interviews of the patients and guardians as well as careful observation of the ability of children to see in dim light (Sommer *et al.*, 1980). This method is suitable for the assessment of early signs of moderate to severe vitamin A deficiency. At the community level, it is useful to enquire if there is a local word for night-blindness. A positive response is highly indicative that the community has or recently had a vitamin A-deficiency problem.

2.5.1.2 Conjunctival impression cytology (*Wittpenn et al., 1986*)

This method involves assessing the morphological appearance of cells from the eye epithelium obtained by pressing a small piece of filter paper onto the conjunctiva. Normally, conjunctival cells resemble epithelial cells and the number of mucin-producing goblet cells is high. In the vitamin A-deficient state, the conjunctival epithelium becomes flattened in appearance and the number of goblet cells is dramatically reduced (WHO, 1996). It has been suggested that this method should be the one for assessing marginal vitamin A deficiency in children (Olson, 1994a). Unfortunately, it is labour-intensive, assessment is dependent on individual skills and the two-month delay for the reading to normalize following treatment of children who previously had low liver reserves of vitamin A and plasma retinol (< 0.7 mol/L) reduces its efficiency in monitoring changes in status (Amédée-Manesme *et al.*, 1988).

2.5.2 Biochemical methods

2.5.2.1 Relative dose response (RDR) (*Underwood, 1990a,b*)

This method is based on release of apo-RBP (i.e. unbound protein, as opposed to holo-RBP, the retinol-bound protein) from the liver to the serum. In individuals with low vitamin A status, apo-RBP accumulates in the liver. Some apo-RBP is released after administration of an oral dose of vitamin A (for example, as retinyl acetate in oil). First, baseline serum retinol (A_0) in a blood sample is measured by high-performance liquid chromatography (HPLC). Five hours after an oral dose of 450–1000 μg retinyl acetate, a second sample is analysed for serum retinol (A_5). An RDR value is calculated from RDR = $(A_5 - A_0) \times 100/A_5$. A value over 20% is a positive indication of vitamin A inadequacy, which indicates a low vitamin A concentration in the liver (≤ 0.07 μmol/g vitamin A) (McLaren & Frigg, 1997).

2.5.2.2 Modified relative dose response (MRDR) (*Tanumihardjo et al., 1990a*)

This method is based on the administration of a single oral dose of 0.53 mmol of 3,4-didehydroretinyl acetate and subsequent analysis of a blood sample 4–6 h later for both 3,4-didehydroretinol and retinol. Vitamin A status is determined by the ratio between 3,4-didehydroretinol and retinol as follows:

MRDR = 3,4-didehydroretinol/retinol

MRDR is considered to be normal when the ratio is below 0.06 (McLaren & Frigg, 1997).

At a population level, the WHO has classified countries as mildly, moderately or severely deficient, based on a prevalence of vitamin A deficiency, as measured by any of these three tests, of < 20%, > 20–30% and > 30%, respectively.

2.5.2.3 Serum retinol

Serum concentrations of retinol can be measured directly by HPLC of an organic solvent extract of a serum sample using reversed-phase chromatography on a C_{18} column and detection by UV absorption at 326 nm (Frolik & Olson, 1984; Catignani & Bieri, 1983; Barua *et al.*, 1993). Since retinol concentrations in serum are under homeostatic control, the values are useful indicators of status only when concentrations are very high or very low. Measurements of serum retinol are most useful at the population level for the assessment of intervention programmes in vitamin A-deficient populations. The concentration of retinol in well nourished adults is 1.8–3.2 μmol/L. The median and range (5–95%) are lower in women (e.g., 1.8 μmol/L; 1.2–2.8 μmol/L) than in men (2.2; 1.4–3.2) (Gregory *et al.*, 1990). The WHO suggests that a serum retinol level of < 0.7 μmol/L in 10% of a population is indicative of a public health problem (WHO, 1996).

The validity of measurements of plasma components is critically dependent on stability during storage. In general, the stability of retinol and its esters is very good when plasma or serum samples are stored in sealed containers at −70 °C. Carotenoids are somewhat less stable than retinoids under similar storage conditions. The stability of retinyl esters in lipoproteins has not been carefully studied. With regard to short-term storage, when serum was left stored overnight at 4°C in the dark, retinol and α-tocopherol concentrations were unchanged, whereas carotenoid concentrations decreased by an average of 5% (Key *et al.*, 1996). To maximize stability for long-term storage at −70°C, serum samples should be prepared as soon as conveniently possible after blood is drawn. The gas space above the sample should be kept as small as possible, and the tube should be hermetically sealed. Degassing the samples before storage is helpful, and filling the gas space, preferably with argon or with oxygen-free nitrogen, is recommended but not essential. Several aliquots of each sample should be prepared to avoid the adverse effects of repeated freezing and thawing at a later time.

2.5.2.4 Vitamin A in food

Determinations of native or supplemental vitamin A in food in the form of provitamin A carotene and retinyl esters are usually performed by reversed-phase high-performance liquid chromatography on a C_{18} column. Foods may or may not have been saponified before the preparation of an organic extract. β-Carotene and other carotenoids are detected by UV absorption at 450 nm and retinol and its esters at 326 nm (Furr *et al.*, 1992). Data in food composition tables on food analyses of retinol and provitamin A carotenoids should be interpreted with care. Values for preformed vitamin A, the form found in foods of animal origin, are usually more accurate than data on carotenoids in vegetable foods. In addition, preformed vitamin A is better and more predictably absorbed than provitamin A sources. Absorption of the latter can vary appreciably depending on food preparation and cooking methods: chopping, heating and the presence of oil tend to increase bioavailability. The methodology used to assess vitamin A status using dietary enquiry methods and food composition tables is described in Section 4.

2.5.2.5 Milk analysis

Human milk contains retinyl esters and provitamin A carotenoids (Canfield *et al.*, 1997; Khachik *et al.*, 1997) in amounts which reflect the vitamin A status of the mother. Therefore, milk analysis provides a non-invasive method of assessing vitamin A status. This analysis includes a saponification step before organic extraction. The extract is then analysed as for serum analysis. A retinol concentration below 1.05 μmol/L in milk is considered by the WHO to reflect vitamin A deficiency and a public health problem is considered to occur when more than 25% of the lactating female population has lower milk levels (McLaren & Frigg, 1997).

3. Metabolism, kinetics, tissue distribution, and inter- and intra-species variation

Much of our knowledge about metabolism and function of vitamin A has been derived from experimental studies with animals, particularly rats (see Section 3.2). In this handbook, recent research studies and current reviews are emphasized. The older literature can be accessed via the reviews cited.

3.1 Human studies

3.1.1 Introduction

Vitamin A is an essential nutrient for humans and other vertebrates (Blomhoff, 1994a; Olson, 1994b; Ross, 1998). Carotenoids that contain at least one unsubstituted β-ionone ring serve as precursors of vitamin A (Blomhoff, 1994; Olson, 1994b; Olson, 1998; Ross, 1998).

Vitamin A is well absorbed by the intestine, transported from the intestine to the liver and other organs in chylomicra, and stored largely in the liver as retinyl esters. Vitamin A functions in vision, cell differentiation, and embryonic development. Many other physiological processes, including growth, reproduction and the immune response, are dependent upon these cellular functions of vitamin A.

3.1.2 Absorption

Preformed vitamin A is present mainly as retinyl esters in the diet. In the small intestine, the esters are hydrolysed by esterases in pancreatic juice and in the brush border of intestinal mucosal cells. Free retinol is incorporated into lipid micelles in the gut lumen and taken up by absorptive epithelial cells of the intestine (Blomhoff, 1994a; Olson, 1994b; Ong, 1994; Ross, 1998). A specific transporter for retinol, identified in rats, may also exist in human intestinal cells (Ong, 1994). Within intestinal cells, retinol, probably as a complex with cellular retinol-binding protein type II (CRBP-II), is re-esterified by transfer of a fatty acid from the α-position of phosphatidyl choline (Ong, 1994). Vitamin A, mainly as retinyl ester, is then incorporated into chylomicra and released into the lymph (Blomhoff, 1994a; Olson, 1994b; Ross, 1998). By analogy with other species, provitamin A carotenoids are mainly cleaved oxidatively to one or two molecules of retinal, which is then enzymically reduced to retinol in intestinal cells (Devery & Milborrow, 1994; Nagao *et al.*, 1996; Olson, 1998). A minor portion of provitamin A carotenoids can be oxidized asymmetrically to β-apocarotenals, by both chemical and enzymatic routes (Krinsky *et al.*, 1993). Under conventional dietary conditions, most absorbed β-carotene is cleaved to vitamin A in the upper part of the human intestine (Parker, 1996), although the liver and other organs also possess this capacity. As β-carotene intake increases, the efficiency of absorption is reduced.

The absorption of preformed vitamin A in healthy humans is quite efficient (60–90%) in the presence of an adequate amount of dietary fat (Blomhoff, 1994a; Olson, 1994b; Ross, 1998). The efficiency of intestinal absorption of retinyl esters from supplement preparations, however, depends on the matrix or carrier present, the rate of release of vitamin A from the preparation, and the types and amounts of solubilizers and stabilizers. The daily dose of retinyl ester that induces signs of toxicity also depends on the nature of the formulation. Intestinal infections reduce the absorption efficiency to only a minor extent (Tanumihardjo *et al.*, 1996). In the absence of bile, as in cholestasis and related disorders, however, vitamin A absorption is markedly reduced (Amédée-Manesme *et al.*, 1988).

Even at doses of vitamin A as high as 200 000 IU (60 mg) in oil, the absorption efficiency is over 50% in healthy humans (Sommer & West, 1996), in contrast to many other nutrients. Indeed, such doses prevent the appearance of signs of vitamin A deficiency in vitamin A-depleted children for periods of up to six months (Underwood & Arthur, 1996).

3.1.3 Transport

Apart from chylomicra, vitamin A is transported in human plasma primarily as all-*trans*-retinol on a specific binding protein, retinol-binding protein (RBP) (Goodman, 1984; Blomhoff, 1994a; Olson, 1994b; Soprano & Blaner, 1994; Ross, 1998). The amino acid sequence and three-dimensional structure of human RBP are known (Goodman, 1984; Soprano & Blaner, 1994; Newcomer, 1995). Its molecular weight is 21 kDa, and it contains a β-barrel as an internal binding-pocket for retinol. RBP is synthesized primarily in parenchymal cells of the liver but also in other organs (Blomhoff, 1994a; Olson, 1994b; Soprano & Blaner, 1994; Ross, 1998). The plasma concentration of the 1:1 retinol–RBP complex (holo-RBP) is finely regulated. As a consequence, liver reserves of vitamin A can vary from relatively high (1 µmol/g) to relatively low (0.07 µmol/g) concentrations without an appreciable change in the plasma concentration (Blomhoff, 1994a; Olson, 1994b; Ross, 1998). The regulatory mechanism, although not fully clarified, seems to depend on three factors: (*a*) the rate of release of retinol from stored retinyl ester in liver cells, (*b*) the release of holo-RBP from liver cells, and (*c*) feedback inhibition of the releasing mechanisms by retinoic acid and other products of metabolism (Blomhoff, 1994a; Olson, 1994b; Ross, 1998). Thus, a dose of retinoic acid lowers plasma retinol level markedly, but in a transient manner, in humans (Barua *et al.*, 1997). Furthermore, an analogue, *N*-(4-hydroxy-phenyl)retinamide (4-HPR), which is being studied as a preventive drug for breast cancer and other cancers, inhibits the release of holo-RBP from liver cells and, as a consequence, markedly lowers plasma retinol in humans (Formelli *et al.*, 1996). In the plasma, holo-RBP is present as a 1:1 complex with tetrameric transthyretin, the binding protein for thyroxine (Blomhoff, 1994a; Olson, 1994b; Ross, 1998).

The plasma concentration of retinol in young children is approximately 60% of that in adults. The level increases during adolescence, however, to reach adult values (Pilch, 1985). Mean values for a healthy population are given in Table 1. Adult males show 12–18% higher values than adult females (Pilch, 1985; Gregory *et al.*, 1990). Steady-state plasma concentrations of retinol may well be affected by genetic factors as well.

Other forms of vitamin A found in human plasma include all-*trans*-retinyl ester, all-*trans*-retinoic acid, 13-*cis*-retinoic acid, all-*trans*-4-oxoretinoic acid, 13-*cis*-4-oxoretinoic acid, all-*trans*-retinyl β-glucuronide all-*trans*-retinoyl β-glucuronide and 13-*cis*-retinoyl β-glucuronide (Blaner & Olson, 1994; Barua, 1997). The plasma concentration of all-*trans*-retinol in healthy adults is about 2 μmol/L, of retinyl ester usually <0.2 μmol/L (10% that of retinol), and that of the other forms approximately 2–20 nmol/L (0.1–1% that of retinol) (Blaner & Olson, 1994; Formelli *et al.*, 1996; Barua, 1997). Retinyl esters are found in chylomicra, in chylomicron remnants and in low-density lipoproteins, whereas retinoic acid forms a complex with albumin. The retinoid glucuronides, although much more water-soluble than vitamin A, are nonetheless bound to plasma proteins (Blaner & Olson, 1994; Formelli *et al.*, 1996; Barua, 1997). Lipoprotein lipase hydrolyses triglycerides present in chylomicra, thereby converting them to chylomicron remnants. Chylomicron remnants, which retain the retinyl esters, are mainly taken up by parenchymal cells of the liver, although other tissues can also remove them from the circulation (Blaner & Olson, 1994).

Table 1. Mean concentrations of serum vitamin A (retinol + retinyl esters) (μg/dL) in humans as a function of age[a]

Age (years)	Percentiles		
	10	50	90
3–5	24.0	35.0	49.1
6–11	27.0	36.1	49.0
12–17	32.0	44.0	59.0
18–44	37.0	54.0	75.1
45–74	42.1	60.0	85.0

[a] Values for all races and both sexes, United States population (Pilch, 1985).

3.1.3.1 Factors affecting plasma retinoid concentrations

Plasma retinol levels are homeostatically controlled. In vitamin A-sufficient persons, therefore, daily intakes of vitamin A of up to 25 000 IU have little or no effect on steady-state serum retinol concentrations (Willett *et al.*, 1983). In some studies with vitamin A-sufficient subjects, however, retinol supplements induced significant, but small, increases in serum retinol concentrations. For example, in a baseline survey of smokers and asbestos workers of both genders, subjects who routinely used commercial supplements of vitamin A (usually 5000 IU/day) showed slightly higher (8%) plasma retinol concentrations than those who did not (Goodman *et al.*, 1996). Similarly, women with low initial serum retinol concentrations who received daily supplements of 10 000 IU showed a significant 9% increase ($p<0.02$) in plasma retinol within four weeks (Willett *et al.*, 1984a). Subjects receiving larger oral supplements of vitamin A (17 000–50 000 IU) daily for 5 or 20 days also showed some increase in plasma retinol levels, but more marked increases in the plasma concentrations of retinyl esters, all-*trans*- and 13-*cis*-retinoic acid and all-*trans*- and 13-*cis*-4-oxoretinoic acid (Eckhoff & Nau, 1990a; Buss *et al.*, 1994). Supplements caused more marked increases in plasma retinoids than the same amount of vitamin A present in calf liver (Buss *et al.*, 1994). This is clearly reflected in the data of Arnhold *et al.* (1996) (see Table 2), from human volunteers consuming a liver meal. The vitamin A was taken up and metabolized very differently to the vitamin provided in a supplement, in particular with regard to its metabolism to all-*trans*-retinoic acid (see for comparison Table 3) (Eckhoff & Nau, 1990a).

Table 2. Plasma retinoids following consumption of fried turkey liver by healthy male volunteers[a]

Retinoid	C_{end} (ng/mL)	Following liver consumption C_{max} (ng/mL)	T_{max} (h)	$AUC_{0\text{-}24\,h}$ (ng x h/mL)
Retinol	641 ± 99	800 ± 105*	9	16822 ± 1982
Retinyl palmitate[b]	32.2 ±19.1	3540 ± 1736*	4	21114 ± 7952
14-Hydroxy-4,14-retroretinol	[c]	3.7 ± 0.9	4	61.7 ± 9.0
All-*trans*-retinoic acid	0.8 ± 0.2	2.0 ± 0.5*	2	19.7 ± 1.7
All-*trans*-4-oxoretinoic acid	[c]	0.8 ± 0.2	10	14.7 ± 6.4
13-*cis*-retinoic acid	1.1 ± 0.2	21.5 ± 4.3*	4	204 ± 35.3
13-*cis*-4-oxoretinoic acid	2.4 ± 0.6	32.1 ± 4.9*	10	435 ± 68.5
9-*cis*-retinoic acid	ND[d]	2.7 ± 1.1	4	10.7 ± 3.4
9,13-di-*cis*-retinoic acid	ND[d]	17.1 ± 5.8	4	68.2 ± 21.6

[a] Values are means ± SD for C_{end}, C_{max} and $AUC_{0\text{-}24\,h}$; medians for T_{max} (n = 10).

[b] Retinyl palmitate data calculated with n = 9 due to one outlier (C_{max} = 14106 ng/mL, and $AUC_{0\text{-}24\,h}$ = 104 858 ng x h/mL).

[c] Endogenously detectable in three samples only; 1.3 ± 0.2 ng/mL (for 14-Hydroxy-4,14-retroretinol), and 0.6 ± 0.3 ng/mL (for all-*trans*-4-oxo retinoic acid).

[d] Not detectable; detection limit; 0.3 ng/mL (for 9-*cis*-retinoic acid), and 0.5 ng/mL (for 9,13-di-*cis*-retinoic acid).

* Significantly higher than C_{end} ($p < 0.001$, Student's *t*-test for paired data).

From Arnhold *et al.* (1996)

Table 3. Retinoic acid concentrations in human plasma following ingestion of a retinyl palmitate supplement

Sample	n[a]	Concentration (ng/mL plasma, mean ± SD) 13-*cis*-4-oxo-RA	13-*cis*-RA	All-*trans*-RA
Normal plasma	10	3.68 ± 0.99	1.63 ± 0.85	1.32 ± 0.46
Max. plasma conc. after 833 IU vitamin A/kg body weight	5	7.60 ± 1.45 [b,c]	9.75 ± 2.18 [c,d]	3.92 ± 1.40[c]

[a] Number of subjects

[b] Highest concentration measured until 6 h after dosing.

[c] Different versus normal plasma $p < 0.01$ (Student's *t*-test).

[d] Different versus maximum of all-*trans*-retinoic acid at $p < 0.01$ (Student's *t*-test).

From Eckhoff and Nau (1990a)

When the vitamin A status is poor, however, serum retinol concentrations are decreased. In such cases, daily doses of vitamin A can markedly increase serum retinol concentrations. For example, retinol concentrations increased 20% as a result of supplementation in a Chinese study (Thurnham *et al.*, 1988) and 13% in an Indian study (Jyothirmayi *et al.*, 1996). Cigarette smoking was associated inversely with plasma concentrations of carotenoids, and to a lesser degree with plasma levels of vitamins C and E, but was positively associated with plasma retinol in Afro-American women (Pamuk *et al.*, 1994). In keeping with this finding, cigarette smoke degraded the carotenoids and α-tocopherol in human plasma to a greater extent than retinol (Handelman *et al.*, 1996). Plasma retinol concentrations were positively associated with alcohol use and physical activity and negatively associated with ingestion of soy products in male Japanese smokers (Kitamura *et al.*, 1997). Adipose tissue concentrations of vitamin A were also positively associated with alcohol and with smoking, but negatively associated with body mass index in European men and women (Virtanen *et al.*, 1996). Plasma α-tocopherol concentrations generally are not depressed by long-term interventions with β-carotene and vitamin A (Goodman *et al.*, 1994).

Diseases also influence plasma retinol concentrations. Values are generally lower in cases of cancer, liver disease, protein-calorie malnutrition and infections and are generally higher in many, but not in all, kidney disorders (Goodman *et al.*, 1994; Soprano & Blaner, 1994; Olmedilla *et al.*, 1996).

3.1.4 Uptake by tissues

Chylomicron remnants contain two apolipoproteins, B48 and E, for which specific receptors exist on the surfaces of parenchymal cells of human liver. Whether such receptors are present on cells of other human tissues is less clear. The uptake of chylomicron remnants is by receptor-mediated endocytosis (Blaner & Olson, 1994; Blomhoff, 1994a; Olson, 1994b; Ross, 1998).

The uptake by tissues of retinol from holo-RBP may proceed by one of two mechanisms: (*a*) interaction with a receptor for RBP on the surface of target cells, or (*b*) dissociation of holo-RBP followed by interaction of free retinol with the membranes of target cells (Blaner & Olson, 1994). The case for a specific receptor has best been shown with bovine retinal pigment epithelial cells, but less convincingly with other tissues, whereas the rate of dissociation of holo-RBP accords with physiological rates of uptake. It is quite possible that both mechanisms occur under different physiological conditions (Blaner & Olson, 1994).

3.1.5 Tissue distribution

All tissues of the human body contain vitamin A. Its distribution in various tissues of generally healthy subjects in Iowa, United States, dying of various causes is shown in Table 4 (Raica *et al.*, 1972). The liver clearly is the major storage organ for vitamin A, although fat and muscle contain significant total amounts, albeit at much lower concentrations. The plasma contains <1% of the total vitamin A in the body of a well nourished adult. Other organs examined contain much smaller amounts. Both the concentrations of vitamin A in tissues and the total amount present in the body vary widely between individuals. The total amount of vitamin A in the body of well nourished individuals (a mean of about 260 mg; Table 4) is catabolized at a slow rate (0.5%/day). Thus, signs of vitamin A deficiency in well nourished persons who ingest a diet very low in total vitamin A appear only after a year or more (Sauberlich *et al.*, 1974).

Nonetheless, different European groups show different concentrations of total retinol (retinol + retinyl esters) in various tissues. For example, middle-aged Norwegian men showed the highest (2.3 μg total retinol/g fatty acids) and middle-aged Spanish women the lowest (0.9 μg/g) mean concentrations of total retinol in adipose tissue biopsies obtained from the buttocks in a study of 1025 subjects in nine European countries (Virtanen *et al.*, 1996). Men tended to show higher mean adipose tissue values than women, except in the Netherlands. Different adipose tissue sites show different mean levels of total retinol. Thus, the mean concentrations of total retinol in breast adipose tissue, while higher than those in buttocks, were essentially the same between premenopausal and postmenopausal women and between those with cancer and those with benign breast disease (Zhu *et al.*, 1995). Mean values in fat were approximately 29 ± 9 mg (SD) of vitamin A/g wet weight, lower than the liver concentration but higher than that of other tissues studied (Table 4). Human colonic epithelial cells contain a mean concentration of 16 ng total retinol/10^7 cells, similar concentrations of various carotenoids and much higher concentrations of vitamin E (Nair *et al.*, 1996). The denser, less mature colonic cells contained most of these nutrients. On average, 10^9 cells are equivalent to 1 g wet weight of tissue. Thus, the mean total retinol concentration would be 1.6 μg/g tissue. Lung tissue of cancer patients contains mean total retinol concentrations of 0.15 μg/g, 60-fold higher α-tocopherol concentrations, and approximately two-fold higher carotenoid concentrations (Redlich *et al.*, 1996). Lung tissue concentrations of total retinol correlated with total retinol levels in bronchoalveolar lavage cells but not with serum values. Mean total retinol concentrations in these cancer patients tended to be lower than those found (0.91 μg/g) in presumably normal lung samples obtained at autopsy (Table 4). The retinoic acid concentration in human prostate carcinoma cells was reduced 5–8-fold relative to normal prostatic cells, whereas the retinol concentrations were the same (Pasquali *et al.*, 1996).

3.1.6 Metabolism

Within the human intestinal mucosa, retinal is readily reduced to retinol by retinal reductase and other similar enzymes. Thus, retinol is the merging point for vitamin A derived both from provitamin A carotenoids and directly from the diet. Because observations in humans are fully consistent with those from other animal species (see Section 3.2), these transformations are only briefly summarized here.

Retinol can be oxidized reversibly to retinal and then further, but irreversibly, to retinoic acid in essentially all organs (Blaner & Olson, 1994). Retinol and retinoic acid, by reaction with uridine diphosphoglucuronic acid, form

Table 4. The distribution of vitamin A (retinol and retinyl esters) in tissues of adult humans

Tissue	Mean vitamin A (μg/g)[a]	Tissue % of body weight[b]	Mean total amount (mg)[c]	% of total amount
Liver	149.00 ± 132.00	2.30	232.44	87.90
Fat	1.46 ± 1.55	18.80	18.69	7.07
Muscle	0.35 ± 0.26	42.80	10.18	3.85
Serum	0.57 ± 0.22[d]	4.90	1.90	0.72
Lung	0.91 ± 1.89	0.73	0.46	0.17
Heart	1.08 ± 1.92	0.42	0.31	0.12
Kidney	0.71 ± 0.61	0.41	0.20	0.08
Spleen	0.89 ± 0.88	0.25	0.15	0.06
Pancreas	0.52 ± 0.28	0.16	0.06	0.02
Testes	1.14 ± 1.23	0.04	0.03	0.01
Adrenal	1.26 ± 0.98	0.02	0.02	<0.01
Thyroid	0.43 ± 0.33	0.04	0.01	<0.01
Prostate	0.32 ± 0.31	0.02	<0.01	<0.01

[a] Mean values ± SD for tissues are taken from Raica *et al.* (1972).
[b] From Long, 1961. Major organs not analysed include bone (11–15%), stomach and intestine (6–10%), skin (7%) and brain (2%).
[c] Based on a reference body weight of 68 kg.
[d] Mean value ±SD, in mg/ml, for adults of both sexes, 18–74 years.

retinyl β-glucuronide and retinoyl β-glucuronide, respectively, in the liver, intestine, and other organs (Blaner & Olson, 1994; Barua, 1997). As already indicated, retinoic acid and these two glucuronides are present in low concentrations in human blood (Blaner & Olson, 1994; Formelli *et al.*, 1996; Barua, 1997). Retinol is esterified by transfer of a fatty acid from the α-position of phosphatidyl choline to yield retinyl esters, most notably in the intestinal mucosa, liver and retinal pigment epithelial (RPE) cells of the eye, but also in other tissues. The major esters formed are palmitate and stearate, with smaller amounts of oleate and of polyunsaturated fatty acids (Blaner & Olson, 1994). In the intestine, retinyl esters are incorporated into chylomicra, in the liver into vitamin A-containing globules of parenchymal cells and stellate cells, and in RPE cells into lipid aggregates. Stellate cells, the major storage cells for vitamin A, have been found in many organs of several species (Wake, 1994).

Retinoic acid can be hydroxylated at the C-4, C-16 and C-18 positions, as well as elsewhere, converted to the 5,6-epoxide, and cleaved at various points in its conjugated chain to form a variety of oxidation products. 4-Hydroxyretinoic acid can be oxidized irreversibly to its 4-oxo derivative. In humans, these oxidation products may also have some biological activity (Blaner & Olson, 1994).

The rate of catabolism of administered retinoic acid has been reported to vary with the presence of some types of carcinoma of the lung. After a large oral dose (45 mg/m^2) of retinoic acid in lipid-rich solution (Ensure®), for example, patients with squamous or large-cell carcinoma were six times more likely to have an area under the concentration–time curve (AUC) greater than 250 ng-h/mL (RR, 5.93; 95% CI, 1.3–27.2) than controls free of cancer. In contrast, these AUC values were inversely associated with adenocarcinomas of the lung (RR, 0.12; 95% CI, 0.02–0.65) (Rigas *et al.*, 1996). The most likely explanation for such differences in retinoic acid catabolism is the activity of cytochrome P450 (CYP) enzymes, which are involved in the 4-hydroxylation of retinoic acid and retinol, as well as in the activation and subsequent inactivation of carcinogens (Leo *et al.*, 1989; Rigas *et al.*, 1996). The conversion of retinol and retinoic acid to their 4-hydroxy metabolites in human liver is catalysed by the CYP2C8 isozyme (Leo *et al.*, 1989).

In RPE cells, a physiologically important enzyme, retinyl ester isomerohydrolase, converts all-*trans*-retinyl ester to 11-*cis*-retinol and a free fatty acid (Rando, 1994). Thereafter, 11-*cis*-retinol can either be esterified in the RPE or oxidized to 11-*cis*-retinal. The latter is transported on a specific protein, the interphotoreceptor retinol-binding protein (IRBP), across the inter-photoreceptor space to the outer segment of rods and cones, where it combines with opsin to form rhodopsin in the rod cells and three types of iodopsins in cone cells (Saari, 1994; Ross, 1998). All-*trans*-retinal, after being released photochemically from rhodopsin and iodopsin, is reduced to retinol, which is then ferried back to the RPE cells on IRBP. Several specific binding proteins, termed cellular retinol-binding proteins (CRBP) and cellular retinoic acid-binding proteins (CRABP), play crucial roles in the enzymatic transformations of vitamin A within cells. Several isoforms of each exist with different tissue distributions and actions. These retinoid-binding proteins may also play important regulatory roles in the overall metabolism of the vitamin (Blaner & Olson, 1994; Napoli, 1996; Ross, 1998).

3.1.7 Function

Vitamin A functions in vision, cell differentiation, immune response and embryonic development (Saari, 1994; Gudas *et al.*, 1994; Semba, 1998; Hofmann & Eichele, 1994). The function most closely associated with cancer is cell differentiation. Most, but probably not all, actions of vitamin A in cell differentiation are induced by retinoic acid via two classes of nuclear retinoid receptor, RAR and RXR (Blomhoff, 1994a; Mangelsdorf *et al.*, 1994; Olson, 1994b; Chambon, 1996; Ross, 1998). Each family has three major subtypes, termed α, β and γ. Because the distribution of each of these subtypes in different cells is different, they are presumed to have distinct cellular functions (Blomhoff, 1994a; Olson, 1994b; Ross, 1998).

Synthetic ligands selective for each of these nuclear receptors are already being tested in clinical trials (Chustecka, 1998).

The nuclear retinoid receptors generally act as heterodimers, of which the most common is the RAR–RXR dimer. To be active, RAR must bind retinoic acid (either the all-*trans* or 9-*cis* isomer), whereas RXR need not. Indeed, in the presence of either 9-*cis*-retinoic acid or a synthetic analogue as a ligand for RXR, the activity of processes dependent on the RAR–RXR dimer is reduced in some systems but is synergistically increased in other in-vitro and in-vivo models (Blomhoff, 1994a; Olson, 1994b; Elmazar *et al.*, 1997; Ross, 1998). RXR also forms hetero-dimers with nuclear receptors for triiodothyronine, 1α,25-dihydroxy-vitamin D_3 (calcitriol), peroxisome proliferator-activated receptors and others (Blomhoff, 1994b; Mangelsdorf *et al.*, 1994; Olson, 1994b; Ross, 1998). Furthermore, the ligand-bound RAR–RXR dimer can attenuate the ability of the jun-fos dimer to activate the AP-1 site of the genome, thereby reducing cell proliferation (Mangelsdorf *et al.*, 1994). Thus, the nuclear retinoid receptors and their ligands, both natural and synthetic, show profound effects on gene expression and on cell differentiation (Blomhoff, 1994b; Mangelsdorf *et al.*, 1994; Olson, 1994; Ross, 1998). The clinical implications of these interactions have been reviewed (Goss & McBurney, 1992; Jetten *et al.*, 1993; Lotan, 1996).

3.1.8 Excretion

Vitamin A (retinol and retinyl esters) in oil is well absorbed (60–90%) from the human intestine and any unabsorbed vitamin A, of course, appears in the faeces. The absorption of provitamin A carotenoids is less (<50%) and is greatly affected both by their bioavailability, which can vary more than ten-fold in different foods, and by the amount ingested (Parker, 1996; Olson, 1998). Absorbed vitamin A is ultimately converted to a variety of inactive products, as previously stated. In healthy individuals, a set of largely undefined products are excreted in the urine in relatively small amounts. During severe bacterial infections, however, holo-RBP is excreted in the urine in amounts that may exceed retinol intake by a large margin (Stephensen *et al.*, 1994). Thus, children can be rapidly depleted of vitamin A as a result of recurrent severe bacterial infections. Light or moderate infestations with intestinal parasites, such as *Ascaris,* do not seem to affect vitamin A absorption much, but heavy infestations do (Tanumihardjo *et al.*, 1996; Olson, 1995).

3.1.9 Kinetics

As noted above, ingested retinyl ester is hydrolysed in the intestinal lumen, resynthesized in the intestinal mucosal cells, and released as a component of chylomicra into the lymph. After entering the plasma, chylomicra are degraded to chylomicron remnants that are removed by the liver and other tissues. Retinyl esters taken up by the liver are hydrolysed to retinol, which is released as holo-RBP back into the plasma. The kinetics of these processes have been carefully investigated, both in rats and in humans (Green & Green, 1994).

The half-life ($t_{1/2}$) for triglyceride removal from human chylomicra is 5–8 min (Karpe *et al.*, 1997). The conversion of chylomicra (S_f > 400) to large chylomicron remnants (S_f 60–400), as measured by the presence of retinyl palmitate in these fractions, is slower (mean $t_{1/2}$ = 51 min), as expected. The kinetic analysis is complicated, however, by the presence of pools of both S_f > 400 and S_f 60–400 species with rapid and slow turn-over. Neither of these larger lipoproteins was detectably converted to smaller ones (S_f 20–60), which ostensibly are of greater concern in the formation of atherosclerotic plaques. The rate of conversion of chylomicra to large chylomicron remnants was inversely related to low-density lipoprotein (LDL)–cholesterol concentrations (Karpe *et al.*, 1997). The initial mean half-life for the clearance of retinyl palmitate-labelled chylomicra and chylomicron remnants was 19 min, within the range (10–53 min) reported in other studies (Berr, 1992). Both monoexponential ($t_{1/2}$ 19 min) and biexponential clearance patterns ($t_{1/2}$ values of 19 min and 123 min) have been noted. Uptake rates are dose-dependent, however, and are saturable at fat intakes of 70–100 g (Berr, 1992).

Investigation of the kinetics of orally ingested vitamin A requires isotopically-labelled vitamin

A to distinguish the dosed molecules from endogenous retinol in the plasma. After a single oral dose of 105 µmol [$^{13}C_3$]retinyl palmitate in coconut oil to fasting male adults, the plasma level of retinyl ester reached a peak of 4.45 µmol/L at a mean of 6.2 h after dosing (Reinersdorff *et al.*, 1996). Baseline retinyl ester concentrations in the plasma are <0.2 µmol/L. The initial half-life for retinyl ester clearance was approximately 1 h, followed by higher values (slower clearance). The composition of the plasma retinyl esters was 70% as the palmitate, 25% as the stearate, and 5% as the oleate. The retinyl ester concentrations returned to baseline values within 36 h. The [$^{13}C_3$]retinol concentrations in plasma rose slowly from 3 to 7 h and then tended to plateau. The appearance of retinol probably represents the release of holo-RBP from the liver. In this regard, the half-life of plasma RBP in healthy male adults is 11–12 h when complexed with transthyretin and 4 h when not complexed (Goodman, 1984). Most RBP (80–90%) is present as holo-RBP in healthy adults, with 96% in the complexed state (Goodman, 1984). Later, the [$^{13}C_3$]retinol concentrations in plasma slowly declined, probably as a result of three factors: (*a*) mixing with total body reserves of vitamin A, (*b*) dilution with dietary vitamin A (although a diet low in vitamin A and fat was prescribed in this study), and (*c*) irreversible loss. The study terminated at four days (Reinersdorff *et al.*, 1996).

The estimated equilibration time for vitamin A in human adults is 12–30 days (Sauberlich *et al.*, 1974; Furr *et al.*, 1989; Haskell *et al.*, 1997), whereas the estimated $t_{1/2}$ value of liver reserves is 126–140 days (Sauberlich *et al.*, 1974; Olson, 1987). Because the dose used (105 µmol) in the Reinersdorff *et al.* (1996) study was approximately 30-fold larger than the normal dietary intake, however, the kinetics observed might differ from those in individuals ingesting a conventional diet.

When [^{14}C]retinol in autologous plasma was intravenously injected into three male adults, the specific activity of retinol in the plasma decreased rapidly for 20–30 days and then tended to plateau (Green & Green, 1994). Kinetic analysis indicated an average transit time of retinol in serum of 5.4 h, an average recycling between tissues and serum of 3 times, an average turnover rate of 6.5 mg/day, and a disposal rate of 1.71 mg/day. The disposal rate (irreversible loss), however, is directly related to total body reserves. Of the retinol turnover rate, 26% was irreversibly utilized and 74% was recycled to the serum. In a devised three-compartment model, the average retinol molecule has been predicted to spend 0.86 days in the serum and 105 days in the whole body pool before being irreversibly lost (Green & Green, 1994). The clearance of retinyl esters is slower ($t_{1/2}$ = 57 min) in persons older than 50 years than in younger individuals ($t_{1/2}$ = 31 min), which may explain the higher mean fasting serum concentrations of retinyl esters (58 nmol/L versus 38 nmol/L) in older persons (Krasinski *et al.*, 1990a).

Labelled vitamin A has also been used to estimate total body reserves in humans by an isotope-dilution procedure. Based on reasonable assumptions concerning intestinal absorption efficiency, portion of the dose stored, equilibration time and catabolic rates, calculated values of total body reserves have been shown to agree well with measurements of vitamin A in liver biopsy specimens (Furr *et al.*, 1989; Haskell *et al.*, 1997).

3.2 Experimental models

3.2.1 Overview

3.2.1.1 Animal models

Most studies of vitamin A physiology have been carried out in the rat. Although far less numerous, studies have also been undertaken in the mouse, guinea-pig, rabbit, ferret, cow, pig, monkey and several non-mammalian species including the chicken and frog. The suitability of any animal model for study of vitamin A uptake, transport, storage and metabolism depends on the physiological context of the work. The processes of hepatic storage and metabolism of vitamin A in man and in other species are generally similar and, consequently, investigations using any of these animal models provides insight relevant to the human situation. In contrast, investigations of the transfer of vitamin A from the mother to the developing fetus may be relevant to humans only if carried out in higher primates, where the gross anatomy of the placenta is similar to that of the human.

The great majority of what is now known regarding vitamin A uptake from the diet, its transport in the circulation and its metabolism and storage has come from investigations carried out in the rat. Recently, arising from the development of transgenic and knock-out mouse models, the mouse has become more widely used for the study of vitamin A physiology.

Although vitamin A physiology in the mouse seems to resemble that of the rat, several striking differences between these species have been observed. One is that mouse lung contains very high concentrations of total retinol (retinol + retinyl ester) compared to the rat (see Section 3.2.6.4). In this regard, the rat closely mimics the human. This difference could raise doubts about the value of the mouse model to study processes in the lung that may be influenced by vitamin A.

It also is clear that the mouse is much more resistant than the rat towards developing vitamin A deficiency. Thus, for a weanling rat maintained continuously on a totally vitamin A-deficient diet, symptoms of vitamin A deficiency are first observed after about two to three months, whereas in the mouse, six months or even much longer are required. In some instances, mice have been maintained on a diet totally lacking vitamin A for two generations before symptoms of vitamin A deficiency were observed. Although it seems possible that the mouse accumulates larger body stores of vitamin A and/or utilizes vitamin A more efficiently, the physiological basis for this difference in sensitivity has not been established. The relevance of this difference in the context of understanding vitamin A physiology in man is not clear.

Although the general processes of vitamin A transport and metabolism are similar across species, concentrations of metabolic intermediates and fluxes through metabolic pathways can be markedly different. Thus, the concentrations of some vitamin A forms can vary substantially from species to species. Such variations are thought to account for known species differences with respect to the teratogenic effects of vitamin A (see also Section 7.2.2.2). It is possible that differences in metabolic fluxes and intermediate concentrations can also influence the chemopreventive actions of vitamin A in different species.

Because most of the published information regarding vitamin A transport and metabolism has come from investigations carried out in the rat, the following review is based largely on rat data. Differences in vitamin A physiology that have been identified between the rat and other species are highlighted as well as strain-specific differences within a species.

3.2.1.2 Vitamin A metabolism and transport

Vitamin A transport and metabolism is highly specialized and complex. These processes involve both very specific intra- and extracellular vitamin A-binding proteins which bind retinol, retinoic acid and retinal and specific enzymes. Vitamin A-binding proteins and enzymes, along with their abbreviated names and proposed physiological functions, are listed in Table 5. The vitamin A-binding proteins can be classified according to whether they bind retinol, retinoic acid or retinal and to whether they are found intra- or extracellularly.

A simplified metabolic scheme for the metabolism of vitamin A from its uptake from the diet to its activation in target cells is presented in Figure 1.

3.2.2 Intestinal uptake and metabolism of dietary vitamin A

Both preformed vitamin A and provitamin A carotenoids undergo metabolism within the intestine (Blaner & Olson, 1994). They undergo a series of metabolic conversions, extracellularly in the lumen of the intestine and intracellularly in the intestinal mucosa, which result in the preponderance of the dietary vitamin A being converted to retinol (vitamin A alcohol). The retinol, along with other dietary lipids in the intestinal mucosa, is packaged as retinyl ester in nascent chylomicra. These are secreted into the lymphatic system, and the bulk of chylomicron vitamin A is eventually taken up (as part of the chylomicron remnants) by the liver, where the majority of the body's vitamin A reserves are stored.

Absorption of vitamin A by the small intestine is markedly influenced by the other constituents of the meal or dietary supplement. An

Table 5. Some vitamin A-binding proteins and enzymes

Protein	Abbreviation	Proposed role(s)
A. Vitamin A-binding proteins		
1. Retinol — Extracellular		
Retinol-binding protein	RBP	Plasma transport of retinol
Interphotoreceptor retinol-binding protein	IRBP	Visual process
2. Retinol — Intracellular		
Cellular retinol-binding protein type I	CRBP-I	Substrate for LRAT reaction Substrate for retinol dehydrogenases Stimulate retinyl ester hydrolase Facilitate cellular uptake of retinol
Cellular retinol-binding protein type II	CRBR-II	Substrate for intestinal retinal reductase Substrate for intestinal LRAT uptake of retinol by the cell
3. Retinoic acid — Intracellular		
Cellular retinoic acid binding protein type I	CRABP-I	Facilitate oxidative metabolism of retinoic acid Delivery/inhibition of delivery of retinoic acid to nucleus
Cellular retinoic acid binding protein type II	CRAPB-II	Facilitate oxidative metabolism of retinoic acid Delivery/inhibition of delivery of retinoic acid to nucleus
Retinoic acid receptor-α	RARα	Regulate transcription of vitamin A responsive genes
Retinoic acid receptor-β	RAR-β	Regulate expression of vitamin A responsive genes
Retinoic acid receptor-γ	RAR-γ	Regulate expression of vitamin A responsive genes
Retinoid X receptor-α	RXR-α	Regulate expression of vitamin A responsive genes
Retinoid X receptor-β	RXR-β	Regulate expression of vitamin A responsive genes
Retinoid X receptor-γ	RXR-γ	Regulate expression of vitamin A responsive genes
4. Retinal — Intracellular		
Cellular retinal-binding protein	CRAIBP	Formation of the visual pigment
B. Enzymes		
Lecithin: retinol acetyltransferase	LRAT	Catalyse retinyl ester formation
Bile salt-independent retinyl ester hydrolase	BSI-REH	Catalyse retinyl ester hydrolysis
Bile salt-dependent retinyl ester hydrolase	BSD-REH	Catalyse retinyl ester hydrolysis
Brush border retinyl ester hydrolase	BB-REH	Catalyse hydrolysis of dietary retinyl ester

accompanying fat load is necessary to assure optimal vitamin A uptake, since both bile salts and free fatty acids are needed to emulsify vitamin A. For supplements, the matrix used to solubilize and/or stabilize the vitamin A can markedly influence the ability of the intestine to take up vitamin A, so that different formulations of vitamin A have markedly different bioavailabilities which must be taken into account in the design and evaluation of chemoprevention trials.

A comprehensive review of the present understanding of dietary vitamin A uptake and metabolism is provided below. All vitamin A

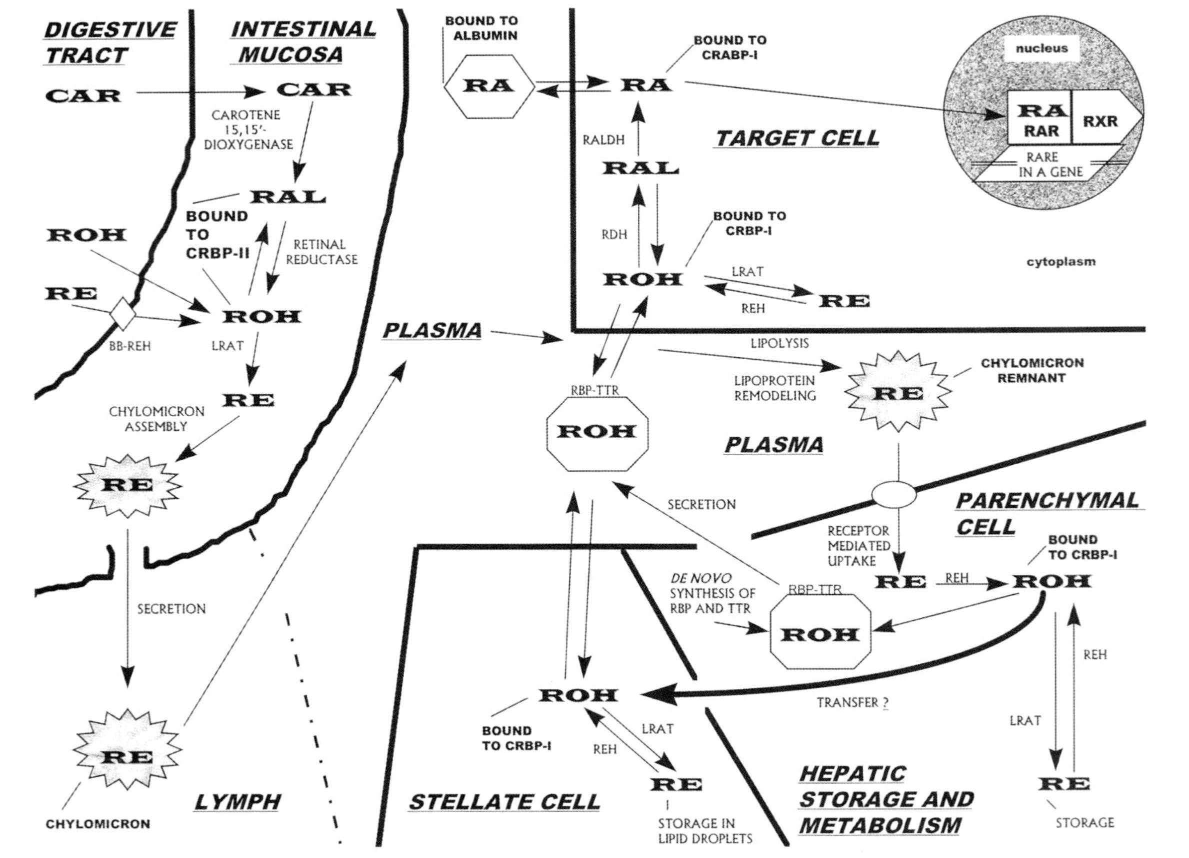

Figure 1. Simplified scheme for the transport and metabolism of retinol and retinyl esters in the digestive tract, the circulation and the liver, and within target cells, applicable to humans and most animal models.
Details of these processes are described in the text. Not all processes, especially those indicated for target cells, necessarily occur in all cells. Abbreviations: CAR, provitamin A carotenoids (including β-carotene); RAL, retinal; ROH, retinol; RE, retinyl esters; RA, retinoic acid; CRBP-I and CRBP-II, cellular retinol-binding protein, types I and II, respectively; CRABP-I, cellular retinoic acid-binding protein; LRAT, lecithin:retinol acyltransferase; BB-REH, brush border retinyl ester hydrolase; REH, retinyl ester hydrolase; RBP, retinol-binding protein; TTR, transthyretin; RAR, retinoic acid receptor; RXR, retinoid X receptor; RARE, retinoic acid response element.

which enters the body must undergo these processes. Since plasma retinol levels are tightly regulated in vitamin A-sufficient individuals, the processes of dietary vitamin A uptake and metabolism probably introduce more variability into the availability of vitamin A to target tissues than does the homeostatically regulated blood retinol pathway.

3.2.2.1 Provitamin A carotenoid uptake and metabolism

Provitamin A carotenoids like β-carotene, α-carotene and β-cryptoxanthin are absorbed intact by the mucosal cells of the proximal small intestine (Blaner & Olson, 1994). Like other neutral lipids in the diet, carotenoids are very insoluble in aqueous environments and must be emulsified with bile salts and free fatty acids within the lumen of the intestine for uptake into the mucosa (Goodman & Blaner, 1984). Within the mucosal cells, β-carotene is cleaved through the action of carotene 15,15′-dioxygenase (also known as the carotene cleavage enzyme) to retinal (vitamin A aldehyde) (Blaner & Olson, 1994). This dioxygenase is known to be cytosolic and influenced by bile salts and vitamin A levels in the diet (van Vliet *et al.*, 1996). In the rat, it is located primarily in mature jejunal enterocytes (Duszka *et al.*, 1996). Although this enzyme was first identified in the mid-1960s (Olson & Hayashi, 1965; Goodman & Huang, 1965), it has never been purified to homogeneity nor has its cDNA or genomic clone been identified. The β-carotene cleavage reaction is a specific oxidation reaction through which molecular oxygen is added across the central double bond (15,15′-double bond) yielding retinal as the sole or preponderant product (Duszka *et al.*, 1996; Nagao *et al.*, 1996). Although some studies suggest that β-carotene can undergo eccentric cleavage at any double bond within the molecule (yielding two of several different β-apocarotenals), it appears that if such cleavage occurs at all, it is not a major pathway (Duszka *et al.*, 1996; Nagao *et al.*, 1996).

Marked species differences exist with respect to carotenoid absorption and/or metabolism (Matsuno, 1991; van Vliet, 1996). No animal model perfectly reflects the human situation for β-carotene metabolism (van Vliet, 1996). Moreover, different commonly studied models show different patterns of β-carotene absorption, storage and conversion into vitamin A (van Vliet, 1996). In man, the majority of absorbed β-carotene (60–70%) is converted to retinal and the remainder is absorbed intact and deposited (or stored) in adipose tissue (Olson, 1990). In addition, humans, unlike most non-primate species, transport β-carotene primarily in the LDL fraction (van Vliet, 1996). Animal models used for study of β-carotene uptake and metabolism include the ferret, the preruminant calf, rodents, the rabbit, the pig and the chicken. The ferret is a poor converter of provitamin A carotenoids to vitamin A (Lederman *et al.*, 1998). Unlike humans, both ferrets and cows have relatively high fasting retinyl ester levels in blood (Ribaya-Mercado *et al.*, 1994; Lederman *et al.*, 1998). Rodents and chickens are very efficient carotenoid converters but they absorb intact carotenoids only when these are provided at high doses (van Vliet, 1996). The pig, in general, is a good model for digestion and absorption of carotenoids, but is not a very efficient converter of β-carotene to vitamin A (Schweigert *et al.*, 1995). Moreover, the pig seems to store most of the absorbed β-carotene in lung and not adipose tissue and liver, two major sites of β-carotene deposition in man (Schweigert *et al.*, 1995). Rabbits similarly do not store carotenoids in fat (van Vliet, 1996). Because of these interspecies differences, it is difficult to formulate from animal studies solely a unified model for β-carotene absorption and its metabolism to vitamin A that is directly applicable to man. The metabolism and conversion of carotenoids into vitamin A is considered in more detail in Volume 2 of the *IARC Handbooks of Cancer Prevention*.

Retinal formed by carotene cleavage is immediately reduced by a microsomal enzyme, retinal reductase, to retinol (Blaner & Olson, 1994). Intestinal retinal reductase requires the participation of a second cytosolic protein, cellular retinol-binding protein, type II (CRBP-II) (Ong *et al.*, 1994). CRBP-II, which binds both retinal and retinol, plays a central role in the processing of dietary vitamin A within the mucosal cell. In the adult rat, CRBP-II is localized solely in the enterocytes of the small intestine and is thought to act solely in dietary vitamin A uptake and metabolism. It is a member of a family of closely related proteins that also includes the intracellular fatty acid-binding proteins and the intracellular retinoid-binding proteins (Ong *et al.*, 1994). CRBP-II shows the highest degree of sequence homology with the widely distributed cellular retinol-binding protein, type I (CRBP-I) but is immunologically distinct (Ong *et al.*, 1994). Retinal, when bound to CRBP-II, is the preferred substrate for reduction to retinol by intestinal retinal reductase. Retinol formed through this pathway is metabolically indistinguishable from retinol arriving in the diet as preformed vitamin A and, hence, undergoes the same subsequent metabolic events as described below for preformed vitamin A.

3.2.2.2 *Preformed vitamin A uptake and metabolism*

Preformed dietary vitamin A consists primarily of retinyl esters and retinol. Within the lumen of the small intestine, some of the esters may be hydrolysed to retinol, which, along with the retinol arriving as such in the diet, is taken up by the mucosal cells. Pancreatic lipases, such as triglyceride lipase and cholesteryl ester hydrolase (also known as carboxy ester lipase and bile-salt-dependent retinyl ester hydrolase) are able to hydrolyse retinyl esters *in vitro* and it has been assumed that these enzymes mediate the luminal hydrolysis of dietary retinyl esters (Goodman & Blaner, 1984; Blaner & Olson, 1994). However, studies in the rat have indicated that a retinyl ester hydrolase activity intrinsic to the brush border membrane of the small intestine plays a central role in this process, making a quantitatively greater contribution to the hydrolysis of dietary retinyl ester than the pancreatic enzymes (Rigtrup & Ong, 1992). The intrinsic brush border retinyl ester hydrolase activity is stimulated by both trihydroxy and dihydroxy bile salts, and preferentially hydrolyses long-chain retinyl esters like retinyl palmitate. This brush border retinyl ester hydrolase from the rat small intestine mucosa is probably identical to the brush border phospholipase B characterized earlier for this tissue (Rigtrup *et al.*, 1994).

Retinol formed through the hydrolysis of dietary retinyl esters or arriving as such in the diet is taken up by the mucosal cells. Unhydrolysed dietary retinyl ester is very poorly absorbed, if at all, from the intestinal lumen. The process of retinol uptake requires emulsification of the retinol by bile salts and free fatty acids (Goodman & Blaner, 1984). In the rat, a retinol transport protein within the plasma membrane of the enterocyte facilitates retinol uptake (Dew & Ong, 1994). Within the intestinal mucosa, all retinol is re-esterified with long-chain fatty acids (primarily palmitic, with smaller amounts of stearic, oleic and linoleic acids) through the action of the enzyme lecithin:retinol acyltransferase (LRAT). The synthesized retinyl esters are packaged along with other dietary lipids into nascent chylomicrons and secreted into the lymphatic system for uptake into the circulation. Intestinal LRAT requires retinol bound to CRBP-II as a substrate (Blaner & Olson, 1994; Ong *et al.*, 1994). Thus, CRBP-II plays a central role in directing or channelling dietary retinol to nascent chylomicra for uptake into the body. Retinal formed by carotene cleavage is also metabolically channelled, through binding to CRBP-II, towards retinyl ester formation and packaging in chylomicra. No information is available concerning the biochemical processes through which the synthesized retinyl ester is packaged by the mucosal cells into nascent chylomicra.

LRAT has been proposed to play a key role in directing the metabolism of retinol throughout the body. This enzyme catalyses the transfer of an α_1 fatty acid from the membrane-associated phosphatidyl choline to all-*trans*-retinol and has been reported to be present in the liver, eye, small intestine and testes (Blaner & Olson, 1994). It is not clear whether the LRAT species in each of these tissues are distinct gene products, but it has been established that hepatic but not intestinal LRAT is actively regulated by vitamin A nutritional status (Randolph & Ross, 1991; Matsuura & Ross, 1993). The biochemical characteristics of LRAT have been summarized by Blaner & Olson (1994). In essence, LRAT utilizes retinol bound to CRBP-II (in intestine) or to CRBP-I (in other tissues) as its preferred substrate. The apparent K_m values of rat intestinal and hepatic LRAT for the retinol-binding protein complexes are in the low micromolar range, a concentration that is physiological (Blaner & Olson, 1994). The properties and roles of hepatic LRAT are discussed in Section 3.2.4.2. Figure 2 provides a schematic view of the uptake and metabolism of pro- and preformed vitamin A by the intestine.

3.2.3 Chylomicron delivery of postprandial vitamin A

3.2.3.1 Overview

Together with triglycerides, cholesteryl esters, phospholipids and other dietary lipids, retinyl esters are incorporated into the apolipoprotein B-48 (apoB48)-containing chylomicra and secreted into the lymphatic system. Once in the general circulation, chylomicra interact with lipoprotein lipase (LPL) bound to the luminal surface of the vascular endothelium and rapid lipolysis of the triglyceride occurs. LPL-catalysed hydrolysis gives rise to free fatty acids and a smaller lipoprotein particle termed a chylomicron remnant. The free fatty acids generated from triglyceride hydrolysis are taken up by extrahepatic tissues, including muscle and adipose tissue, where they are ultimately used as substrates for energy metabolism (Cooper, 1997). The chylomicron remnants acquire apolipoprotein E (apoE) either in the plasma or in the space of Disse, where apoE can

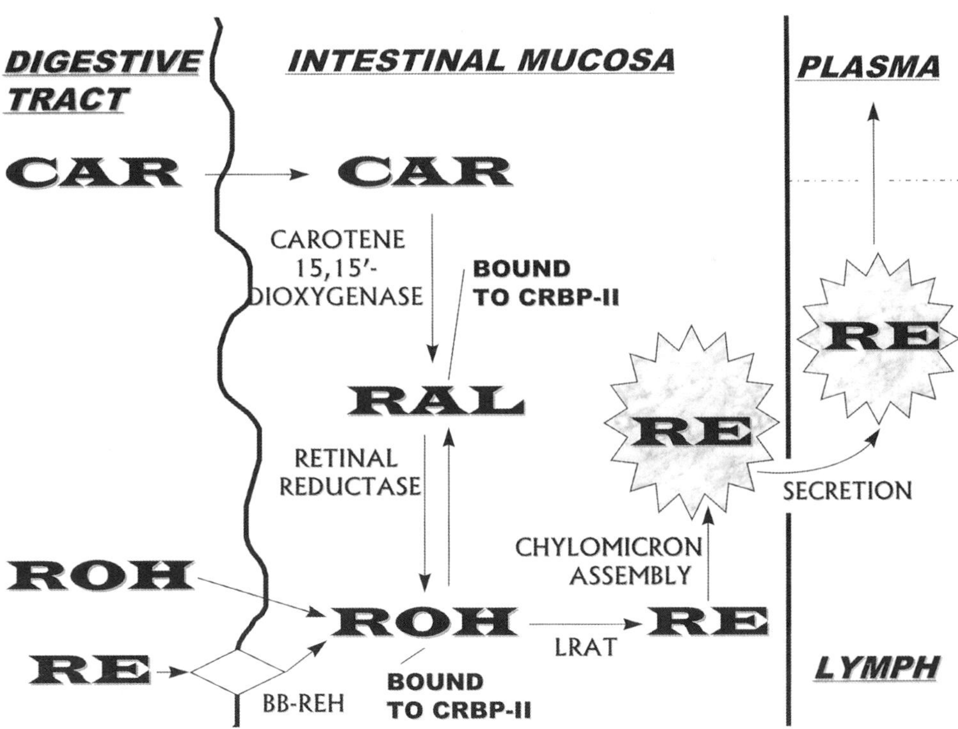

Figure 2. Simplified scheme for the uptake and metabolism of retinol and retinyl esters in the digestive tract applicable to humans and many animal models.
However, many animal species do not take up and/or metabolize carotenoids well. Details of these processes and specific species differences are described in the text.
For key to abbreviations, see Figure 1.

accumulate after its secretion from hepatocytes (Williams *et al.*, 1985; Hamilton *et al.*, 1990; Ji *et al.*, 1994, 1995). The acquisition of apoE by the remnant particles is essential for their clearance by the liver (Cooper, 1997). The importance of apoE in chylomicron remnant clearance is underscored by the fact that apoE-deficient mice clear postprandial cholesterol very slowly (Ishibashi *et al.*, 1994, 1996; Mortimer *et al.*, 1995). These mice also show very high circulating levels of total cholesterol and retinyl esters, even in the fasting state. Data accumulated from studies carried out over the past 35 years consistently show that approximately 75% of chylomicron retinyl ester is removed from the circulation by the liver and the remaining 25% by extrahepatic tissues, including skeletal muscle, adipose tissue, heart, spleen and kidney (Goodman *et al.*, 1965).

Most species seem to process and metabolize dietary lipids in a similar manner. In general, dietary vitamin A uptake and its clearance from the circulation are not thought to be very different in rats, mice, rabbits and humans. However, one major exception to this generalization can become important in disease states that lead to decreased rates of clearance of dietary lipids. Specifically, some species, including rodents, totally lack plasma cholesteryl ester transfer protein, which catalyses the transfer within the circulation of cholesteryl esters and retinyl esters from triglyceride-rich lipoproteins like chylomicra to low-density lipoprotein (LDL) and high-density lipoprotein (HDL) (Tall, 1995). Thus, in both man and rabbits, which express cholesteryl ester transfer protein, some postprandial retinyl ester is transferred to these lipoprotein fractions if lipid clearance is impaired as the result of either disease or experimental intervention (Goodman & Blaner, 1984; Blaner & Olson, 1994). The retinyl ester transferred to LDL or HDL would then be processed as a component of these lipoproteins. In most healthy individuals the amount of postprandial retinyl ester transferred by cholesteryl ester transfer protein to LDL and/or HDL is very small. Nevertheless, this process may be significant in some pathological states which involve delayed plasma lipid clearance.

3.2.3.2 Hepatic clearance

ApoE is required for uptake of chylomicron remnants by the liver, but the exact mechanisms involved are still unclear. Several distinct cell surface receptors that are able to bind apoE-containing lipoproteins may well be involved in the uptake of chylomicron remnants by hepatocytes. Among these are the LDL receptor (LDL-R), the LDL receptor-related protein (LRP) and the lipolysis-stimulated receptor (LSR) (Cooper, 1997). In addition, heparin sulfate proteoglycans (HSPG), located on the surface of hepatocytes, may also be responsible for the initial interaction of remnants with the cells of the liver (Cooper, 1997). Roles for LPL and hepatic lipase in hepatic uptake have also been suggested (Shafi *et al.*, 1994; Beisiegel *et al.*, 1991).

Gene targeting of the LDL-R has provided evidence for the involvement of the LDL-R in chylomicron remnant clearance by hepatocytes. In a mouse strain totally lacking this receptor (LDL-R$^{-/-}$), the rate of plasma clearance of chylomicron remnants was unaffected, but endocytosis of the remnant by the hepatocyte was delayed (Mortimer *et al.*, 1995; Ishibashi *et al.*, 1994, 1996; Herz *et al.*, 1995). Thus, the rate of clearance of chylomicron remnant cholesteryl ester from the circulation was comparable to that of wild-type mice, but uptake of chylomicron remnant lipids into the liver of LDL-R$^{-/-}$ mice was significantly delayed (Mortimer *et al.*, 1995; Herz *et al.*, 1995). In double mutant mice totally lacking both the LDL-R and apoE, chylomicron remnants accumulated in the circulation to levels comparable to those observed in apoE-deficient mice carrying the wild-type LDL-R alleles (Ishibashi *et al.*, 1996). Overall, these data imply that the LDL-R contributes to hepatic uptake of chylomicron remnants, but suggest that chylomicron remnants are also taken up by the liver through alternative apoE-dependent processes which are distinct from the LDL-R pathway and can compensate for absence of the LDL-R pathway.

One such alternative apoE-dependent process may involve LRP, a 600 kDa calcium-dependent multifunctional receptor protein that is a member of the LDL-R protein family. LRP is identical to the receptor reported to be the activated receptor form of the α_2-macroglobulin receptor and therefore also is known as α_2-macroglobulin receptor/LRP. It is known to interact with various ligands that are present in the circulation (Cooper, 1997). These include apoE, activated α_2-macroglobulin, LPL, lactoferrin, receptor-associated protein (RAP) and various serum proteases. The involvement of LRP in chylomicron remnant metabolism is supported by studies using RAP, a 39 kDa protein that binds to LRP in the presence of calcium ions and upon binding suppresses binding of other ligands to LRP (Cooper, 1997). For mice totally deficient in RAP ($RAP^{-/-}$), no difference in the rate of chylomicron remnant clearance was observed; however, in double mutants lacking both LDL-R and RAP, chylomicron remnants (as assessed by apoB48 concentrations) accumulated in the circulation to high levels (Willnow *et al.*, 1995). Overexpression of RAP in mice leads to accumulation of apoB48- and apoE-containing particles in the circulation of $LDL\text{-}R^{-/-}$ mice (Willnow *et al.*, 1994). Thus, it would appear that LRP, like the LDL-R, is not essential for clearance of chylomicron remnants by the liver. However, like the LDL-R, LRP contributes to hepatic clearance of chylomicron remnants in a manner that can be compensated for through the actions of other receptors.

A third receptor proposed to be present on hepatocytes, the LSR, is distinct from the LDL-R and LRP and may also contribute to uptake of chylomicron remnants by hepatocytes (Bihain & Yen, 1992; Yen *et al.*, 1994; Mann *et al.*, 1995). The role of this protein in chylomicron remnant clearance has been studied in both human and rat cells. LSR activity seems to depend on two distinct but interacting membrane proteins (Bihain & Yen, 1992; Yen *et al.*, 1994). Free fatty acids are thought to activate the LSR by causing a conformational shift that reveals cryptic binding sides for apoE and apoB. LSR binds to lipoproteins (preferentially triglyceride-rich particles) and to RAP at high concentrations. Unlike lipoprotein particle binding to the LDL-R and LRP, binding of ligands is calcium-independent (Yen *et al.*, 1994). Whether LSR contributes to chylomicron remnant clearance *in vivo* remains to be established.

While internalization of chylomicron remnants by hepatocytes is mediated by cell surface receptors, initial binding of the remnant to the surface of the hepatocyte may involve the actions of cell-surface HSPGs, which are especially abundant in the space of Disse. Data supporting a role for HSPGs in facilitating hepatocyte removal of chylomicron remnants has been obtained from studies in mice. Following intravenous administration of heparinase to mice, the rate of removal of apoE-rich remnant particles by the liver was greatly reduced for both wild-type and $LDL\text{-}R^{-/-}$ mice (Ji *et al.*, 1995; Mortimer *et al.*, 1995). It seems reasonable to speculate that remnant binding to hepatocyte HSPGs helps increase the residence time of apoE-containing remnant particles at the cell surface, thus allowing time for the remnant to bind to receptors like the LDL-R and/or LRP.

In summary, apoE plays an essential role in the uptake of chylomicron remnants by the liver. It seems likely that initially the chylomicron remnants are sequestered in close proximity to the hepatocytes through binding to HSPGs in the space of Disse. Subsequently, the remnant is able to interact with a cell surface receptor that mediates endocytosis of the remnant particle. Both the LDL-R and LRP appear to be important cell surface receptors for the uptake of chylomicron remnants. De Faria *et al.* (1996), employing RAP or antibodies against the LDL-R, have estimated that approximately 55% of chylomicron remnants are cleared through the LDL-R-mediated pathway and approximately 25% through the LRP-mediated pathway. Ishibashi *et al.* (1996) estimated that approximately 75% of chylomicron remnants are cleared through the LDL-R pathway. Although the role of LSR in chylomicron remnant clearance by the liver has not been fully established, this receptor too may contribute substantially to the process.

3.2.3.3 Extrahepatic tissue clearance

Early work by Goodman *et al.* (1965) indicated that in rats approximately 25% of postprandial retinyl ester is taken up by extrahepatic tissues. Following intravenous injection of doses of rat mesenteric chylomicra containing [^{14}C]retinyl ester, a substantial portion of the ^{14}C-label was detected in skeletal muscle, depot fat, heart, spleen and kidney. Neither the physiological significance nor the biochemical basis for the observation that some chylomicron or chylomicron remnant retinyl ester is taken up by extrahepatic tissues has been systematically investigated until recently. It now appears that LPL plays an important role in facilitating uptake of postprandial vitamin A by extrahepatic tissues.

Blaner *et al.* (1994) established that after most of the chylomicron triglyceride has been hydrolysed, chylomicron retinyl esters become substrates for LPL-catalysed hydrolysis. The hydrolysis of chylomicron retinyl ester enhances the uptake of chylomicron vitamin A by cultures of murine BFC-1β adipocytes (Blaner *et al.*, 1994). This led to the hypothesis that LPL plays an important role *in vivo* in facilitating clearance of dietary vitamin A by extrahepatic tissues. Study of three mouse strains having different patterns of expression of mouse and human LPL (wild-type mice, LPL-null mice overexpressing human LPL in skeletal muscle and wild-type mice overexpressing human LPL in skeletal muscle) have provided support for this hypothesis. Mice overexpressing human LPL in skeletal muscle took up approximately two-fold more chylomicron vitamin A than did wild-type mice. The data from these studies and from other studies in rats are consistent in that the level of expression of LPL activity in skeletal muscle, adipose tissue and heart directly correlates with the amount of chylomicron vitamin A taken up by the tissues. Thus, it seems that the level of LPL activity in skeletal muscle, adipose tissue and heart is a key determinant of the amount of postprandial vitamin A taken up by these tissues.

Other important findings regarding the clearance of chylomicron retinyl esters have come from studies in primates (marmosets) and rabbits (Cooper, 1997). Mahley and Hussain (1991) reported that the bone marrow of rabbits and of marmosets takes up substantial amounts of chylomicra. Chylomicron uptake by rabbit bone marrow was 50–100% of that of the liver. Unlike rabbit liver, where LPL helps facilitate uptake of the chylomicron and its remnant, rabbit bone marrow takes up chylomicron retinyl ester in the total absence of LPL activity (Hussain *et al.*, 1997). It is thus clear that bone marrow too plays a dynamic role in the overall metabolism of postprandial vitamin A.

The LXR nuclear receptor, a member of the steroid–thyroid–retinoid superfamily of receptors, is thought to be involved in regulating expression of a variety of genes believed to be important in the metabolism and transport of cholesterol and triglycerides (Janowski *et al.*, 1996). The ligand for LXR is proposed to be a sterol metabolite. LXR must form a heterodimer with RXR to be active. Thus, vitamin A may play a role, along with sterol, in regulating its own uptake and transport following a vitamin A-containing meal.

3.2.4 Hepatic storage and metabolism of vitamin A

The liver is the major organ in the body for the storage and metabolism of vitamin A. The preponderance of the body's vitamin A reserves is stored as retinyl esters in hepatic stellate cells (also called Ito cells, fat-storing cells, perisinusoidal cells and lipocytes; described more fully in Section 3.2.4.4), although other tissues including adipose tissue, lung and kidney contain significant vitamin A stores and/or are active in vitamin A metabolism (see Section 3.2.6) (Blaner & Olson, 1994). The processes of vitamin A storage and metabolism in the liver are complex and many details regarding these processes and their regulation are still not fully understood. Hepatic vitamin A metabolism is mediated by enzymes such as LRAT, which esterifies retinol with long-chain fatty acids, and retinyl ester hydrolase, which hydrolyses retinyl esters to retinol, and by CRBP-I (Blaner & Olson, 1994). To meet tissue needs for vitamin A, retinol is secreted from hepatic parenchymal cells bound to its specific plasma transport protein, RBP (Soprano & Blaner, 1994). Like hepatic vitamin A storage and metabolism, the factors and processes which regulate retinol mobilization from the liver are not fully understood. It is clear, however, that for well nourished animals the concentrations of vitamin A stored in liver are both species- and strain-dependent. Thus, hepatic vitamin A levels are different in rats, mice and rabbits, the best studied animal models. Similarly, different strains of rats maintained on diets providing the same levels of vitamin A show different hepatic vitamin A concentrations.

3.2.4.1 Hepatic processing of dietary vitamin A

Chylomicron remnants are thought to be internalized solely by hepatocytes (Cooper, 1997). Confirming earlier work, Mortimer *et al.* (1995), used confocal microscopy to show that fluorescent-labelled cholesteryl ester derivatives arriving in chylomicron remnants accumulated solely in hepatocytes and not in other hepatic cell types. Very shortly after endocytosis by hepatocytes, the chylomicron remnant retinyl esters are hydrolysed to retinol (Blaner & Olson, 1994). Harrison *et al.* (1995) showed that the newly endocytosed retinyl esters co-localize with a retinyl ester hydrolase in early endosomes. The esters are hydrolysed to retinol at this stage of endocytosis, before the remnant particle has reached the lysosome (Harrison *et al.*, 1995). At this point in the uptake process, the metabolism of dietary vitamin A diverges from that of dietary cholesterol. The retinol formed by retinyl ester hydrolysis is bound to apo-CRBP-I, which is found in relatively high concentrations in hepatocytes (see Table 6). CRBP-I-bound retinol may be delivered to newly synthesized apo-RBP, leading to secretion of holo-RBP into the circulation. The amount of newly endocytosed retinol that is secreted from the liver depends on the vitamin A nutritional status of the animal, more of the newly arrived retinol being secreted from hepatocytes of animals with poor nutritional status (Batres & Olson, 1987). An alternative fate for newly absorbed retinol is storage as retinyl ester in hepatocytes or in stellate cells following transfer from the hepatocyte. The mechanism through which retinol is transferred from hepatocytes to hepatic stellate cells

Table 6. Distribution of retinol, retinol-binding protein (RBP), cellular retinol-binding protein type I (CRBP-I), cellular retinoic acid-binding protein type I (CRABP-I), bile-salt-dependent retinyl ester hydrolase (BSD-REH), bile-salt-independent retinyl ester hydrolase (BSI-REH), and lecithin:retinol acyltransferase (LRAT) in isolated rat liver parenchymal and stellate cells[a,b]

Parameter	Parenchymal cells	Stellate cells
Total retinol	5.2 ± 2.4 nmol/10^6 cells 2.6 ± 1.2 nmol/mg protein	293 ± 107 nmol/10^6 cells 1558 ± 569 nmol/mg protein
RBP	6.6 ± 0.3 pmol/10^6 cells 0.34 ± 0.16 pmol/mg protein	0.04 ± 0.02 pmol/10^6 cells 0.18 ± 0.09 pmol/mg protein
CRBP-I	30.1 ± 15.8 pmol/10^6 cells 16.2 ± 8.2 pmol/mg protein	15.7 ± 5.9 pmol/10^6 cells 83.3 ± 31.8 pmol/mg protein
CRABP-I	0.37 ± 0.26 pmol/10^6 cells 0.19 ± 0.22 pmol/mg protein	0.58 ± 0.37 pmol/10^6 cells 29.3 ± 20.0 pmol/mg protein
BSD-REH	826 ± 47 pmol FFA/h/10^6 cells 427 ± 24 pmol FFA/h/mg protein	1152 ± 144 pmol FFA/h/10^6 cells 6129 ± 768 pmol FFA/h/mg protein
BSI-REH	Not determined	10.98 ± 1.08 nmol FFA formed/h/mg protein
LRAT	158 ± 53 pmol retinyl ester formed/min/mg microsomal protein	383 ± 54 pmol retinyl ester formed/min/mg microsomal protein

FFA, free fatty acid

[a] Values are taken from Blaner *et al.* (1985), Blaner *et al.* (1990) and Friedman *et al.* (1993)

[b] One gram of rat liver is taken to consist of 108 × 10^6 parenchymal cells, 16 × 10^6 stellate cells, 19 × 10^6 endothelial cells, and 9 × 10^6 Kupffer cells. Parenchymal cells were determined to contain 1934 ± 161 mg protein/10^6 cells and stellate cells 188 ± 80 mg protein/10^6 cells (Blaner *et al.*, 1985).

has not been fully established. The specific events important to hepatic vitamin A storage and metabolism that occur in hepatocytes and stellate cells are summarized below for each cell type, and are represented diagrammatically in Figure 3.

3.2.4.2 Vitamin A storage and metabolism in hepatocytes

The hepatocyte is an important site of vitamin A storage and metabolism. Hepatocytes have relatively high concentrations of total retinol (retinol + retinyl ester), CRBP-I, LRAT, bile-salt-stimulated and bile-salt-independent retinyl ester hydrolases, retinol dehydrogenases and retinal dehydrogenases, as well as other enzymes that catalyse the oxidative, conjugative and/or catabolic metabolism of retinoic acid. The cellular concentrations or specific activities of some of these components in both rat hepatocytes and hepatic stellate cells are shown in Table 6.

Hepatocytes from rats fed a control diet contain total retinol concentrations of 5.2 ± 2.4 nmol retinol per 10^6 hepatocytes (2.6 ± 1.2 nmol retinol/mg hepatocyte total protein). Approximately 95–99% of this total retinol is present as retinyl esters, primarily the esters of palmitic, stearic, oleic and linoleic acids (Blaner *et al.*, 1985). It has been estimated that approximately 5–30% of the total retinol in the livers of rats maintained on a control diet is present in

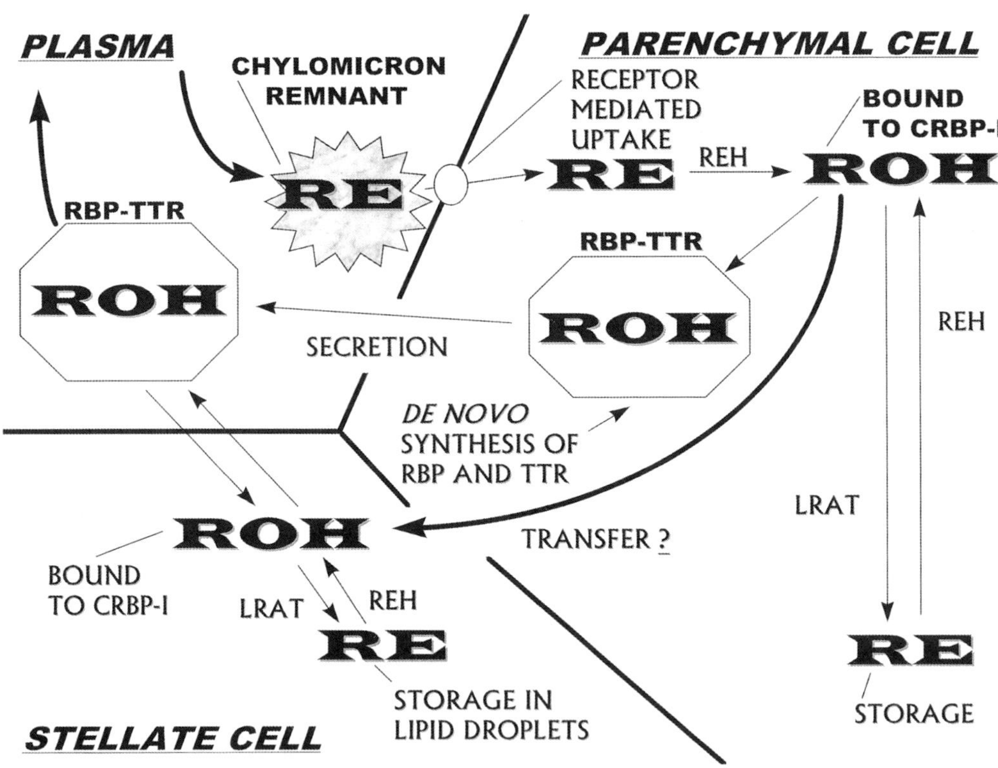

Figure 3. Simplified scheme for the uptake, transport, metabolism and storage of retinol and retinyl esters in the liver, applicable to humans and most animal models.
Details of these processes are described in the text.
For key to abbreviations, see Figure 1.

hepatocytes (Blaner *et al.*, 1985; Batres & Olson, 1987), with the remainder in stellate cells. The relative abundance of total retinol in hepatocytes is thought to be inversely related to the level of hepatic stores (Batres & Olson, 1987). Thus, as hepatic vitamin A stores decline, the proportion of vitamin A in hepatocytes increases relative to hepatic stellate cells. Since the hepatocyte is the site of RBP synthesis in the liver (Soprano & Blaner, 1994), this may imply that hepatocyte total retinol levels remain relatively constant in order to regulate circulating retinol–RBP levels.

Chylomicron remnant retinyl esters are hydrolysed through the action of a bile-salt-independent retinyl ester hydrolase that is present in the hepatocyte plasma membrane (Harrison *et al.*, 1995). This hydrolase in rats is identical to carboxylesterase ES-2, which was first described as a thiol esterase (Sun *et al.*, 1997). The activity of rat liver bile-salt-independent retinyl ester hydrolase *in vitro* is reported to be markedly influenced by the presence of *N*-(4-hydroxyphenyl)retinamide, all-*trans*-retinoic acid or 13-*cis*-retinoic acid in the assay mixture (Ritter & Smith, 1996). The enzyme was identified originally as a bile-salt-independent retinyl ester hydrolase as opposed to the bile-salt-stimulated retinyl ester hydrolase from rat liver that was characterized in the late 1970s. It had been believed that the bile-salt-stimulated retinyl ester hydrolase was the key enzyme responsible for hydrolysis of retinyl ester before its mobilization from the liver (Goodman & Blaner, 1984; Harrison, 1993). Later work demonstrated that in rats this enzyme is identical to cholesteryl ester hydrolase (Chen *et al.*, 1997a), a lipid hydrolase that is expressed in both liver and pancreas (as described in Section 3.2.2.2). Although rat hepatocytes possess both bile-salt-stimulated and bile-salt-independent retinyl ester hydrolases, the bile-salt-stimulated enzyme is not required for hepatic retinyl ester hydrolysis. The physiological actions of this enzyme in the liver are redundant with those of other enzymes. Whether the bile-salt-independent retinyl ester hydrolase plays a unique and irreplaceable role in retinyl ester hydrolysis within hepatic cells remains to be demonstrated. However, it is thought that this enzyme is important for hydrolysing chylomicron remnant retinyl ester and it may also be involved in the hydrolysis of hepatocyte retinyl ester stores to provide retinol to newly synthesized RBP.

CRBP-I concentrations in hepatocytes are relatively high, and it has been estimated that approximately 90% of the CRBP-I present in the liver is localized in hepatocytes (Blaner *et al.*, 1985). In rat liver and testis, CRBP-I is present at concentrations in excess of those of retinol, suggesting that all retinol present within these tissues is bound to CRBP-I (Harrison *et al.*, 1987). CRBP-I plays an important role in retinol metabolism (Ong *et al.*, 1994). Holo-CRBP-I has been reported to deliver retinol to LRAT for esterification (Ong *et al.*, 1994) and to provide retinol to retinol dehydrogenases which catalyse the first of two oxidation steps needed for formation of retinoic acid. Both LRAT (Blaner & Olson, 1994) and several retinol–CRBP-I-utilizing retinol dehydrogenases (Napoli, 1996) are present in hepatocytes. In addition, apo-CRBP-I has been reported to enhance hepatic bile-salt-independent retinyl ester hydrolase activity (Blaner & Olson, 1994). It also has been postulated that holo-CRBP-I delivers retinol to newly synthesized RBP for secretion from the liver into the circulation (Blaner & Olson, 1994). Finally, based on the binding characteristics of retinol to CRBP-I, it has been proposed that CRBP-I plays an important role in facilitating retinol uptake by cells from the circulating retinol–RBP complex. Thus, CRBP-I serves as an intracellular transporter of retinol, linking and facilitating the processes of retinol uptake, metabolism and mobilization within the hepatocyte.

Hepatic LRAT is present in both hepatocytes and stellate cells, but its specific activity is highest in the latter (Blaner *et al.*, 1990; Matsuura *et al.*, 1997). However, because of the large size and the number of hepatocytes, approximately 85% of the hepatic LRAT activity is present in hepatocytes (Blaner *et al.*, 1990). As outlined in Section 3.2.2.2, retinol bound to CRBP-I is the preferred substrate for hepatic LRAT, which shows an apparent K_m of 2.2 μmol/L for retinol–CRBP-I. LRAT has not been purified from any tissue or cell and its cDNA and gene have not been cloned. Using radiation inactivation analyses, Ross and Kempner (1993) estimated that hepatic LRAT has a molecular size of approximately 52 ± 10 kDa. In rats, hepatic but not intestinal LRAT activity is regulated by vitamin A nutritional status (Randolph & Ross, 1991). Hepatic LRAT activity falls progressively during vitamin A depletion and within eight hours after repletion of vitamin A-deficient rats with retinol, hepatic LRAT activity starts to rise, reaching control levels within 24 hours after the start of repletion. Repletion with retinoic acid also increased hepatic LRAT activity in vitamin A-deficient rats, but this effect could be abolished if hepatocytes were pre-treated with inhibitors of gene transcription and protein synthesis. Taken together, these data suggest that hepatic LRAT expression is regulated by retinoic acid and consequently vitamin A availability. This provides a convenient regulatory mechanism through which retinol, in times of sufficient intake, can be converted to retinyl ester for storage or, in times of insufficient intake, can remain in the unesterified form to serve as a substrate for retinoic acid synthesis.

3.2.4.3 Transfer of vitamin A between hepatocytes and stellate cells

For vitamin A homeostasis to be maintained, interactions between hepatocytes and stellate cells must be tightly regulated. However, little is known about how hepatocytes and stellate cells communicate or about how vitamin A is transferred between the two cell types. Blaner and Olson (1994) reviewed mechanisms that have been proposed to explain the movement of vitamin A between hepatocytes and stellate cells. Although it is clear that chylomicron remnant retinyl ester must be hydrolysed before it is transferred from hepatocytes to stellate cells, the specific roles of RBP, CRBP-I and/or intercellular contacts between hepatocytes and stellate cells in the transfer process have not been definitively established. It is widely believed that vitamin A transfer involves the action of RBP and bulk movement through the extracellular space, but the possibility that movement of free retinol, retinol–CRBP-I or retinyl ester occurs via intercellular contacts between hepatocytes and stellate cells has not been ruled out (Blaner & Olson, 1994).

Early studies supporting the participation of RBP in the uptake process demonstrated that RBP is taken up by rat stellate cells both *in vivo* and *in vitro* (Blomhoff *et al.*, 1988; Senoo *et al.*, 1993). This was taken to indicate that RBP is important for the delivery of retinol from hepatocytes to stellate cells (Senoo *et al.*, 1993). Furthermore, in a perfused rat liver model, transfer of newly absorbed retinol between hepatocytes and stellate cells was effectively blocked when the animals were perfused with antibodies against RBP (Blomhoff *et al.*, 1988; Senoo *et al.*, 1990). Support for a role of RBP in the uptake process has come from studies of the transfer of RBP between co-cultured human HepG2 hepatoma cells, which are known to secrete RBP, and rat hepatic stellate cells. After co-culture for 18 hours, human RBP was identified by indirect immunolabelling on the surface, in coated pits and in vesicles in the stellate cells, suggesting movement of hepatocyte-secreted human RBP to the stellate cells. The amount of human RBP associated with the stellate cells was significantly reduced when antibodies against human RBP were added to the culture medium (Blomhoff *et al.*, 1988). The intracellular pool of vitamin A within stellate cells influences the amount of retinol that is esterified when retinol–RBP is added to the cell medium but not when free retinol is added (Trøen *et al.*, 1994). A need for RBP in intercellular transfer was not supported, however, by the finding that while stellate cells may take up RBP and retinol bound to RBP, the uptake of retinol into stellate cells does not depend on RBP (Matsuura *et al.*, 1993a,b). Thus, it remains unclear whether RBP plays an essential role in the transfer of retinol from hepatocytes to stellate cells.

3.2.4.4 Vitamin A storage and metabolism in hepatic stellate cells

In the vitamin A-sufficient adult rat, 70–95% of hepatic vitamin A is stored as retinyl ester in lipid droplets of stellate cells (Blaner & Olson, 1994). Hepatic stellate cells are non-parenchymal cells located perisinusoidally in the space of Disse, in recesses between parenchymal cells (Geerts *et al.*, 1994). They comprise about 5–8%

of total rat liver cells, and 1% of the total liver mass (Geerts *et al.*, 1994) and are the major cellular site of vitamin A storage in the body. Approximately 99% of the vitamin A present in stellate cells is present as retinyl ester. The lipid droplets are located in the cytoplasm of the stellate cells and represent the characteristic morphological feature of these cells. They are larger (up to 8 μm in diameter) than those in rat parenchymal cells (up to 2.5 μm in diameter) (Geerts *et al.*, 1994). The size and number of the lipid droplets in stellate cells is markedly influenced by dietary vitamin A intake (Wake, 1980; Kudo, 1989) and intraportal injection of retinol (Wake, 1980).

Stellate cell lipid droplets are formed through vacuolization of cisternae of the rough endoplasmic reticulum and exist in membrane-bound and non-membrane-bound forms (Wake, 1980). There is general agreement regarding the lipid composition of these droplets (Blaner, 1994). One study reported that the lipid of droplets isolated from vitamin A-sufficient rats consisted of approximately 42% retinyl ester, 28% triglyceride, 13% total cholesterol (free + ester) and 4% phospholipid (Yamada *et al.*, 1987). The retinyl esters in the droplets consisted of approximately 70% retinyl palmitate, 15% retinyl stearate, 8% retinyl oleate, 4% retinyl linoleate and smaller percentages of other long-chain retinyl esters (Yamada *et al.*, 1987). A later study showed that the lipid composition of the droplets is markedly affected in rats by dietary retinol intake, but not by dietary triglyceride (calorie) intake (Blaner & Olson, 1994).

The mechanism by which vitamin A regulates and maintains the lipid composition of the lipid droplets in stellate cells is not understood. However, it has been suggested that retinoic acid may be important (Yumoto *et al.*, 1989). Because retinoic acid has a sparing effect on hepatic retinol levels, intracellular retinoic acid may well influence hepatic retinol secretion (Shankar & DeLuca, 1988). Although the liver contains some retinoic acid (Kurlandsky *et al.*, 1995), its cellular distribution has not been determined. Because retinoic acid receptors-α, -β, and -γ (RAR-α, -β and -γ) and retinoid X receptor-α (RXR-α) are all expressed in stellate cells (Weiner *et al.*, 1992; Friedman *et al.*, 1993), retinoids may well play a role in regulating the state of differentiation and metabolism within stellate cells.

As seen in Table 6, stellate cells are highly enriched in CRBP-I and the enzymes which are able to hydrolyse (bile-salt-dependent and bile-salt-independent retinyl ester hydrolases) and to synthesize retinyl esters (LRAT). In addition, the stellate cells contain an intracellular binding protein for retinoic acid, cellular retinoic acid-binding protein, type I (CRABP-I). However, stellate cells contain very little RBP (Blaner & Olson, 1994).

In vivo, rat liver stellate cells exhibit a dual phenotype, that is, a quiescent phenotype in normal healthy liver and an activated phenotype in chronically diseased liver (Geerts *et al.*, 1994). The quiescent phenotype is characterized by lipid droplets rich in vitamin A, a low proliferative rate and low levels of collagen synthesis. In contrast, the activated or myoblast-like phenotype is distinguished by loss of vitamin A-containing lipid droplets, increased cell proliferation and increased synthesis of collagen. The activated form predominates in liver fibrosis (Friedman, 1993) and is observed in livers of rats experiencing vitamin A toxicity. Although these observations suggest a possible link between stellate cell vitamin A storage and liver disease, the underlying pathophysiological mechanisms remain unclear. It has been established that retinoic acid exacerbates rat liver fibrosis by inducing activation of latent transforming growth factor-β (TGF-β) (Okuno *et al.*, 1997), the major cytokine implicated in the pathogenesis of liver fibrosis and cirrhosis (Friedman, 1993). This action of retinoic acid on TGF-β activity could be an important process linking vitamin A toxicity and hepatic fibrosis.

In culture, stellate cells isolated from healthy control rats rapidly lose their *in vivo* quiescent phenotype and become activated. One characteristic of this activated phenotype observed in cultured rat stellate cells is the rapid loss of their capability to store retinyl ester (Trøen *et al.*, 1994). Freshly isolated rat stellate cells contain about 144 nmol retinol/mg cellular protein;

this concentration declines to 33 nmol/mg after two days in culture (Trøen *et al.*, 1994) and continues to decline until no vitamin A remains. Therefore, the many *in vitro* studies utilizing primary cultures of rat stellate cells may not be relevant for understanding normal hepatic vitamin A physiology, since these cells have the activated rather than quiescent phenotype.

3.2.4.5 Hepatic mobilization and plasma transport of retinol: retinol-binding protein

The transport of retinol from vitamin A stores in the liver to target tissues is accomplished exclusively by means of its specific plasma transport protein, RBP (Goodman, 1984; Soprano & Blaner, 1994). In the circulation, the retinol–RBP complex is bound to another plasma protein, transthyretin (TTR).

The liver is the major site of synthesis of RBP, which occurs primarily in the parenchymal cells (Goodman, 1984; Soprano & Blaner, 1994). Initial immunocytochemical studies indicated that RBP distribution within the liver was restricted to the parenchymal cells. Likewise, examination by specific and sensitive radioimmunoassay procedures of highly purified fractions of parenchymal cells, Kupffer cells, endothelial cells and stellate cells revealed RBP only in the purified parenchymal cell preparations (Blaner *et al.*, 1985). Subsequent investigations have established that RBP mRNA is localized solely in parenchymal cells and not in stellate cells (Yamada *et al.*, 1987; Weiner *et al.*, 1992; Friedman *et al.*, 1993). High resolution immunoelectron microscopy similarly did not reveal immunoreactive RBP in any hepatic cell type other than parenchymal cells (Suhara *et al.*, 1990). However, after a large dose of human RBP (corresponding to about twice the amount of RBP present in the entire circulation of a rat) was injected into the circulation of rats, a very small amount of human RBP was detected by immunohistochemical techniques in the stellate cells (Senoo *et al.*, 1990). Nevertheless, the great majority of RBP of hepatic origin, if not all, seems to be synthesized by parenchymal cells.

RBP secretion from the liver is a highly regulated process that is still not fully understood. The factors and processes that regulate RBP secretion are primarily localized to the endoplasmic reticulum (Goodman, 1984; Soprano & Blaner, 1994). It seems that retinol availability within the cell is the most critical factor regulating the secretion of RBP. In addition, other hormonal and physiological factors probably play roles in regulating the efflux of RBP from cells. It has long been known, for instance, that when retinoic acid is provided chronically in the diet to rats, plasma retinol–RBP concentrations decline by 25–50% (Shankar & DeLuca, 1988). Recent data suggest that the retinol-RBP:TTR complex forms in the hepatocyte before being secreted into the circulation (Soprano & Blaner, 1994). However, it remains uncertain what biochemical signals or processes are important for regulating the transcription of RBP, for retaining RBP within cells or conversely, for allowing the secretion of RBP. It is not yet known if the information needed to bring about secretion of RBP is internal in the RBP primary sequence or if this information resides in some other still undescribed molecule.

In vitamin A deficiency, apo-RBP accumulates in the liver to levels which are 3–10-fold higher than those observed in corresponding control livers (Goodman, 1984; Soprano & Blaner, 1994), while liver RBP mRNA levels show no difference between the two nutritional states (Soprano & Blaner, 1994). It is clear that retinol-deficiency specifically inhibits the secretion of RBP from the liver. Several biochemical studies have shown that retinol deficiency largely prevents the movement of newly synthesized RBP from the endoplasmic reticulum to the Golgi apparatus (Suhara *et al.*, 1990). RBP concentrations in endoplasmic reticulum fractions isolated from retinol-deficient rat livers were substantially elevated over levels in similar fractions from normal rat livers (Soprano & Blaner, 1994). In cultured hepatocytes prepared from retinol-deficient rats, pulse-labelled RBP accumulated in the endoplasmic reticulum and was not secreted into the cell medium. Interestingly, the transit of RBP through the endoplasmic reticulum of cultured hepatocytes prepared from normal rats is relatively slow compared to the transit times for albumin and transferrin. Studies investigating the subcellular localization of plasma RBP in normal, retinol-deficient, and retinol-repleted retinol-deficient rats using electron microscopic techniques have provided additional information regarding the RBP secretory pathway (Suhara *et al.*, 1990). In the normal liver parenchymal cell, RBP was localized in synthetic and secretory structures, including endoplasmic reticulum, Golgi complex and secretory vesicles. This distribution changed markedly with retinol depletion. A heavy accumulation of RBP in the endoplasmic reticulum accompanied by a marked decrease in RBP-positive Golgi complex and secretory vesicles was observed in the parenchymal cells of retinol-deficient rats. After repletion of deficient rats with retinol, the RBP from the endoplasmic reticulum appeared to move rapidly through the Golgi complex and the secretory vesicles to the surface of the cell.

3.2.4.6 Hepatic retinoic acid formation and metabolism

The liver is a site for both synthesis of retinoic acid from retinol and oxidative metabolism of retinoic acid. This oxidative metabolism may be activating in nature, since some retinoic acid metabolites such as the 4-hydroxy and 4-oxo derivatives are active in transactivation assays (Mangelsdorf *et al.*, 1994; Hofmann & Eichele, 1994; Gudas *et al.*, 1994) or may be catabolic in nature, generating products which will be eliminated from the body (Blaner & Olson, 1994).

(a) Retinoic acid formation

Many studies of the formation of retinoic acid from retinol have been carried out using enzyme preparations from rat liver, as described in detail in Section 3.2.7.1. As outlined below, hepatocytes are especially rich in both cytosolic and membrane-bound enzymes that catalyse the oxidation of retinol to retinal (Blaner & Olson, 1994). In addition, hepatocytes are rich in retinal dehydrogenases that catalyse oxidation of retinal to retinoic acid (Blaner & Olson, 1994). It is clear that many different enzymes in the liver are able to catalyse the oxidation of retinol or retinal *in vitro*, but there is as yet no consensus regarding the physiological relevance of each of these in intact animals.

An important question for understanding the metabolism of vitamin A within the intact organism concerns whether retinoic acid is specifically synthesized in some tissues for export into the circulation to other tissues. Although there is very little information addressing this possibility, it is assumed by some investigators that some of the retinoic acid synthesized in the liver is secreted into the circulation for delivery to other tissues. Considering the great capacity of hepatic enzymes to catalyse retinol and retinal oxidation *in vitro*, this may be reasonable, but it remains to be established experimentally.

(b) Retinoic acid metabolism

The liver also possesses enzymatic machinery that is able to metabolize retinoic acid. Metabolites of all-*trans*-retinoic acid generated *in vivo* include 13-*cis*-retinoic acid, 9-*cis*-retinoic acid, retinoyl β-glucuronide, 5,6-epoxyretinoic acid, 4-hydroxyretinoic acid, 4-oxoretinoic acid and 3,4-didehydroretinoic acid (Blaner & Olson, 1994). Some of these metabolites may be active in mediating retinoic acid function, whereas others are probably catabolic products destined for export from the body. The formation of many of these metabolites seems to be catalysed by enzymes of the cytochrome P450 system. Aspects of retinoic acid metabolism and the role of the cytochrome P450 system are described in Section 3.2.7.3.

3.2.5 Plasma transport of vitamin A

In the fasted state, the predominant form of vitamin A in the circulation is retinol, bound to RBP. It is thought that retinol accounts for more than 99% of the vitamin A present in the circulation of fasted rats (Goodman, 1984; Soprano & Blaner, 1994). However, low levels are also present of all-*trans*-retinoic acid, 13-*cis*-retinoic acid, glucuronides of both retinoic acid and retinol, some retinyl ester bound to lipoproteins and possibly some other metabolites of retinol and retinoic acid. The same seems to hold for most other animal species which have been investigated, although the relative abundance of each of the vitamin A metabolites may vary among species. Nevertheless, these other forms of vitamin A in the circulation may be important sources of vitamin A for some tissues under some physiological and/or pathological conditions. The different vitamin A species present in the fasting circulation are considered separately below and in Section 7.2.

3.2.5.1 Retinol delivery to target tissues

The sole plasma transport protein for retinol is RBP. This is a single polypeptide chain with a molecular weight of about 21 000 and has one binding site for one molecule of all-*trans*-retinol. In the blood, RBP circulates as a 1:1 molar complex with another serum protein, transthyretin (formerly called prealbumin). Studies of transthyretin-deficient mice have demonstrated that the formation of the complex reduces the glomerular filtration and renal catabolism of RBP. Normal levels of serum retinol and RBP in healthy well nourished Caucasian populations are about 2–3 μM (Goodman, 1984; Soprano & Blaner, 1994). The levels are slightly lower (1–2 μM) in the circulations of well nourished rats, mice and rabbits (Goodman, 1984; Folman *et al.*, 1989; Soprano & Blaner, 1994; Wei *et al.*, 1995). Since essentially all retinol in the circulation is bound to RBP, serum retinol and RBP levels are highly correlated in well nourished humans as well as vitamin A-sufficient rats and mice (Goodman, 1984). Erythrocytes contain only very small amounts of vitamin A (Bieri *et al.*, 1979). Treatment of humans and rats with *N*-(4-hydroxyphenyl)retinamide markedly lowers serum retinol concentrations (Formelli *et al.*, 1996).

Circulating levels of retinol–RBP remain very constant except in response to extremes in vitamin A, protein, calorie and zinc nutrition, or hormonal factors or stress or as a consequence of some disease states (Goodman, 1984; Soprano & Blaner, 1994). The physiological process responsible for maintaining and regulating retinol–RBP levels in the circulation are not well characterized. Plasma retinol–RBP levels could be maintained through regulation of RBP synthesis and/or secretion from the hepatocyte, through regulation of retinol–RBP plasma clearance and catabolism, or through a combination of these mechanisms. RBP synthesis and secretion from hepatocytes is a regulated process that is still not fully understood (Soprano & Blaner, 1994). Hormonal and physiological factors probably play roles in regulating the efflux of RBP from hepatocytes, but it remains uncertain which biochemical signals or processes are important for retaining RBP within hepatocytes or conversely, for allowing the secretion of RBP. Similarly, there is very little information regarding the catabolism of RBP or its regulation. It is believed that the kidney plays an important role, since human patients and rats with chronic renal failure show elevated plasma RBP levels (Goodman, 1984). However, it is not understood how the kidney or other organs influence or regulate RBP turnover.

Plasma retinol homeostasis in the rat has been extensively studied (Sundaresan, 1977; Keilson *et al.*, 1979; Underwood *et al.*, 1979; Lewis *et al.*, 1981, 1990; Green *et al.*, 1985, 1987; Gerlach & Zile, 1990, 1991), leading to the conclusion that a feedback control mechanism regulates mobilization and/or release of retinol–RBP from hepatic stores. It has been proposed that in response to peripheral tissue needs for vitamin A, a signal is sent from the periphery to the liver to regulate retinol–RBP release (Vahlquist *et al.*, 1973; Sundaresan, 1977; Green *et al.*, 1985, 1987; Lewis *et al.*, 1990). Although this feedback signal has not been identified, circulating retinoic acid levels may provide such a signal (Sundaresan, 1977; Keilson *et al.*, 1979; Underwood *et al.*, 1979; Lewis *et al.*, 1981). A regulatory linkage between plasma retinol and retinoic acid levels is suggested by the finding that plasma retinol levels are lower in animals receiving relatively high amounts of retinoic acid in the diet (Keilson *et al.*, 1979; Lewis *et al.*, 1981; Shankar & DeLuca, 1988). Others have suggested that apo-RBP levels (Vahlquist *et al.*, 1973; Sundaresan, 1977; Green *et al.*, 1985, 1987; Lewis *et al.*, 1990) or a modified form of circulating RBP (Keilson *et al.*, 1979; Underwood *et al.*, 1979) may serve as such a signal. At present, though, the identity and nature of such a signal from the periphery to the liver remain elusive.

Even though data have been lacking, there also have been suggestions that the magnitude of vitamin A uptake from the diet may play some role in influencing or possibly regulating plasma retinol–RBP levels (Keilson *et al.*, 1979; Lewis *et al.*, 1990). Among other possibilities, Underwood *et al.* (1979) suggested that the rate of release of retinol from retinyl esters in the liver from newly absorbed vitamin A may be important for regulating plasma retinol levels. Lewis *et al.* (1990) suggested that when RBP synthesis is not compromised, the rate-limiting factor for retinol secretion from the liver is the appropriate positional availability of unesterified retinol near the intracellular site of RBP synthesis. They also suggested that an acute influx of a reasonable load of diet-derived vitamin A will increase hepatocyte retinol–RBP secretion up to some saturation point at which apo-RBP availability becomes rate-limiting.

The biochemical mechanism through which cells take up retinol from plasma RBP is central for understanding vitamin A metabolism and actions within cells, but has not yet been identified. The possible existence of a cell surface receptor for RBP has been extensively explored (Soprano & Blaner, 1994), but only very limited data characterizing a plasma membrane protein implicated as an RBP receptor have appeared. Thus, even though many cellular systems have been characterized as having cell surface RBP-binding activity, the biochemical nature of such a putative plasma membrane receptor remains unclear. Other studies failed to demonstrate a cell surface receptor for RBP in isolated cells or found that such a receptor is not necessary to ensure the cellular uptake of retinol from RBP. Overall, the recent reports concerning this topic can be divided into two groups based on the nature of the studies. One group consists of reports which characterize the binding (or lack of binding) of RBP to tissue minces, cultured cells or plasma membrane vesicles and the uptake of retinol from RBP by them. The second group examines retinol transfer from RBP (or other proteins able to bind retinol) to liposomes or isolated membrane systems. Two opposing views have been derived from these studies. One proposes the involvement of a cell surface receptor for RBP in the process of internalization of retinol by cells. The other view suggests that retinol is internalized by cells from RBP through a non-receptor-mediated uptake process. It is also possible that some cell types require retinol through a cell surface receptor whereas others do not; these two uptake possibilities can possibly coexist within the body.

In hypervitaminosis A (vitamin A toxicity), it is postulated that toxicity arises due to the inability of RBP to pick up and transport vitamin A 'leaking' from overfilled hepatic storage sites. Essentially, the available RBP is overwhelmed with excessive vitamin A and is unable to bind all the retinol in need of uptake and transport. The retinol not bound to RBP would then be free to associate with lipoproteins which non-specifically deliver it to cells and subcellular locations that do not usually process retinol. The retinol-containing lipoproteins would accumulate within cellular lysosomes. Here the retinol is thought to have a disrupting effect on the lysosomal membranes, causing release of lysosomal enzymes into the cell that could be the underlying cause of the pathology associated with hypervitaminosis A (Goodman, 1984).

In hypovitaminosis A (vitamin A deficiency), plasma retinol–RBP levels drop only after hepatic total retinol stores become depleted. Studies in the rat indicate that RBP is synthesized by the hepatocyte normally, but, in the absence of retinol, the apo-RBP is not secreted from the hepatocyte (Goodman, 1984). In hypovitaminosis A, apo-RBP levels in the liver rise. If retinol becomes available again, this RBP rapidly binds the retinol and is immediately secreted into the circulation for delivery to target tissues.

3.2.5.2 Plasma retinoic acid

In plasma, retinoic acid circulates bound to albumin (Blaner & Olson, 1994). The fasting plasma level of retinoic acid is very low, in the range of 1–14 nmol/L in humans (about 0.2–0.7% of plasma retinol levels) (De Leenheer *et al.*, 1982; Eckhoff & Nau, 1990a; Arnhold *et al.*, 1996) and 1–7 nmol/L in rats (Cullum & Zile, 1985; Napoli *et al.*, 1985; Tzimas *et al.*, 1995). It is not known if the retinoic acid present in the circulation arises solely from the diet (i.e., is of intestinal origin) or if some arises through export of retinoic acid from tissues which synthesize it from retinol. The possibility that the kidney is a site of synthesis and export of retinoic acid has been raised (Bhat *et al.*, 1988a,b); however, at present, no data are available to support the possibility that some tissues (except for the intestine after dietary intake of carotenoids or retinoids) are able to provide retinoic acid to the circulation for delivery to other tissues.

Retinoic acid is taken up efficiently by cells. No cell surface receptor specific for the all-*trans* acid is known. Retinoic acid, although fully ionized in aqueous solutions at pH 7.4, is uncharged when within a lipid environment (Noy, 1992a,b). In the uncharged state, it moves rapidly between the outer and inner leaflets of the plasma membrane and can thus traverse cellular membranes and rapidly enter the cell.

The concentration of retinoic acid in the blood can be markedly influenced by recent uptake of vitamin A. For example, in monkeys different vitamin A supplement formulations had marked effects on plasma levels of retinol, retinyl esters, all-*trans*-, 13-*cis*-, all-*trans*-4-oxo- and 13-*cis*-4-oxoretinoic acid and retinyl-β-glucuronide and retinoyl-β-glucuronide. Plasma levels of these compounds were much higher when the vitamin A was in a Tween 20-containing aqueous preparation as compared to a soybean oil-based vehicle (Eckhoff *et al.*, 1991a). The vitamin A present in a liver meal (see Section 3.1.3.1 and Tables 2 and 3) is handled differently by humans as compared to vitamin A present in a supplement, in particular with regard to the metabolism of all-*trans*-retinoic acid (see also Section 7.2.2).

Kurlandsky *et al.* (1995) explored the contribution of plasma retinoic acid to tissue pools of this compound in chow-fed male rats, and reported the tissue levels (Table 7). Using a steady-state tracer kinetic approach, these authors determined how much of the retinoic acid in each tissue was derived from the circulation. For the liver and brain, more than 75% was derived from the circulation (88.4% in brain and 78.2% in liver). The seminal vesicles, epididymis, kidney, epididymal fat, perinephric fat, spleen and lungs derived, respectively, 23.1%, 9.6%, 33.4%, 30.2.%, 24.5%, 19.0% and 26.7% of their all-*trans*-retinoic acid from the circulation. In the pancreas and eyes, only 2.3% and 4.8%, respectively, was contributed by the circulation. The testes did not take up any (<1%) retinoic acid from the circulation. The authors also reported a fractional catabolic rate for retinoic acid in plasma of 30.4 plasma pools/h and an absolute catabolic rate for retinoic acid of 640 pmol/h. These rates are very rapid compared with those of the only other naturally occurring form of vitamin A studied under normal physiological conditions, all-*trans*-retinol (Lewis *et al.*, 1990). Very little 9-*cis*- or 13-*cis*-retinoic acid was detected in any of these tissues. These data demonstrate that plasma all-*trans*-retinoic acid is a significant source of all-*trans*-retinoic acid for some, but not all, tissues; this suggests, by inference, that tissues have different capacities for the conversion of retinol to retinoic acid.

In rabbits, the β-carotene content of the diet influences serum levels of retinoic acid (Folman *et al.*, 1989). In female rabbits given graded doses of β-carotene in their diet for nine weeks, β-carotene intake was associated with higher serum concentrations of retinoic acid.

3.2.5.3 Plasma 13-cis-retinoic acid

Cullum and Zile (1985) reported that 13-*cis*-retinoic acid is an endogenous retinoid present in the intestinal mucosa, intestinal muscle and

Table 7. All-*trans*-retinoic acid concentrations in various rat tissues [a,b]

Tissue	All-*trans*-retinoic acid (pmol/g tissue)
Liver	11.3 ± 4.7
Brain	6.8 ± 3.3
Testis	10.7 ± 2.7
Seminal vesicles	12.0 ± 7.0
Epididymis	4.2 ± 1.6
Kidney	8.3 ± 4.0
Pancreas	29.3 ± 16.3
Epididymal fat	15.7 ± 12.3
Perirenal fat	12.7 ± 8.7
Spleen	12.7 ± 12.0
Eyes	125 ± 37.3
Plasma	1.8 ± 0.7[c]

[a] From Kurlandsky *et al.* (1995)
[b] Each value is given as the mean ± 1 standard deviation for separate measurements employing eight individual 400–450 g male Sprague-Dawley rats.
[c] pmol/mL plasma.

plasma of vitamin A-sufficient rats. When a dose of all-*trans*-retinoic acid was administered by intrajugular injection into vitamin A-depleted rats, 13-*cis*-retinoic acid appeared in the plasma and small intestine within 2 min after dosing. The endogenous plasma concentrations of all-*trans*- and 13-*cis*-retinoic acid in vitamin A-sufficient rats were reported to be 9.7 and 3.0 nmol/L, respectively. The authors concluded that 13-*cis*-retinoic acid is a naturally occurring metabolite of all-*trans*-retinoic acid. Napoli *et al.* (1985) similarly demonstrated that 13-*cis*-retinoic acid is a naturally occurring form of retinoic acid in rat plasma. Bhat and Jetten (1987) demonstrated that cultures of rabbit tracheal epithelial cells can convert all-*trans*-retinoic acid to 13-*cis*-retinoic acid, and Tang and Russell (1990) confirmed that 13-*cis*-retinoic acid is an endogenous component in human serum. Fasting serum levels of all-*trans*- and 13-*cis*-retinoic acid determined in 26 human volunteers ranged from 3.7 to 6.3 nmol/L and from 3.7 to 7.2 nmol/L, respectively (Tang & Russell, 1990), levels similar to those observed for the rat. Plasma levels of all-*trans*- and 13-*cis*-retinoic acid levels rose 1.3- and 1.9-fold, respectively, above fasting levels, in human subjects who had received a physiological dose of retinyl palmitate (Tang & Russell, 1991). Similarly, Eckhoff *et al.* (1991b) demonstrated that 13-*cis*-retinoic acid is an endogenous component of human plasma and that administration of an oral dose of retinyl palmitate elevated plasma levels of 13-*cis*-retinoic acid.

3.2.5.4 Plasma 9-cis-retinoic acid

The existence of 9-*cis*-retinoic acid in cells was reported simultaneously by Levin *et al.* (1992) and Heyman *et al.* (1992). Using a nuclear receptor-dependent ligand-trapping technique to identify 9-*cis*-retinoic acid, Levin *et al.* (1992) demonstrated that this stereoisomer is an activating ligand for RXR-α in COS-1 cells. Heyman *et al.* (1992) similarly reported that 9-*cis*-retinoic acid is a ligand for the human nuclear retinoid receptor, RXR-α and estimated that the concentrations of 9-*cis*-retinoic acid in mouse liver and kidney were 13 and 100 pmol/g tissue, respectively. Mangelsdorf *et al.* (1992) showed that 9-*cis*-retinoic acid is able to transactivate gene expression through the actions of mouse RXR-α, RXR-β and RXR-γ.

3.2.5.5 Retinoid glucuronides

When all-*trans*-retinoic acid is orally administered to rats, all-*trans*-retinoyl β-glucuronide is secreted into the bile in significant amounts (Blaner & Olson, 1994). This metabolite is synthesized from retinoic acid and uridine diphosphoglucuronic acid in the liver, intestine, kidney and other tissues by several of the 40 or more identified microsomal β-glucuronyl transferases (Genchi *et al.*, 1996, 1998). Of various tissues, the intestinal mucosa seems to be the most active in synthesizing and retaining retinoyl β-glucuronide. When 13-*cis*-retinoic acid is administered, all-*trans*-retinoyl β-glucuronide is a major metabolite in rats *in vivo*. Isomerization to all-*trans*-retinoic acid probably, but not necessarily, occurs before conjugation. The extent of retinoyl β-glucuronide formation from retinoic acid, as assessed from pharmacokinetic measurements, is dependent on both the isomer administered and the species, although retinoyl β-glucuronide is formed in all species studied. Orally administered retinoyl β-glucuronide is hydrolysed only slowly *in vivo* in vitamin A-sufficient rats, but more rapidly in vitamin A-deficient rats (Kaul & Olson, 1998).

Retinol is also conjugated with glucuronic acid *in vivo* and *in vitro* to form retinyl β-glucuronide (Blaner & Olson, 1994). Like retinoyl β-glucuronide, retinyl β-glucuronide is present in human plasma at a mean concentration of 6.8 nmol/L (Blaner & Olson, 1994). Retinyl β-glucuronide is hydrolysed *in vivo* to retinol, however, which is esterified and stored in the liver.

3.2.5.6 Other metabolites of retinol

In 1990, Buck *et al.* showed that human lymphoblastoid cells in culture are dependent for growth on a constant supply of retinol. In the absence of retinol, these cells perished within days. Retinoic acid was unable to prevent cell death. Employing sensitive trace-labelling techniques, Buck *et al.* (1991a) did not detect retinoic acid and 3,4-didehydroretinoic acid as metabolites of retinol in activated B lymphocytes. Nevertheless, B lymphocytes formed several other metabolites of retinol, which were able to sustain B cell growth in the absence of an external source of retinol (Buck *et al.*, 1991a). Buck *et al.* (1991b) found one of these active metabolites to be optically active 14-hydroxy-4,14-retro-retinol, identified as a direct biosynthetic product of retinol in 5/2 lymphoblastoid cells. This metabolite was isolated, by reverse-phase HPLC, from cells of the lymphoblastoid line 5/2 which were grown in the presence of [^{3}H]retinol–RBP complex; it was active in sustaining the growth of cells of the lymphoblastoid line 5/2 (and of T cell lines) in the absence of retinol. In confirmation of their initial studies, retinoic acid was not active in these growth assays. Thus, in addition to the retinoic acid pathway, a second pathway of retinol metabolism mediates the actions of retinoids in cellular growth and differentiation, at least in specific cells. In mouse skin, retinol was also converted to 14-hydroxy-4,14-retro-retinol (Sass *et al.*, 1996).

Another metabolite of all-*trans*-retinol proposed to have biological activity is all-*trans*-4-oxoretinol. Achkar *et al.* (1996) identified this metabolite as being essentially involved in maintaining F9 cell differentiation after its induction with all-*trans*-retinoic acid. The possible importance of 4-oxoretinol *in vivo* remains to be established.

3.2.5.7 Lipoprotein-bound retinyl ester

Low levels of retinyl ester can be found in the very low-density lipoprotein (VLDL), LDL and HDL plasma fractions from fasting humans (Krasinski *et al.*, 1990b). It is possible that this arises through the actions of cholesteryl ester transfer protein, which can transfer retinyl ester between triglyceride-rich chylomicrons and other lipoprotein fractions (Goodman & Blaner, 1984; Krasinski *et al.*, 1990b; Blaner & Olson, 1994; Tall, 1995). Alternatively, human hepatocytes may package and secrete some retinyl ester in nascent VLDL.

In the rabbit, the liver does not secrete retinyl ester in VLDL; all of the retinyl ester present in the circulation appears to ultimately arise from transfer of chylomicron retinyl ester to other lipoprotein fractions (Thompson *et al.*, 1983). However, this is not the case for all animal species. Fasting blood of some species, especially ferrets and dogs, contains high levels of retinyl ester in VLDL, LDL and HDL (Wilson *et al.*, 1987; Schweigert, 1988; Ribaya-Mercado *et al.*, 1994; Lederman *et al.*, 1998). In both dogs and ferrets, retinyl ester is the major form of vitamin A in the fasting circulation. In dogs, lipoprotein-bound retinyl ester in the fasting circulation may arise from hepatic secretion of retinyl ester in VLDL (Wilson *et al.*, 1987).

Overall, different species show very distinct patterns of distribution of retinyl ester in fasting blood. The level of retinyl ester present in fasting rodent and rabbit blood closely resembles the level in fasting human blood. However, since rodents do not express cholesteryl ester transfer protein and since rabbits do not secrete retinyl ester in VLDL, one must apply caution when trying to extrapolate from these species to man.

3.2.6 Extrahepatic vitamin A storage and metabolism

Peripheral tissues other than the liver play important roles in the storage and mobilization of retinol. Four lines of evidence support this conclusion. (*a*) Kinetic modelling studies (Lewis *et al.*, 1981, 1990; Green *et al.*, 1985, 1987) initially suggested that, in both vitamin A-sufficient and -deficient rats, retinol is extensively recycled among the liver, plasma, interstitial fluid and peripheral tissues. A multicompartment model of whole-body retinoid metabolism (Green *et al.*, 1985) provides an excellent means for understanding the dynamics of retinoid transport and storage in liver and peripheral tissues. According to this model, extrahepatic tissues of rats with normal plasma retinol levels but with very low total liver stores (< 0.35 μmol of vitamin A), should contain 44% of whole-body vitamin A. (*b*) The sole mechanism for plasma transport of retinol from the liver to tissues is by complexing with RBP (see Section 3.2.5.1). Although most RBP is thought to be synthesized in the liver, Soprano *et al.* (1986) have demonstrated that a variety of tissues, including the kidney, lung, heart, spleen, skeletal muscle and adipose tissue express RBP; thus, these tissues may well play a role in the recycling of retinol back to the liver. (*c*) Retinol and retinyl esters as well as enzymes that are able to esterify retinol and to hydrolyse retinyl esters are found in most peripheral tissues. (*d*) Many rat tissues, including lung, kidney and small intestine, contain cells which morphologically and structurally resemble hepatic stellate cells (Nagy *et al.*, 1997). These extrahepatic stellate-like cells contain lipid droplets which resemble those of hepatic stellate cells and both their size and number increase in response to administration of excess dietary vitamin A. Limited biochemical data suggest that these cells contain relatively high concentrations of vitamin A, which increase in response to dietary vitamin A intake (Nagy *et al.*, 1997), supporting a role for these 'extrahepatic stellate cells' in vitamin A storage and metabolism.

Figure 4 represents the transport and metabolism of retinol and its metabolites within target cells.

Table 8 provides a summary of total retinol levels reported in the literature for adipose tissue, kidney, testis, lung, bone marrow and eye cups for some species. For some tissues, the range of total retinol levels reported by different investigators is large. Presumably, this reflects species and strain differences and the physiological status (age, sex and dietary

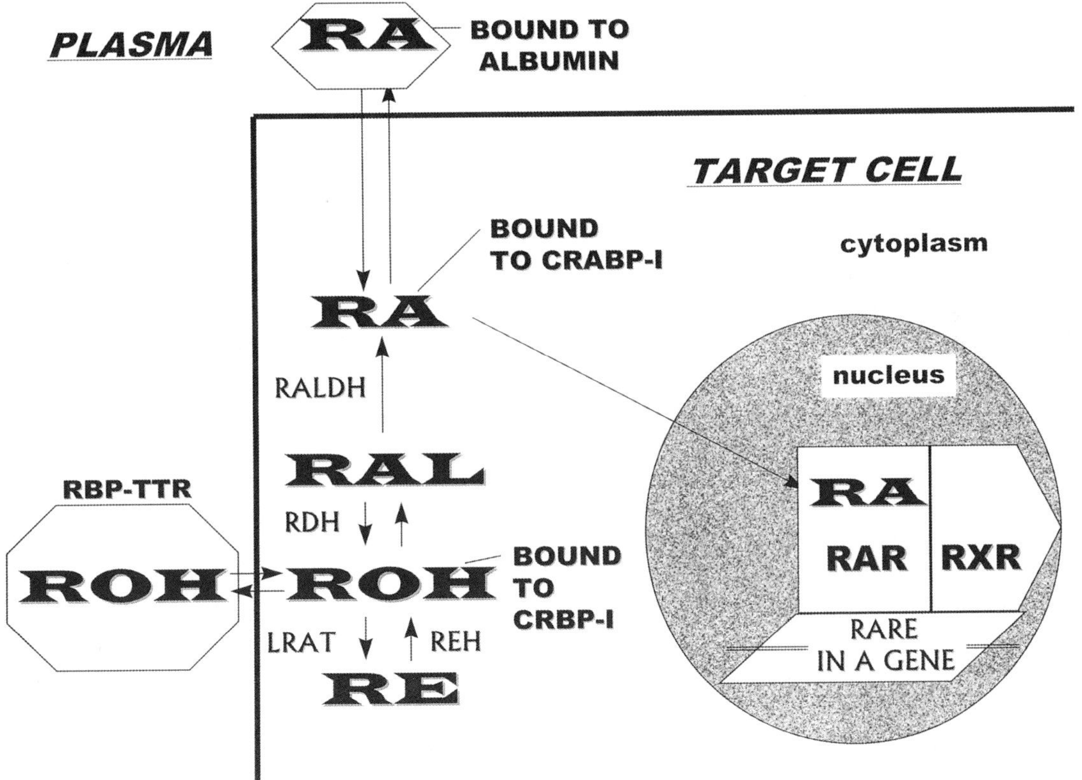

Figure 4. Simplified scheme for the transport and metabolism of retinol and retinyl esters within target cells, applicable to humans and most animal models.
Details of these processes are described in the text. Not all processes necessarily occur in all cells. For key to abbreviations, see Figure 1.

Table 8. Reported total retinol levels in extrahepatic tissues for various animal species

Tissue	Species	Vitamin A concentration (nmol/g tissue)	Reference
Adipose tissue	Rat	20 ± 8	Tsutsumi *et al.* (1992)
	Rabbit	8.0	Blaner *et al.* (1993)
	Ferret	34 ± 4	Ribaya-Mercado *et al.* (1992)
Kidney	Rat	40.9	Bhat & Lacroix (1983)
	Rat	6.6	Napoli *et al.* (1984)
	Rat	10.0	Gerlach *et al.* (1989)
	129sv mouse	1.4 ± 0.7	Wei *et al.* (1995)
	Ferret	87.1 ± 14.4	Schweigert *et al.* (1995)
Testis	Rat	20.3	Bhat & Lacroix (1983)
	Rat	4.2	Gerlach *et al.* (1989)
	129sv mouse	2.8 ± 1.4	Wei *et al.* (1995)
Lung	Rat	21.5	Bhat & Lacroix (1983)
	Newborn rat pups	53.6	Shenai & Chytil (1990)
	C57BL mouse	700 – 1400	Ribaya-Mercado *et al.* (1992)
Bone marrow	Rabbit	13	Blaner *et al.* (1993)
	Rabbit	2.3	Skrede *et al.* (1993)
Eye	Eye cup of 129sv mouse	1.9 ± 0.6	Wei *et al.* (1995)

status) of the animals employed. A difficulty in compiling Table 8 arose from differences in how investigators report tissue vitamin A levels. Some report concentration of retinol (vitamin A) per g tissue wet weight, as given in Table 8. However, other investigators have reported tissue retinol levels per g tissue dry weight or per mg tissue total protein and consequently, it is not always possible to reconcile all of the reported tissue vitamin A concentrations.

3.2.6.1 Adipose tissue

Vitamin A has long been known to be present in adipose tissue (Moore, 1957). Tsutsumi *et al.* (1992) reported similar retinoid levels in six anatomically different adipose depots(inguinal, dorsal, mesenteric, epididymal, perinephric, and brown adipose tissue) of chow-fed rats, averaging approximately 20 nmol retinol/g adipose tissue. About two thirds of the retinoid present in adipose tissue was reported to be present as retinol and the remainder as retinyl ester. In these studies, hepatic vitamin A levels were approximately 520 nmol/g liver. Because adipose tissue and liver in mature rats represent approximately 15% and 4%, respectively, of the total body mass, the total amount of vitamin A in adipose tissue was approximately 14% of that in the liver. Thus, adipose tissue contributes substantially to total body retinoid stores. Tsutsumi *et al.* (1992) also identified the adipocyte (and not the stromal-vascular cells) as the cellular site of retinoid storage in adipose tissue. Adipocytes from the epididymal, perinephric and brown adipose depots contained between 2 and 3 nmol retinol per 10^6 cells. Primary rat hepatocytes contain between 0.35 and 1.2 nmol vitamin A per 10^6 cells (Blaner *et al.*, 1985; Yamada *et al.*, 1987), whereas rat liver stellate cell isolates contain 38 nmol vitamin A per 10^6 cells (Yamada *et al.*, 1987). Thus, rat adipocytes and liver parenchymal cells contain similar levels of vitamin A. From this perspective, the adipocyte should be considered as important for retinoid storage.

Zovich *et al.* (1992) demonstrated that murine BFC-1β preadipocytes during their differentiation to adipocytes take up and esterify retinol, primarily to retinyl palmitate and oleate. Whether retinol esterification in adipocytes occurs via an acyl coenzyme-A-dependent or -independent process (involving the actions of LRAT) has not been defined. However, the esterification process seems to depend on the state of adipocyte differentiation in BFC-1β cells. This is also true for expression of RBP, which is not expressed in undifferentiated preadipocytes, but highly expressed in BFC-1β adipocytes. LPL, which is synthesized and secreted by BFC-1β adipocytes and binds to the surface of these cells, is active in hydrolysing chylomicron retinyl ester after much of the chylomicron triglyceride has been first hydrolysed (Blaner *et al.*, 1994). Therefore LPL may play a role in facilitating uptake of postprandial vitamin A by extrahepatic tissues. Hormone-sensitive lipase, a cAMP-stimulated lipase which also hydrolyses both triglycerides and cholesteryl esters, catalyses the hydrolysis of the retinyl esters present in BFC-1β adipocytes (Wei *et al.*, 1997). Hydrolysis of adipocyte retinyl ester catalysed by hormone-sensitive lipase seems to be regulated through cAMP-signalling pathways. Taken together, these results demonstrate that the adipocyte is dynamically involved in vitamin A uptake, storage and metabolism.

The role of adipose tissue in retinol storage has also been investigated in other species. Perinephric and epididymal fat from rabbits fed a control diet have been reported to contain 8.0 and 8.7 nmol total retinol/g tissue, respectively (Blaner *et al.*, 1993). For ferrets receiving control diets, subcutaneous adipose tissue is reported to contain 21.4 ± 6.4 nmol retinyl ester and 6.8 ± 3.1 nmol retinol/g tissue (Ribaya-Mercado *et al.*, 1992). In ferrets receiving the same diet supplemented with β-carotene (80 μg/g wet weight) for three weeks, subcutaneous adipose tissues contained less retinyl ester (13.4 ± 2.3 nmol/g) and more retinol (20.6 ± 1.8 nmol/g) than the control-fed ferrets (Ribaya-Mercado *et al.*, 1992). The mechanistic basis for this effect of β-carotene on total retinol levels in ferret adipose tissue was not established.

3.2.6.2 Kidney

Bhat and Lacroix (1983) reported that retinyl ester levels in normal rat kidney tissue are 40.9 nmol/g tissue. The retinyl esters consisted of 94.2% palmitate, 3.8% stearate, 1.0% linoleate and 1.0% palmitoleate. The concentration of 9-*cis*-retinol in rat kidney was reported to be approximately 10% of that of all-*trans*-retinol. The kidney of vitamin A-deficient rats given a single intraperitoneal injection of vitamin A (consisting of 53 μg retinol) accumulated progressively more vitamin A as the liver was progressively depleted (Bhat, 1997). This finding, along with the identification and localization of a retinal dehydrogenase, which is able to oxidize either 9-*cis*- or all-*trans*-retinal to the corresponding retinoic acid isomer in the kidney, led these investigators to propose that the kidney is able to synthesize all-*trans*-retinoic acid and 9-*cis*-retinoic acid from the all-*trans*- and 9-*cis*-retinol present in the tissue. They further proposed that the newly synthesized retinoic acid isomers are carried from the kidney in the blood to fill the needs of other tissues for retinoic acid (Bhat *et al.*, 1988a,b; Bhat, 1997).

Napoli *et al.* (1984) reported rat kidney retinol levels of 6.6 nmol/g of tissue. Of the total retinol localized in kidney, 74% was present as retinyl ester, with the remainder as retinol. In rats maintained on an α-tocopherol-free diet, the levels of retinol remained approximately the same (5.2 nmol retinol/g tissue), but retinyl esters markedly decreased (2.2 nmol/g tissue or only 30% of the total vitamin A present). A bile-salt-dependent retinyl ester hydrolase in normal rat kidney homogenates has a specific activity in the range 154–180 pmol/h/mg protein (Napoli *et al.*, 1984; Napoli & Beck, 1984). This hydrolase was inhibited by addition of 250 μmol/L α-tocopherol to the assay mixture (Napoli *et al.*, 1984). A microsomal bile-salt-independent retinyl ester hydrolase, which is unable to hydrolyse cholesteryl oleate, is also present in rat kidney (Napoli *et al.*, 1989).

Gerlach *et al.* (1989) reported that kidney from vitamin A-sufficient rats contains an average of approximately 10 nmol vitamin A/g dry weight of tissue. Of the total vitamin A present, half each consisted of non-esterified retinol and of various retinyl esters.

Ribaya-Mercado *et al.* (1992) reported that kidney from ferrets fed a control diet contains 87.1 ± 14.4 nmol retinyl ester/g tissue and 15.1 ± 9.8 nmol retinol/g tissue. Maintaining ferrets on the same diet supplemented with β-carotene (80 μg/g diet) for three weeks led to an approximately four-fold reduction in renal retinyl ester content and 2.3-fold increase in renal retinol content. Kidney from five-week-old female pigs is reported to contain 61.5 ± 11.5 nmol total retinol/g tissue (Schweigert *et al.*, 1995). The relative distribution of this total retinol as retinyl ester and retinol was not reported.

3.2.6.3 Testis

Rajguru *et al.* (1982) demonstrated by autoradiographic techniques that vitamin A is primarily localized in three cellular sites within the adult rat testis, namely, the macrophages of the interstitial tissue, the lipid droplets of the Sertoli cells, and the spermatids in association with Golgi saccules. In rats receiving a control diet, the testes have been reported to contain retinyl ester at a concentration of 20.3 nmol/g tissue (Bhat & Lacroix, 1983). Approximately 98% was retinyl palmitate, the remainder consisting of the stearate, linoleate and palmitoleate (Bhat & Lacroix, 1983). Gerlach *et al.* (1989) reported that rat testis contained approximately 4.2 nmol vitamin A/g dry weight of tissue, retinol accounting for approximately 50% of the total vitamin A (retinol + retinyl ester) present. Studies by Chaudhary and Nelson (1985, 1986), exploring the metabolism of all-*trans*-retinyl acetate in rat testes, demonstrated that non-esterified retinol accounts for approximately 50% of the total vitamin A present in the testes, with the remainder present primarily as retinyl palmitate.

When retinol was provided to rat Sertoli cell cultures as [^{3}H]retinol–RBP:TTR, retinol was rapidly taken up and largely converted to retinyl ester (Bishop & Griswold, 1987). Within 28 h after the labelled retinol was applied, 83% of the labelled retinoids found in the Sertoli cells was accounted for as retinyl ester (64% of the ester was the palmitate). The endogenous retinol concentrations in isolated rat Sertoli cells averaged 75 ± 13 pmol/mg cellular protein.

Although both the acyl coenzyme-A-dependent and -independent retinyl ester synthase activities are present in rat Sertoli cell microsomes, LRAT is the physiologically important activity in the Sertoli cell (Shingleton *et al.*, 1989). A bile-salt-dependent retinyl ester hydrolase has also been reported to be present in rat testis homogenates, with a specific activity of 38–97 pmol/h/mg protein (Napoli *et al.*, 1984).

3.2.6.4 Lung

Bhat and Lacroix (1983) reported retinyl ester levels of 21.5 nmol vitamin A/g tissue in lungs of vitamin A-sufficient rats. Retinyl palmitate accounted for 62% of the total retinyl ester and the remainder was mainly retinyl stearate (Bhat & Lacroix, 1983). Napoli *et al.* (1984) reported substantially higher values; namely total vitamin A levels of 53.6 nmol/g tissue, with approximately 81% of the retinol present as retinyl ester. The palmitate and oleate together accounted for 53% of lung retinyl ester (Napoli *et al.*, 1984).

Within 24 h of the oral administration of retinol to pregnant rats, the concentrations of retinyl esters in the lungs of fetuses and of newborn pups were significantly (1.7–7.1-fold) higher than in the lungs of the control group (Shenai & Chytil, 1990). In untreated rats, prenatal levels of retinyl ester ranged between 7 and 14 nmol/g tissue, and postnatal levels, from birth to 14 days, consistently averaged around 3.5 nmol/g tissue. In contrast, after pregnant mothers were given a single intragastric dose of 52 μmol retinyl palmitate, retinyl ester levels in prenatal lungs ranged between 28 and 38 nmol/g tissue. During a 14-day postnatal period, however, vitamin A concentrations continuously declined. Thus, vitamin A concentrations in fetal lung clearly are responsive to prenatal administration of a single large dose of retinol to the mother.

Zachman *et al.* (1992) reported retinyl palmitate levels in alveolar Type II cells of 21 ± 3.5 pmol/mg protein and 8 ± 4.2 pmol/mg protein in cells isolated from control and vitamin A-deficient rats, respectively. When added to a monolayer of Type II cells, [^{3}H]retinol was converted, in a time-dependent manner, to retinyl palmitate. Interestingly, cultured Type II cells are also able to synthesize retinoic acid from exogenous retinol (Zachman *et al.*, 1992).

Nagy *et al.* (1997) have reported that rat lung contains stellate-like cells which seem to take up and store vitamin A when rats are fed excess vitamin A. This finding is consistent with an earlier report of the isolation in high yield and high purity of retinol-storing cells from rat lung and their subsequent culture *in vitro* (Okabe *et al.*, 1984). These isolated cells apparently possess the overall morphology, including lipid droplets, that is characteristic of the retinol-storing cells found in lung tissues.

Levels of total retinol in lung tissue from three-month-old male C57BL mice fed a chow diet range between 700 and 1400 nmol of retinol per g tissue wet weight, compared with liver levels of 2100–2800 nmol. In these mice, the total retinol concentration in lung, when normalized per g tissue weight, is between 25 and 50% of that in the liver. Since the weight of a mouse lung is approximately 50% of the weight of the liver from the same animal, this implies that lung tissue of mice contains approximately 12.5 to 25% of the total retinol that is present in the mouse liver. Male Sprague-Dawley rats three months of age maintained on a chow diet have lung concentrations of total retinol ranging between 7 and 17.5 nmol retinol per g wet weight and liver levels ranging between 350 and 1050 nmol retinol per g wet weight. In the rat, when normalized per tissue weight, the lung contains approximately 1 to 5% of the total retinol present in the liver (Nagy *et al.*, 1997).

In ferrets receiving a control diet, retinyl ester concentrations in lung have been reported to be 4.3 ± 0.9 nmol/g tissue and lung retinol levels 0.31 ± 0.15 nmol/g tissue (Ribaya-Mercado *et al.*, 1992). Supplementation of the diet with β-carotene for three weeks resulted in an approximately two-fold increase in both lung retinyl ester and retinol concentrations.

3.2.6.5 Bone marrow

As outlined in Section 3.2.3.3, bone marrow of rabbits and of primates takes up substantial amounts of chylomicra. Chylomicron uptake by rabbit bone marrow is 50–100% of that of the liver. Rabbit bone marrow contains some stored retinol (Blaner *et al.*, 1993; Skrede *et al.*, 1993), one report indicating a level of 13 nmol total retinol/g tissue and another 2.3 nmol total retinol/g tissue. These reports agree that most if not all of the retinol present in bone marrow is unesterified. By comparison, rabbit perinephric and epididymal fat were reported to contain 8.0 and 8.7 nmol total retinol/g tissue, respectively (Blaner *et al.*, 1993) and the mean total retinol level for control rabbit liver (n = 3) was 429 nmol/g tissue (Skrede *et al.*, 1993). Interestingly, rabbit bone marrow also expresses RBP (Blaner *et al.*, 1993). Thus, bone marrow may well play a dynamic role in the overall metabolism of vitamin A.

It has been proposed that the vitamin A stored in bone marrow is important for maintaining normal blood cell differentiation (Twining *et al.*, 1996). Rats receiving a totally vitamin A-deficient diet reached a state where both hepatic and serum retinol concentrations were less than 1% of those of rats fed a control diet, but bone marrow from the vitamin A-deficient rats contained four times more retinol than that of control-fed animals. This suggests that bone marrow vitamin A stores are among the last tissue stores to be mobilized in the face of inadequate vitamin A intake. The vitamin A sequestered in the bone marrow of vitamin A-deficient rats may be important for the survival of the animal, since it will be needed to maintain the differentiation of myeloid cells to neutrophils.

3.2.6.6 Eye

The eye is an important site for vitamin A metabolism and action. Retinyl ester levels in cells of fresh retinal pigment epithelium (RPE) from human eyes range between 3.5 and 14 nmol per 10^6 cells (Flood *et al.*, 1983). This retinyl ester consists of 11-*cis*-retinyl palmitate, 11-*cis*-retinyl stearate, all-*trans*-retinyl palmitate (the major component), all-*trans*-retinyl stearate and all-*trans*-retinyl oleate. The post-mortem human pigment epithelium–choroid contains 36 ± 25 nmol vitamin A/g tissue (7.9 ± 4.5 nmol vitamin A/eye) (Blaner & Olson, 1994). Retinas contained 15.3% of the retinoid present in the whole pigment epithelium–choroid complex. Most of the retinoid in the eye was esterified (98.3% in the pigment epithelium–choroid complex; 79.3% in the retina).

The lacrimal gland contains retinyl esters and both acyl-coenzyme A:retinol acyltransferase (ARAT) and retinyl ester hydrolase activities (Blaner & Olson, 1994). By cannulation of the lacrimal gland ducts of rabbits and rats, retinol was shown to be present in the tear fluid. When microsomes prepared from rabbit lacrimal gland were incubated with [^{3}H]retinol in the presence of an acyl-coenzyme A generating system, a mixture of retinyl esters, including the laurate, linoleate, palmitate and stearate, was formed. In the presence of 180 μmol/L [^{3}H]retinol and 100 μmol/L palmitoyl-coenzyme A, retinyl palmitate was synthesized at 175–220 pmol/mg/min and the reaction displayed Michaelis–Menten kinetics. Thus, the lacrimal gland seems to synthesize retinyl esters via an acyl-coenzyme A-dependent process. A bile-salt-independent retinyl ester hydrolase which is present in microsomes of rat lacrimal gland has a pH optimum of 7 and a maximum specific activity of 1073 pmol/mg/h.

A crucial step in the visual cycle is the isomerization of all-*trans*- to 11-*cis*-retinol, which occurs primarily, if not solely, in the RPE (Shi & Olson, 1990; Winston & Rando, 1998). All-*trans*-retinol is first acylated by LRAT, followed by a concerted hydrolysis and isomerization reaction to yield 11-*cis*-retinol (Winston & Rando, 1998).

In addition to having a complex pattern of vitamin A metabolism, the eye is possibly the most sensitive organ with regard to vitamin A availability. An early symptom of vitamin A deficiency is night-blindness. Well nourished patients receiving *N*-(4-hydroxyphenyl)retinamide (4HPR) also display night-blindness as a side-effect of the drug. 4HPR-induced night-blindness appears to arise from a competition between 4HPR and retinol for apo-RBP in liver cells, thereby markedly reducing the plasma concentration of holo-RBP (Ritter & Smith, 1996).

3.2.6.7 Other tissues and species

Many other tissues take up and store retinol. In addition to those discussed above, Gerlach *et al.* (1989) reported that trachea, intestine and spleen of vitamin A-sufficient rats contain retinyl esters. In the guinea-pig, Biesalski (1990) found significant concentrations of retinyl esters in the kidney, lung, testes, epididymis, vas deferens, trachea, nasal mucosa, tongue and inner ear. It seems likely that other tissues will also be found to store vitamin A. These local stores may be used to meet both local tissue demands as well as total body needs.

3.2.7 Retinoic acid metabolism

Although it is generally accepted that all-*trans*- and 9-*cis*-retinoic acid facilitate most of the actions of vitamin A in mammalian tissues, other forms of vitamin A, including all-*trans*-3,4-didehydroretinoic acid and 4-oxo-all-*trans*-retinoic acid are reported to bring about RAR interaction with RXRs and may be important for facilitating retinoid actions in birds and amphibians *in vivo* (Hofmann & Eichele, 1994; Mangelsdorf *et al.*, 1994). Each of these vitamin A forms, however, must be derived from all-*trans*-retinol. A metabolic scheme for the formation of these active retinoid forms from all-*trans*-retinol is given in Figure 5. The pathways shown are for the most part hypothetical, since data supporting some of the conversions are extremely limited. Only the enzymatic processes responsible for the formation of all-*trans*-retinal from all-*trans*-retinol and for the oxidation of all-*trans*-retinal to all-*trans*-retinoic acid have been much studied. Even the processes by which all-*trans*-retinoic acid is enzymatically formed within tissues by oxidation of all-*trans*-retinol have not been unequivocally established (Duester, 1996; Napoli, 1996). The currently prevailing hypothesis is that retinol is first oxidized to retinal, which in turn is oxidized to retinoic acid, a process analogous to the oxidation of ethanol to acetaldehyde and on to acetic acid. This process is represented diagramatically in Figure 5.

3.2.7.1 Retinoic acid formation in tissues

It has long been known that the relatively nonspecific alcohol dehydrogenase of liver can catalyse the oxidation of retinol to retinal (Blaner & Olson, 1994; Duester, 1996: Napoli,

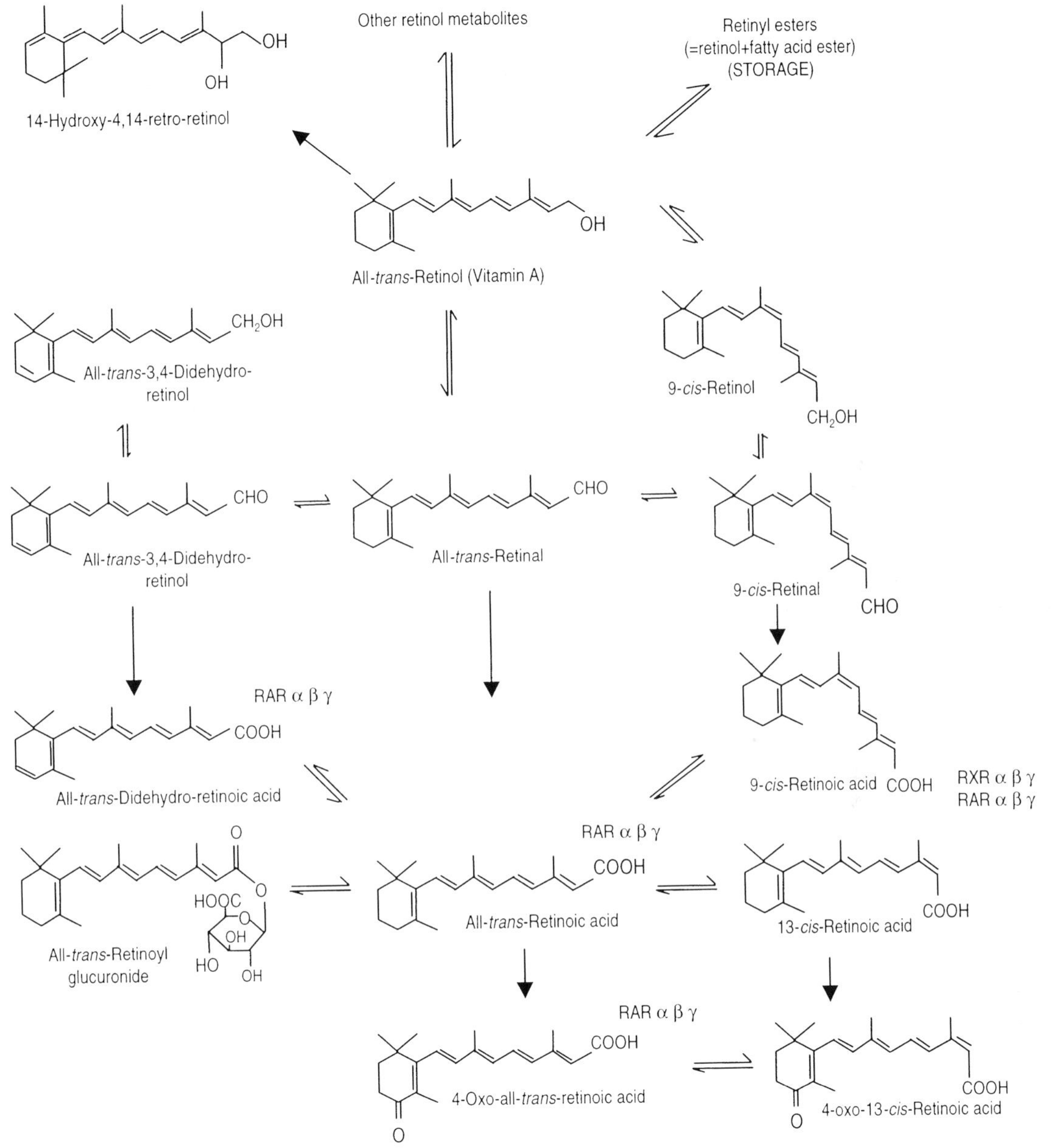

OH

OH

14-Hydroxy-4,14-retro-retinol

Other retinol metabolites

Retinyl esters
(=retinol+fatty acid ester)
(STORAGE)

OH

All-*trans*-Retinol (Vitamin A)

CH_2OH

All-*trans*-3,4-Didehydro-
retinol

9-*cis*-Retinol

CH_2OH

CHO

All-*trans*-3,4-Didehydro-
retinol

CHO

All-*trans*-Retinal

9-*cis*-Retinal

CHO

RAR α β γ

COOH

All-*trans*-Didehydro-retinoic acid

9-*cis*-Retinoic acid COOH

RXR α β γ
RAR α β γ

O

O

HOOC

O

OH

HO

OH

All-*trans*-Retinoyl
glucuronide

RAR α β γ

COOH

All-*trans*-Retinoic acid

COOH

13-*cis*-Retinoic acid

RAR α β γ

COOH

4-Oxo-all-*trans*-retinoic acid

O

COOH

O

4-oxo-13-*cis*-Retinoic acid

Figure 5. Hypothetical scheme for the metabolism of all-*trans*-retinol.
Although all of the metabolite interconversions indicated in this scheme have not been unequivocally demonstrated experimentally, all of these transformations of vitamin A species have been postulated in the literature to take place in some living organism. The reader should especially focus on the metabolic transformations described in the body of the text. These are the most extensively studied transformations and involve the oxidative metabolism of retinol to retinoic acid and the oxidative and conjugative transformations of retinoic acid to more polar metabolites. Less well understood are the *cis-trans* isomerizations proposed in the figure.

1996) and that aldehyde oxidase can convert retinal to retinoic acid (Duester, 1996; Napoli, 1996). Because retinoic acid in tiny amounts shows such potent physiological actions, however, one must question the role of abundant enzyme systems (such as alcohol dehydrogenase, aldehyde dehydrogenase and aldehyde oxidase), which possess relatively broad substrate specificities, in forming retinoic acid. This issue is now a focus of much research and debate.

(a) Oxidation of retinol

The enzymes which catalyse the formation of retinal from retinol have not been unequivocally established. Members of two distinct families of enzymes have been proposed as being important. Several members of the family of cytosolic alcohol dehydrogenases catalyse retinol oxidation *in vitro* (Boleda *et al.*, 1993; Duester, 1996; Napoli, 1996), and much circumstantial evidence supports the idea that some of these are importantly involved in retinoic acid formation *in vivo*. Members of a second family of enzymes, the short-chain alcohol dehydrogenase family, have also been proposed as being physiologically relevant for catalysing retinol oxidation (Duester, 1996; Napoli, 1996). The members of this enzyme family, which are known to catalyse retinol oxidation, are present in cells and tissues at relatively low concentrations and are associated with membrane fractions. Several of the short-chain alcohol dehydrogenases which oxidize retinol prefer as a substrate, over unbound retinol, retinol bound to vitamin A-binding proteins (CRBP-I or cellular retinal-binding protein (CRalBP)) (Saari, 1994; Duester, 1996; Napoli, 1996). This is unlike the cytosolic alcohol dehydrogenases, which require unbound retinol as substrate (Duester, 1996; Napoli, 1996). It remains unclear whether all or only some of the enzymes reported to be important for retinoic acid formation are indeed physiologically essential.

Both class I and class IV alcohol dehydrogenases catalyse the oxidation of all-*trans*-retinol to all-*trans*-retinal (Duester, 1996; Napoli, 1996). In developing mouse embryos, the pattern of expression of a class IV alcohol dehydrogenase overlaps both temporally and spatially with the pattern of retinoic acid distribution (Ang *et al.*, 1996). A class IV alcohol dehydrogenase purified from rat stomach is able to catalyse both the oxidation of omega-hydroxy fatty alcohols and of free retinol (Boleda *et al.*, 1993). Nevertheless, since most retinol within a cell is bound to CRBP-I and since class I and IV alcohol dehydrogenases only catalyse the oxidation of free retinol, these authors were not convinced as to whether this class IV alcohol dehydrogenase is physiologically important for retinoic acid formation (Duester, 1996; Napoli, 1996).

Other reports indicate that oxidation of all-*trans*-retinol to all-*trans*-retinal is catalysed by microsomal enzymes that use all-*trans*-retinol bound to CRBP-I as substrate. Napoli and colleagues have cloned and characterized three microsomal retinol dehydrogenases from rat liver (termed retinol dehydrogenase, type I, type II and type III). Each of these recognizes all-*trans*-retinol bound to CRBP-I as substrate (Posch *et al.*, 1991; Boerman & Napoli, 1995; Chai *et al.*, 1995, 1996). Since most retinol within cells is bound to CRBP-I, this substrate specificity suggests that these enzymes are physiologically relevant for retinol oxidation. Sequence analysis indicates that these enzymes are 82% identical to each other and are members of the class of short-chain alcohol dehydrogenases. Each requires $NADP^+$ as an electron acceptor and is expressed most prominently in liver. Retinol dehydrogenase type I is the best studied isoform and is reported to be present also in kidney, brain, lung and testis, but at levels less than 1% of that in liver (Boerman & Napoli, 1995). Retinol dehydrogenase type II is expressed in kidney, brain, lung and testis at levels which are 25, 8, 4 and 3%, respectively, of that observed in liver, whereas retinol dehydrogenase type III is expressed only in liver (Chai *et al.*, 1996). Interestingly, retinol dehydrogenase type I does not oxidize 9-*cis*-retinol (Posch *et al.*, 1991; Boerman & Napoli, 1995). The substrate specificity of the type II and III enzymes for different retinol isomers has not been reported (Chai *et al.*, 1995, 1996). The properties of these three enzymes suggest that they are physiologically involved in the oxidation of all-*trans*-retinol to all-*trans*-retinal.

17β- and 3α-hydroxysteroid dehydrogenases cloned from rat and human prostate share a high degree of primary sequence homology with rat retinol dehydrogenase type I, suggesting that the microsomal retinol dehydrogenases might also use hydroxysteroids as substrates (Biswas & Russell, 1997). Indeed, recombinant rat retinol dehydrogenase type I and recombinant protein generated from the newly cloned human homologue of this enzyme both catalyse the oxidation of 5α-androstan-3,17-diol to dihydrotestosterone, with the same apparent K_m value 0.1 μM (Biswas & Russell, 1997) (as compared to approximately 2 μM for retinol–CRBP-I for rat retinol dehydrogenase type I (Boerman & Napoli, 1995)). Thus, the microsomal retinol dehydrogenases may play important roles both in the generation of active forms of vitamin A and in the generation of active steroids.

In ocular tissue, the interconversion of retinol and retinal is an essential part of the visual cycle. Several membrane-bound dehydrogenases catalyse this oxidation–reduction process (Saari, 1994). One such enzyme, present in the rod outer segments, catalyses the interconversion of all-*trans*-retinol and all-*trans*-retinal. In the eye, soluble alcohol dehydrogenases, although present, may not play a major role in retinoid metabolism (Saari, 1994).

In the RPE, a different membrane-bound dehydrogenase, which is a member of the short-chain alcohol dehydrogenase family, has been reported to catalyse the stereospecific interconversion of 11-*cis*-retinol and 11-*cis*-retinal (Saari, 1994). Interestingly, 11-*cis*-retinal bound to CRalBP is reduced reversibly by this RPE enzyme to 11-*cis*-retinol (Saari, 1994). Simon *et al.* (1995) and Driessen *et al.* (1995) independently described the isolation, cloning and characterization of this stereospecific 11-*cis*-retinol dehydrogenase from bovine RPE. Like the enzymes characterized by Napoli and colleagues (Boerman & Napoli, 1995; Chai *et al.*, 1995, 1996), this dehydrogenase is a member of the family of short-chain alcohol dehydrogenases. However, unlike Napoli's enzymes, it does not employ all-*trans*-retinol as a substrate and requires NAD^+ and not $NADP^+$ as an electron acceptor. The bovine 11-*cis*-retinol dehydrogenase shows a 54% amino acid sequence homology with rat liver retinol dehydrogenase type II (Chai *et al.*, 1995, 1996). Northern blot analysis of total RNA from bovine RPE, liver, kidney, adrenal, lung, testis, brain and muscle indicates that the 11-*cis*-retinol dehydrogenase is present only in the RPE, supporting the idea that this enzyme is important for providing 11-*cis*-retinal for visual pigment formation (Simon *et al.*, 1995; Driessen *et al.*, 1995).

Edwards *et al.* (1992) reported that cultured rabbit Müller cells are able to synthesize retinoic acid from [^{3}H]retinol. [^{3}H]Retinoic acid initially accumulated slowly, but by 30 min, retinoic acid was rapidly released into the medium. Extracellular retinoic acid exceeded the intracellular amount after 30 min of incubation. Thus, some cells of the vertebrate retina have the capacity to synthesize retinoic acid from retinol and to release retinoic acid into the medium.

Shih and Hill (1991) have reported that an NADPH-dependent oxidase is present in rat liver microsomes, with an optimal pH between 8.2 and 8.7, which converts retinol to retinal. This oxidase was induced by 3-methylcholanthrene and inhibited by citral, ketoconazole and α-naphthoflavone, but was unaffected by the dehydrogenase inhibitor pyrazole. This enzyme seems to be distinct from previously characterized cytosolic and microsomal enzymes.

(b) Oxidation of retinal

Lee *et al.* (1991a) explored the ability of the 13 aldehyde dehydrogenases known at the time to be present in mouse tissues to catalyse the oxidation of all-*trans*-retinal to all-*trans*-retinoic acid. Three of the six aldehyde dehydrogenases present in mouse liver cytosol were able to catalyse this oxidation. One of these, ALDH-2, was estimated to catalyse about 95% of the oxidation of retinal to retinoic acid in the liver. The apparent K_m of ALDH-2 for all-*trans*-retinal was 0.7 μM. None of the aldehyde dehydrogenases present in the particulate fractions of mouse liver were able to catalyse retinal oxidation significantly. Based on these data, the authors concluded that the enzymes responsible for retinoic acid formation from retinal are cytosolic, NAD-linked, substrate-non-specific dehydrogenases.

Other investigators have demonstrated that cytosol preparations from rat kidney, testis and lung can catalyse the oxidation of retinal to retinoic acid (Bhat *et al.*, 1988a,b). The enzyme responsible seems to be an oxidase, inasmuch as the oxidative formation of retinoic acid was stimulated by the addition of NADPH and blocked by inhibitors of aldehyde oxidase (Bhat *et al.*, 1988a). An enzymatic activity present in rat liver cytosol catalyses the formation of retinoic acid from retinal, showing linear kinetics with respect to protein concentration (0–2.4 mg/mL) and time (0–30 min), a broad pH maximum of 7.7 to 9.7, and an apparent K_m of 0.25 mmol/L for all-*trans*-retinal (Hupert *et al.*, 1991).

An aldehyde dehydrogenase present at high levels in the basal forebrain of mice has been reported to catalyse the formation of retinoic acid (McCaffery & Dräger, 1995; Zhao *et al.*, 1996). This enzyme, now termed RALDH-2, is expressed very early in embryonic development and levels of expression decline later in development (McCaffery & Dräger, 1995; Niederreither *et al.*, 1997). In mouse embryos, a teratogenic dose of all-*trans*-retinoic acid at embryonic day 8.5 results in downregulation of expression of this enzyme (Niederreither *et al.*, 1997). Bhat and Lacroix have purified and characterized a cytosolic retinal dehydrogenase from rat kidney which is NAD^+-dependent and catalyses the oxidation of both all-*trans*- and 9-*cis*-retinal to the corresponding retinoic acid isomer (Labrecque *et al.*, 1993, 1995). A similar retinal dehydrogenase has been partially purified from rat liver cytosol and characterized by El Akawi and Napoli (1994). This enzyme also catalyses the oxidation of both all-*trans*- and 9-*cis*-retinal in an NAD^+-dependent manner. Presence of CRBP-I decreases the rate of all-*trans*-retinoic acid synthesis by the rat liver retinal dehydrogenase (El Akawi & Napoli, 1994). Thus, these and other studies (Blaner & Olson, 1994) strongly support a role for cytosolic retinal dehydrogenases in the formation of retinoic acid *in vivo*.

Roberts *et al.* (1992) reported that CYP1A2 and CYP3A6 from rabbit liver microsomes oxidize retinal to retinoic acid. No work exploring the roles of cytosolic retinal dehydrogenases in formation of retinoic acid in the rabbit has been reported. Thus, it is possible that retinoic acid formation and metabolism in other mammalian species may differ from that in rodents or humans.

*(c) 9-*cis*-Retinoic acid formation*

9-*cis*-Retinoic acid acting through RARs and RXRs is an essential vitamin A form for regulating retinoid-responsive gene activity. The genes regulated by retinoids are very diverse and are involved in regulating a wide array of cellular functions. Thus, any factor which influences 9-*cis*-retinoic acid availability to or within a cell will have a broad impact on retinoic acid signalling pathways and cellular responses.

There is still only very limited information on how 9-*cis*-retinoid isomers are formed. For the visual process, the isomerization of all-*trans*-retinoids to 11-*cis*-retinoids is catalysed by a specific enzyme and the isomerization takes place at the level of the retinols and not the aldehydes (Saari, 1994). Since the first reports in 1992 that 9-*cis*-retinoic acid is a ligand for the RXRs, several studies have explored possible pathways for 9-*cis*-retinoic acid formation. Urbach and Rando (1994) reported that membranes prepared from bovine liver catalyse non-enzymatically the isomerization of all-*trans*-retinoic acid to 9-*cis*-retinoic acid. This isomerization depends on free sulfhydryl groups present in the microsomes and does not involve the participation of an enzyme. Hébuterne *et al.* (1995) reported that 9-*cis*-β-carotene serves as a precursor for 9-*cis*-retinoic acid *in vivo* in the rat. The rate of cleavage of 9-*cis*-β-carotene, however, is only 6–7% of that of all-*trans*-β-carotene (Nagao & Olson, 1994). Furthermore, since rats maintained on carotenoid-free diets display normal health, the conversion of 9-*cis*-β-carotene to 9-*cis*-retinoic acid cannot be an essential pathway for formation of this retinoic acid isomer. The ability of retinal dehydrogenases in rat kidney (Labrecque *et al.*, 1993, 1995) and rat liver (El Akawi & Napoli, 1994) to catalyse the oxidation of 9-*cis*-retinal to 9-*cis*-retinoic acid was taken to suggest that a pathway starting with 9-*cis*-retinol may be important for 9-*cis*-retinoic acid formation. The presence of 9-*cis*-

retinol in rat kidney at approximately 10% of the level of all-*trans*-retinol (Labrecque *et al.*, 1993, 1995) supports this possibility. Although each of these reports is individually convincing, it still is unclear whether any or all of these possibilities are important for 9-*cis*-retinoic acid formation *in vivo*.

An NAD-dependent retinol dehydrogenase which specifically oxidizes 9-*cis*-retinol but not all-*trans*-retinol has recently been cloned from a human mammary tissue cDNA library and characterized upon its expression in CHO cells (Mertz *et al.*, 1997). This enzyme, a member of the short-chain alcohol dehydrogenase enzyme family, is expressed in adult human mammary tissue, kidney, liver and testis. Mertz *et al.* (1997) proposed that this enzyme may play an important role in the synthesis of 9-*cis*-retinoic acid. Interestingly, this enzyme, termed 9-*cis*-retinol dehydrogenase, is expressed in kidney, a tissue which has been reported to contain significant quantities of 9-*cis*-retinol (Labrecque *et al.*, 1993, 1995). However, it remains to be established whether this enzyme is physiologically important for generating active forms of vitamin A like 9-*cis*-retinoic acid.

A second *cis*-retinol dehydrogenase, also a member of the short-chain alcohol dehydrogenase family, has been described by Napoli and colleagues (Chai *et al.*, 1997). The cDNA for this mouse liver enzyme, termed the *cis*-retinol/3α-hydroxysterol short-chain dehydrogenase, encodes a 317-amino acid-containing enzyme which recognizes 9-*cis*- and 11-*cis*-retinol, 5α-androstan-3α,17β-diol and 5α-androstan-3α-ol-17-one as substrates. The apparent K_m values for these substrates indicate that the *cis*-retinol dehydrogenase has a greater affinity for the sterol substrates. This mouse enzyme, which is most similar to mouse retinol dehydrogenase isozymes types 1 and 2 (86% and 91% homology, respectively), uses NAD^+ as its preferred cofactor. It is expressed in liver, kidney, small intestine, heart, RPE, brain, spleen, testis and lung. Chai *et al.* (1997) proposed that this multifunctional enzyme is important for generating both 9-*cis*-retinoic acid and bioactive androgens. It is possible that this enzyme provides a link between the actions of vitamin A and androgens.

(d) Summary

The extent to which soluble, relatively nonspecific, enzymes such as alcohol dehydrogenase, aldehyde dehydrogenase or aldehyde oxidase are involved in the enzymatic formation of retinoic acid from retinol is unclear. The oxidation of retinol to retinal is most likely catalysed by a microsomal enzyme or enzymes, which use retinol bound to CRBP-I as substrate. Whether the oxidation of retinal to retinoic acid is also CRBP-I-dependent or is catalysed by a soluble aldehyde dehydrogenase and/or aldehyde oxidase is still uncertain. Nonetheless, multiple enzymatic activities clearly are involved in the conversion of retinol to retinoic acid.

3.2.7.2 Synthesis of retinoic acid from carotenoids within tissues

In 1988, Napoli and Race reported that cytosol preparations from rat tissues could catalyse the formation of retinoic acid from β-carotene. The rate of retinoic acid synthesis from 10 μmol/L β-carotene ranged from 120 to 224 pmol/h/mg protein for intestinal cytosol, and from 334 to 488 pmol/h/mg protein for cytosols prepared from kidney, lung, testes and liver. Retinol that was generated during β-carotene metabolism was determined not to be the major substrate for retinoic acid synthesis. Retinal was not detected as a free intermediate in this process, but retinal might be tightly bound by the enzyme. Alternatively, β-carotene might be oxidized to a 15,15′-enediol before dioxygenase cleavage, by analogy with the conversion of catechol to *cis,cis*-muconic acid. Other mechanisms for producing retinoic acid from β-carotene without yielding retinal are possible, but as yet no intermediates have been characterized.

Wang *et al.* (1991) reported that homogenates of liver, lung, kidney and fat from monkey, ferret and rat formed retinoic acid upon incubation with 2 μmol/L β-carotene, with a pH optimum of 7.0. Because citral, which inhibits the conversion of retinal to retinoic acid, did not affect retinoic acid formation from β-carotene or β-apocarotenals, Wang *et al.* (1992) concluded that retinoic acid is formed through a biochemical process that does not involve retinal as an intermediate.

3.2.7.3 Metabolism of retinoic acid

Metabolites of all-*trans*-retinoic acid generated *in vivo* include 13-*cis*-retinoic acid, 9-*cis*-retinoic acid, retinoyl β-glucuronide, 5,6-epoxyretinoic acid, 4-hydroxyretinoic acid, 4-oxoretinoic acid, and 3,4-didehydroretinoic acid (Blaner & Olson, 1994). Some of these metabolites retain activity in mediating retinoic acid function, whereas others seem to be inactive catabolic products.

The cytochrome P450 system is active in metabolizing retinoic acid. Roberts *et al.* (1979) reported that the formation of polar metabolites of retinoic acid was catalysed by an activity present in the microsomal fraction of rat intestine and liver homogenates. This activity required NADPH and oxygen, and was strongly inhibited by carbon monoxide. In addition, the activity was markedly induced by retinoids, but only to a minor extent by phenobarbital or 3-methylcholanthrene. Roberts *et al.* (1979) concluded that the enzyme responsible for the formation of polar metabolites of retinoic acid is a member of a class of mixed function oxidases containing the cytochrome P450s. Leo *et al.* (1984) reported that rats fed a diet containing a 100-fold excess of retinyl acetate, for two to three weeks, showed an increase in hepatic microsomal cytochrome P450 content. When microsomes were isolated from the livers of the treated rats, the conversion of all-*trans*-retinoic acid to more polar metabolites, including 4-hydroxy- and 4-oxoretinoic acid, was enhanced. Purified rat liver CYP2C7 and CYP2B1 catalysed the conversion of retinoic acid to polar metabolites, including 4-hydroxy-retinoic acid (Leo *et al.*, 1984). The isozyme CYP2C8 of human liver microsomes oxidizes retinoic acid to 4-hydroxyretinoic acid and 4-oxoretinoic acid (Leo *et al.*, 1989). Roberts *et al.* (1992) reported that many rabbit liver CYP isoforms, including 2A4, 1A2, 2E1, 2E2, 2C3, 2G1 and 3A6, catalyse the 4-hydroxylation of retinoic acid, as well as of both retinol and retinal, but not the conversion of 4-hydroxy-retinoids to the corresponding 4-oxoretinoids. Van Wauwe *et al.* (1992) showed that oral administration of a dose (40 mg/kg body weight) of liarozole, a 1-substituted imidazole derivative which inhibits cytochrome P450 activity, enhances the endogenous plasma concentrations of retinoic acid from less than 1.7 nmol/L to 10–15 nmol/L. Thus, the cytochrome P450 system seems to play an important role in retinoic acid metabolism and homeostasis.

Novel cytochrome P450s of the CYP26 family (termed P450RA from P19 cells and P450RAI from the zebrafish), which are able to metabolize retinoic acid, were recently cloned (Fujii *et al.*, 1997; White *et al.*, 1997a). One cDNA clone (P450RA) was obtained from a subtraction library prepared from retinoic acid-treated and untreated murine P19 embryonic carcinoma cells (Fujii *et al.*, 1997). When expressed, the murine P450RA cDNA catalysed the oxidation of all-*trans*-retinoic acid to 5,8-epoxy-all-*trans*-retinoic acid. Both 13-*cis*- and 9-*cis*-retinoic acid are also substrates for P450RA. This cytochrome P450 is expressed in a stage- and region-specific fashion in mouse development, but expression does not appear to be inducible by excess retinoic acid. In the adult mouse, P450RA is expressed only in liver (Fujii *et al.*, 1997). White *et al.* (1997a) reported the isolation and characterization of a cDNA for cytochrome P450RAI expressed during gastrulation of the zebrafish. P450RAI was expressed normally during gastrulation and in a defined pattern in epithelial cells of the regenerating caudal fin in response to administration of exogenous all-*trans*-retinoic acid. When the cDNA for P450RAI was expressed in COS-1 cells, all-*trans*-retinoic acid was rapidly metabolized to more polar metabolites, two of which were identified as 4-oxo-all-*trans*-retinoic acid and 4-hydroxy-all-*trans*-retinoic acid. P450RAI, which is induced upon retinoic acid exposure, catalyses the oxidative metabolism of retinoic acid. It is tempting to speculate that the oxidative metabolism catalysed by P450RAI and P450RA is an important and common mechanism through which cells and tissues regulate levels of this active form of vitamin A; however, this possibility requires further studies.

Livers from aryl hydrocarbon receptor-null ($AHR^{-/-}$) mice possess total retinol levels which are approximately three-fold higher than those of wild-type mice (Andreola *et al.*, 1997). In addition, $AHR^{-/-}$ mice show a reduced capability to oxidize retinoic acid and significantly decreased hepatic mRNA levels for both retinal dehydrogenase types 1 and 2. Interestingly, expression of P450RAI was not different in AHR-deficient and wild-type mice. These results strongly suggest that the aryl hydrocarbon receptor plays an important role in vitamin A homeostasis within the body. This is in keeping with observations that mice and rats given 2,3,7,8-tetrachlorodibenzo-*p*-dioxin show a rapid decline in hepatic total retinol levels (Brouwer *et al.*, 1985; Chen *et al.*, 1992a). Thus, it would appear that there is a direct link between xenobiotic exposure and metabolism and vitamin A metabolism and homeostasis in mice and rats. Although the potential pathological consequences of such a link are clear, the underlying biochemical processes and mechanisms still need to be resolved.

A direct role for CRABP-I in the oxidative metabolism of retinoic acid has been proposed by Fiorella and Napoli (1991). Microsomal enzymes of rat testes catalyse the conversion of CRABP-I-bound all-*trans*-retinoic acid to 3,4-didehydro-, 4-hydroxy-, 4-oxo-, 16-hydroxy-4-oxo- and 18-hydroxy-retinoic acids. Thus, CRABP-I may well play a direct role in the oxidative metabolism of all-*trans*-retinoic acid. Furthermore, the binding of all-*trans*-retinoic acid to CRABP may provide a mechanism for discriminating metabolically between all-*trans*- and 13-*cis*-retinoids.

4. Preventive effects

4.1 Humans

4.1.1 Epidemiological studies

The proportion of total vitamin A intake that is contributed by preformed vitamin A (retinol and its esters) varies between populations, depending on a number of factors, including the balance of animal and plant foods and the prevalence of dietary supplements. In the United States, for example, preformed vitamin A makes up about 50% of the total dietary intake of vitamin A (Tee, 1992). Restricting this review to studies that separated the preformed vitamin A and carotenoid components would cause a number of potentially informative investigations to be omitted. Therefore, the Working Group chose to include studies that reported only total vitamin A (preformed and provitamin A) in the diet, but to present and discuss the findings separately from studies that specifically identified preformed vitamin A intake.

The review does not cover all studies that have reported on associations of vitamin A intake and cancer at any site. The Working Group chose to include cancer sites that have been reported in at least two studies and to exclude studies that were based on a small number of cases.

4.1.1.1 Methodological issues

(a) Case–control studies

Most of the studies relating vitamin A intake to cancer in humans are case–control studies. In these studies, individuals with cancer are compared with persons sampled from the general population with respect to prior consumption of vitamin A, or of foods rich in vitamin A. Advantages of such studies include efficiency and the capacity to study multiple exposures related to a single disease outcome. Often, studies of this kind provide the only information that is available. However, several methodological problems limit the ability of case–control studies to provide strong evidence for causal relations with vitamin A intake. Biased estimates of the relationship between vitamin A intake and disease may result if the controls are not representative of the population which gave rise to the cases (selection bias). For a case series at a hospital, for example, it may be difficult to define this underlying population, and even more difficult to sample it randomly, although in some instances hospital-based controls may give unbiased estimates of effect.

It may be difficult to obtain accurate information on past diet from cases and controls. In cancer studies, epidemiologists are usually interested in the diet of the cases months or years before the time the diagnosis is made. Estimates of diet at some time in the past are likely to be imprecise. Moreover, cases may differ systematically from controls in the accuracy of their description of their past diet (recall bias), particularly in view of the prominence given to diet–cancer hypotheses in some countries. For rapidly fatal cancers such as lung cancer, cases may be dead or too ill to participate by the time they are contacted, and information can be obtained only from a proxy respondent, such as the spouse. This approach may yield unreliable data, particularly for a complex exposure such as dietary habits. These and other sources of error are important when studies are searching for small effects. In many studies of vitamin A, for instance, relative risks between the highest and lowest categories of intake are expected to be small and may be obscured by a relatively minor degree of bias.

The usual measure of effect in case–control studies is the odds ratio (OR; the relative odds of exposure among cases compared with the odds of exposure among controls). In a population-based case–control study, it can be shown that the odds ratio is an unbiased estimate of the measure of effect used in cohort studies (the relative risk (RR), i.e., the ratio of the incidence rate of the outcome among the exposed compared with the incidence rate in the unexposed). For simplicity, in this chapter, the term relative risk is used throughout.

(b) Cohort studies

In a cohort (prospective or follow-up) study, a group of persons whose dietary intake has been ascertained is followed over time with respect to disease incidence. Subsequent cases of cancer are compared with subjects who did not develop cancer, with respect to initial diet. The major advantage is that diet is assessed before the occurrence of disease, and thus should not be influenced by it. Selection bias should not occur, as the comparison group for the cases is explicit (the non-cases in the cohort). The major limitation of cohort studies is that a very large number of people (typically thousands or tens of thousands) must be enrolled and followed for many years to generate enough cancer diagnoses to achieve statistical power. For relatively uncommon cancer types or sites, a prospective study may never accrue enough cases. In addition, most cohort studies are limited to exposure data collected at the beginning of the study (unless blood or tissue samples are stored). Nonetheless, for vitamin A and the major cancers, prospective data are available, and generally constitute the best available sources of non-experimental evidence.

(c) Nested case–control studies

A common strategy in prospective studies using biomarkers of exposure is to employ a nested case–control design. It is usually prohibitively expensive and wasteful of samples to analyse all samples in a cohort. In a nested case–control study, typically most or all of the cases and a sample of non-cases (controls) are analysed. The study has the advantages of a prospective design, as the specimens providing the exposure data were collected before the diagnosis of cancer.

4.1.1.2 Assessment of exposure

The quality of the data on vitamin A and cancer in humans depends not only on study designs used, but also on the validity of the measurements of vitamin A intake. In general, intake can be measured by diet assessment (combining information on an individual's average intake of foods with the average vitamin A content of the foods), history of supplement use, or by measuring vitamin A (either retinol and/or retinyl esters) in the blood or other tissues.

(a) Diet assessment

Because certain foods (e.g., liver) are particularly rich sources of vitamin A, day-to-day variation in vitamin A intake is high. In many countries, certain foods such as milk are fortified with preformed vitamin A, and for some individuals, these foods account for a substantial proportion of their intake on some days. Thus, it is particularly important to assess intake of these foods over weeks or months, since one or a few days of intake (obtained for instance from 24-hour or three-day recalls) may be highly unrepresentative of long-term intake. Thus, many investigators use food frequency questionnaires, which generally seek to obtain information on average intake of foods over months or a year. The available data suggest that these instruments measure vitamin A intake reasonably well, although the effectiveness of questionnaires varies depending on the quality of the survey instrument, the circumstances in which information is sought and the skills and understanding of the study participants. For instance, the correlation between total vitamin A intake estimated from a 61-item food frequency questionnaire compared with four weeks of diet records, in a population of women in the United States, was $r = 0.5$ ($p < 0.05$) (Willett *et al.*, 1985).

Many studies, particularly earlier ones, were not able to differentiate between preformed vitamin A (retinol and retinyl esters) and carotenoids with vitamin A activity, and thus reported data for total vitamin A, not preformed vitamin A specifically.

In contrast to some nutrients such as carotenoids (Ascherio *et al.*, 1992), validation of estimates of dietary intake of preformed vitamin A by comparison with serum levels is not feasible (see Section 4.1.1.2(*b*)).

A further issue is potential confounding of vitamin A by other nutrients in vitamin A-rich foods. For instance, dairy products are major sources of preformed vitamin A, but also have high levels of saturated fats. Thus, an artefactual positive association with preformed vitamin A may be observed at sites where cancer has a positive relation with saturated fat. Similarly, whenever total vitamin A intakes reflect intake of provitamin A-rich vegetables, confounding by other potentially anti-carcinogenic nutrients in these vegetables is a concern.

In the evaluation of dietary intake of retinol, it is worth distinguishing populations, chiefly North American ones, who have a relatively high probability of having been taking vitamin supplements, from other populations (e.g., southern Europe, Asia), where this practice is uncommon. When the use of vitamin supplements (mostly multivitamin preparations) has been specifically evaluated, this is mentioned in the description of the specific studies.

(b) Biochemical markers

Although serum retinol levels are depressed when vitamin A intake is sufficiently low to produce clinical deficiency, over the range of intake in generally well nourished populations serum retinol levels are only minimally related to vitamin A intake. For example, no material increase in blood retinol level was observed in a study in which 25 000 IU of preformed vitamin A (more than five times the usual dietary intake) was taken as a daily supplement for eight weeks (Willett *et al.*, 1983). Similarly, large supplements of β-carotene had no notable effect on blood retinol levels. Even among women with initially low values of plasma retinol, a daily supplement of 10 000 IU of vitamin A (fish-liver extract) increased blood levels only by 9%, although this was significant ($p < 0.02$) (Willett *et al.*, 1984a). Thus, serum retinol is not a valid indicator of vitamin A intake in vitamin A-sufficient subjects.

Case–control studies are particularly problematic for another reason: cancer and cancer treatment usually reduce retinol levels from pre-treatment values. Consequently, case–control studies that relied solely on blood retinol measures have been omitted from this review.

(c) Preformed vitamin A supplement use

In principle, users of preformed vitamin A supplements constitute a useful population to test the hypothesis that preformed vitamin A intake influences cancer risk. In practice, however, there are major limitations to this approach. In most populations, use of single vitamin A supplements is relatively rare; most preformed vitamin A supplements are taken in conjunction with other supplements, or in the form of multivitamins. This obviously limits the interpretation of information on preformed vitamin A supplement use. Vitamin supplements may also be used for relatively short periods, or in variable amounts, which further complicates interpretation of observational studies. Furthermore, supplement users tend to differ from non-supplement users in their exposure to established cancer risk factors (such as tobacco use) and socioeconomic status, suggesting that residual confounding due to these variables may remain even after statistical adjustment.

Patterson *et al.* (1997) reviewed vitamin supplement use and cancer risk in observational studies. Of eight prospective studies examining vitamin A supplement use and cancer at multiple sites, the only significant inverse association observed was for colon cancer among women, but not men, in a cohort in California, United States (Shibata *et al.*, 1992). Among case–control studies, the upper aerodigestive tract was the only site at which more than one study reported a significant inverse association of cancer with vitamin A supplement use (see Table 10) (Patterson *et al.*, 1997). Patterson *et al.* (1997) concluded that further observational studies of supplement use 'appear warranted; however, methodological problems ... impair the ability to assess supplement use ... and cancer risk.' Because of the low prevalence of preformed vitamin A supplement use in most of the available studies, combined with the other methodological concerns, the Working Group did not systematically review the limited observational evidence relating supplement use to cancer risk.

4.1.1.3 Vitamin A and specific cancer sites

In the following review of the evidence relating vitamin A intake to specific cancers, studies are included which have presented data comparing relative risks for subjects according to categories of total and preformed vitamin A intake (high versus low). Details of these studies are presented in Tables 9–17. Studies that presented data only as a difference in mean vitamin A intake or blood retinol levels for cases and controls have been largely excluded, as were studies that reported only total cancer incidence as an endpoint.

(a) Lung cancer

The largest body of evidence on vitamin A and a specific cancer site exists for lung cancer (Table 9). Most of the case–control studies have reported an inverse association between total vitamin A intake and lung cancer, although some notable exceptions exist (Ziegler *et al.*, 1984; Jain *et al.*, 1990). In the study of Jain *et al.* (1990), increased consumption of vegetables was associated with significantly decreased risk, but the association was strongest for vegetables which are poor sources of vitamin A.

In general, among studies that have examined preformed vitamin A and carotenoid intake separately, no association or only a weak inverse association with preformed vitamin A is evident. In contrast, most of these studies have observed an inverse association with increased carotenoid consumption.

Prospective data are relatively sparse, with only four studies reporting more than 100 cases. Bjelke (1975) reported on 36 incident cases among 8278 Norwegian men who had earlier completed a mailed dietary questionnaire. Kvåle *et al.* (1983), in the further follow-up of the extended cohort (168 cases), observed a relative risk of 0.5 for high versus low intake of total vitamin A. This inverse association was mostly attributable to intake of carrots and other vegetables, with some additional contribution from milk. Thus, this study is more consistent with a beneficial effect of carotenoid sources of vitamin A than one of preformed vitamin A.

Shekelle *et al.* (1981) reported data on the independent associations of carotenoids and preformed vitamin A. In 19 years of follow-up of 2107 men, 33 cases occurred. Preformed vitamin A intake was weakly positively associated with disease risk, but a strong inverse association was observed for carotenoid intake, which was similar in magnitude for smokers and non-smokers. Paganini-Hill and colleagues (1987) observed little protective effect of total vitamin A or preformed vitamin A, but a modest decrease in lung cancer risk among both men and women in the upper tertile of carotenoid intake. Knekt *et al.* (1991a), in a follow-up of Finnish men, observed a weak positive relationship with preformed vitamin A among smokers. Yong *et al.* (1997) observed little evidence of any association with total vitamin A (based on 24-h recall estimates of dietary intake), and a relative risk of 1.3 for high versus low intake of preformed vitamin A.

As discussed earlier, blood retinol levels are poor indicators of preformed vitamin A intake. However, blood carotenoids do reflect carotenoid intake. A protective effect of being in the highest category of blood β-carotene level or total carotenoid intake has been a remarkably consistent finding in the nested case–control studies. In none of the nested case–control studies was a significant association with blood retinol levels observed.

In summary, the observational studies, including both case–control and prospective evidence, support a protective effect of higher intakes of foods containing carotenoids on risk of lung cancer. The possibility that other components of carotenoid-rich foods may be

Table 9. Studies of vitamin A intake and lung cancer

Reference, site	No. of cases[a]	Categories[b]	Total vitamin A[c] RR	Total vitamin A[c] 95% CI	Preformed vitamin C[c] RR	Preformed vitamin C[c] 95% CI	Vit. supp.[d]	Proxies (% cases)	Adjusted for
Case–control studies									
Mettlin *et al.* (1979), USA	292 M	Three	[0.6]	$p < 0.05$	–	–	N	0	Age, smoking
Gregor *et al.* (1980), UK	78 M	Three	[0.5]	p, trend < 0.05	–	–	Y	0	Unadjusted
	22 F		[1.9]	p, trend < 0.05					
Hinds *et al.* (1984), USA	364	Quartiles	[0.7]	[0.5–1.1]	–	–	Y	24%	Age, ethnicity, sex, smoking, cholesterol intake, occupation
Ziegler *et al.* (1984), USA	763 M, white	Quartiles	[1.1][f]	p, trend = 0.30	[1.3]	p, trend = 0.11	Y	60%[e]	Age, race, residence, smoking
Byers *et al.* (1984), USA	427 M	Tertiles	1.2[g]	p, trend = 0.73	–	–	N	0	Age, smoking
			0.7[d]	p, trend = 0.07					
			0.6[h]	p, trend = 0.09					
Samet *et al.* (1985), USA	332 Anglo	Tertiles	[0.6]	[0.4–1.0]	[1.1]	[0.7–1.7]	Y	47%	Age, ethnicity, sex, smoking
	125 Hispanic		[1.1]	[0.6–2.0]	[1.7]	[0.8–3.3]			
Wu *et al.* (1985), USA	220 F	Quartiles	–	–	[0.8]	[0.4–2.0]	Y	0	Age, residence, smoking
		Dichotomous			[1.0]	[0.4–2.5]			
Byers *et al.* (1987), USA	296 M	Quartiles	[0.7]	p, trend = 0.12	–		N	0	Age, smoking
	154 F		[0.8]	p, trend = 0.4	–				
Pastorino *et al.* (1987), Italy	47 F	Tertiles	–	–	[0.3]	[0.1-1.2]	N	0	Age, smoking, serum cholesterol, triglycerides
Fontham *et al.* (1988), USA	1253	Tertiles	–	–	0.9	0.7–1.1	N	27%	Age, race, sex, smoking
Koo (1988), Hong Kong	88 F, Chinese non-smokers	Three	–	–	[0.4]	p, trend = 0.02	N	0	Age, parity, education
Ho *et al.* (1988), Singapore	50 M, Chinese	Quartiles	[0.6]	[0.2–2.0]	–	–	Y	0	Age, ethnicity, sex
Le Marchand *et al.* (1989), USA	230 M	Quartiles	[0.6]	p, trend = 0.003	[1.1]	p, trend = 0.70	Y	29%	Age, ethnicity, smoking
	102 F		[0.4]	p, trend = 0.14	[1.0]	p, trend = 0.75			
Dartigues *et al.* (1990), France	106	< 3 330 IU	–	–	[0.2]	[0.1–0.4]	N	0	Age, residence, sex, smoking, alcohol, occupation
Jain *et al.* (1990), Canada	839	Quartiles	1.2	p, trend = 0.46	1.2	p, trend = 0.54	Y	34%	Age, residence, sex, smoking
Kalandidi *et al.* (1990), Greece	91 F, non-smokers	Quartiles	–	–	1.3	0.98–1.8	N	0	Age, education, energy
Candelora *et al.* (1992), USA	124 F non-smokers	Quartiles	–	–	1.2	0.6–2.4	Y	0	Age, education, energy

Table 9. (contd)

Reference, site		No. of cases[a]	Categories[b]	Total vitamin A[c]		Preformed vitamin A[c]		Vit. supp.[d]	Proxies (% cases)	Adjusted for
				RR	95% CI	RR	95% CI			
Cohort studies	Cohort size									
Kvåle *et al.* (1983), Norway	16 713 M	153	Four	[0.6]	*p*, trend < 0.04	–	–	N	0	Unadjusted
Paganini-Hill *et al.* (1987), USA	10 473	37 M	Tertiles	[0.9]	*p*, trend > 0.05	[0.8]	*p*, trend > 0.05	Y	0	Age
		18 F		[0.9]	*p*, trend > 0.05	[0.7]	*p*, trend > 0.05			
Knekt *et al.* (1991a), Finland	4538 M		Tertiles					Y	0	Age, smoking
	non-smokers	18		–	–	[0.7]	*p*, trend = 0.72			
	smokers	99		–	–	[1.4]	*p*, trend = 0.08			
Yong *et al.* (1997), USA	10 068	248	Quartiles	1.0	0.7–1.5	1.3	0.9–1.8	Y	0	Age, race, education, activity, body mass index, family history, energy, smoking, alcohol

Reference, site	No. of cases	No. of controls	Categories	Blood retinol[c]		Adjusted for
				RR	95% CI	
Prospective blood-based studies						
Friedman *et al.* (1986), USA	151	302	Quintiles	0.8	*p*, trend = 0.94	Age, sex, skin colour, smoking
Menkes *et al.* (1986), USA	99	196	Quintiles	1.1	*p*, trend = 0.68	Age, sex, race, smoking
Knekt *et al.* (1990), Finland	108 M	204	Quintiles	1.5	0.3–1.3	Age, sex, residence, smoking
	6 F	12		1.4	0.2–10.0	
Eichholzer *et al.* (1996), Switzerland	87 M	2173	Octiles			Age, smoking, lipids
	> 60 y			[0.4]	[0.8–8.1]	
	≤ 60 y			[0.7]	[0.3–1.7]	

[a] Study populations include both men and women unless otherwise stated

[b] Number of categories used (if quantiles not used); otherwise number of quantiles used for categorization

[c] Relative risk for highest versus lowest category

[d] Vitamin supplement use assessed (Y) or vitamin supplement use not assessed, or unclear if it was assessed (N)

[e] For cases and controls combined

[f] Adenocarcinoma

[g] Squamous-cell carcinoma

[h] Small cell carcinoma

responsible for an apparent effect of carotenoids deserves further exploration. The data support the conclusion that dietary intake of preformed vitamin A does not influence lung cancer risk.

(b) Upper aerodigestive tract cancer

Five case–control studies (four from the United States and one from Australia) (Table 10) evaluated the relationship between dietary intake of total vitamin A or preformed vitamin A and the risk of cancer of the oral cavity and pharynx. Two studies (McLaughlin *et al.*, 1988; Gridley *et al.*, 1990) found direct associations which were significant in males. These included the largest investigation on the topic (831 cases and 979 controls) which yielded RRs of 1.6 in men (*p*, trend = 0.007) and 1.4 (*p*, trend = 0.27) in females in the highest quartile of intake (McLaughlin *et al.*, 1988). In one study (Marshall *et al.*, 1982), a significantly reduced risk was reported for the highest tertile for vitamin A intake. The relationship between cancer of the oesophagus and retinol intake was evaluated in eight case–control studies. Approximately two-fold elevated RRs were reported in four investigations, including the largest from Calvados, France (743 cases and 1975 controls) (Tuyns *et al.*, 1987) and another from the United States, where adjustment for total energy intake was possible (Graham *et al.*, 1990a). No study suggested risk reduction in individuals who reported high retinol intake. For cancer of the larynx, three case–control investigations suggested either an elevated risk after allowance for total energy intake (Freudenheim *et al.*, 1992) or no effect on risk modification (Mackerras *et al.*, 1988; Estève *et al.*, 1996). The latter was a large collaborative European study (1147 cases and 3057 controls), where cancer of the hypopharynx was also evaluated and an RR of 0.6 was observed in the highest quartile for preformed vitamin A intake.

A prospective study of postmenopausal women in Iowa, United States, reported an RR of 0.9, (95% CI, 0.4–2.2) based on 33 cases of cancer of the oral cavity, pharynx and oesophagus (Zheng *et al.*, 1995).

Nomura *et al.* (1997a) evaluated the association between serum levels of various micronutrients and cancer incidence in a cohort of 6832 American men of Japanese ancestry. Serum levels were measured on average six years before the diagnosis of cancer of the oral cavity and pharynx (16 cases), oesophagus (28) or larynx (23). Mean levels of retinol and total retinoids were very similar in cancer cases and 138 controls.

Among the studies listed in Table 10, four reported RRs for intake of vitamin A supplements and/or multivitamin preparations. These tended to be systematically below unity. Gridley *et al.* (1992), in an expanded re-evaluation of the study by McLaughlin *et al.* (1988) on 1114 cases of cancer of the oral cavity and pharynx and 1268 controls, reported an RR of 0.4 (95% CI, 0.2–0.8) for 10 or more years of vitamin A supplement use. This was seen consistently in men and women but after adjustment for vitamin E intake (the strongest protective factor) became 0.6 (95% CI, 0.3–1.4).

(c) Gastric cancer

Almost all the published epidemiological data on the relationship between vitamin A and gastric cancer are from case–control studies (Table 11). Stehr *et al.* (1985) observed a positive association between total vitamin A intake, as reported by next-of-kin of deceased gastric cancer cases, and gastric cancer risk; the use of proxy interviews increases the likelihood of misclassification and bias in this study. Risch *et al.* (1985) observed a strong inverse association with β-carotene but not preformed vitamin A; inverse associations with β-carotene but not retinol have been reported by La Vecchia *et al.* (1987a), You *et al.* (1988), Buiatti *et al.* (1990), Gonzalez *et al.* (1994) and Hansson *et al.* (1994). A strong positive association with preformed vitamin A intake was reported by Graham *et al.* (1990b), along with a significant inverse association with β-carotene. In a study in Milan, Italy by La Vecchia *et al.* (1994), preformed vitamin A intake was not associated with cancer risk.

In a prospective study, Nomura *et al.* (1995) observed essentially no relationship between serum retinol levels and subsequent risk of gastric cancer, but a modest inverse trend with β-carotene levels.

Table 10. Total vitamin A and retinol intake and risk of upper aerodigestive cancers

Reference, site	Cancer site	No. of cases[a]	Categories[b]	Total vitamin A[c] RR	Total vitamin A[c] 95% CI	Preformed vitamin A[c] RR	Preformed vitamin A[c] 95% CI	Vit. supp.[d]	Proxies (% cases)	Adjusted for
Case-control studies										
Marshall *et al.* (1982), USA	Oral cavity	425	Tertiles	0.5	p, trend < 0.05	–	–	N	0	Age, alcohol, smoking
McLaughlin *et al.* (1988), USA	Oral cavity and pharynx	871	Quartiles	–	–	M 1.6 F 1.4	p, trend = 0.007 p, trend = 0.3	Y	0	Smoking, alcohol
Rossing *et al.* (1989), USA	Pharynx	166	Quartiles	–	–	1.1	0.6–2.0	Y	52%	Age, smoking, alcohol
Gridley *et al.* (1990), USA	Oral cavity and pharynx	190	Quartiles	–	–	M 4.5 F 0.6	p, trend = 0.001 p, trend = 0.8	N	29%	Alcohol, smoking, energy
Kune *et al.* (1993), Australia	Oral cavity and pharynx	41	Tertiles	–	–	0.6	0.3–1.4	N	0	Age
Ziegler *et al.* (1981), USA	Oesophagus	120	Tertiles	0.7	p, trend > 0.05	–	–	N	100%	Alcohol
Tuyns *et al.* (1987), France	Oesophagus	743	4 levels	1.0	0.7– 1.6	2.1	1.5–3.0	N	0	Alcohol, smoking
Brown *et al.* (1988), USA	Oesophagus	207 M	Tertile	–	–	1.9	1.0–3.5	N	0 (diet)	Smoking, alcohol
Decarli *et al.* (1987), Italy	Oesophagus	105	Three	–	–	2.3	1.1–4.5	Y	0	Age, education, social class, body mass index, alcohol, smoking
Graham *et al.* (1990a), USA	Oesophagus	176	Quartiles	2.1	1.1–4.0	3.0	1.6–5.8	N	0	Age, education, alcohol, tobacco, energy

Table 10. (contd)

Reference, site	Cancer site	No. of cases[a]	Categories[b]	Total vitamin A[c]		Preformed vitamin A[c]		Vit. supp.[d]	Proxies (% cases)	Adjusted for
				RR	95% CI	RR	95% CI			
Gao *et al.* (1994), China	Oesophagus	902	Quartiles	–	–	M 0.9 F 1.3	*p*, trend = 0.8 *p*, trend = 0.1	N	0	Age, education, birth place, tea, smoking, alcohol, energy
Hu *et al.* (1994), China	Oesophagus	196	Quartiles	–	–	1.3	0.7–2.4	Y		Alcohol, smoking, occupation
Tavani *et al.* (1994), Italy	Oesophagus	46	Tertiles	–	–	1.1	0.5–2.7	Y	0	Education, age, smoking
Mackerras *et al.* (1988), USA	Larynx	151	Tertiles	[0.8]	[0.4–1.4]	[1.1]	[0.6–2.5]	N	0	Age, smoking, alcohol
Freudenheim *et al.* (1992), USA	Larynx	250 M	Quartiles	0.6	0.3–1.04	2.8	1.4–5.6	N	0	Education, alcohol, smoking, total energy
Estève *et al.* (1996), Europe, six regions	Larynx Hypopharynx + epilarynx	727 M 399 M	Five	–	–	1.0 0.6	0.7–1.4 0.4–0.9	N	0	Age, alcohol, smoking, centre
Cohort studies	Cancer site	Cohort size								
Zheng *et al.* (1995), USA	Mouth, pharynx, oesophagus	34691 33	Tertiles	–	–	0.9	0.4–2.2	Y	0	Age, smoking, energy

[a] Study populations include both men and women unless otherwise stated

[b] Number of categories used (if quantiles not used); otherwise number of quantiles used for categorization

[c] Relative risk for highest versus lowest category

[d] Vitamin supplement use assessed (Y) or vitamin supplement use not assessed, or unclear if it was assessed (N)

Table 11. Studies of vitamin A intake and gastric cancer

Reference, site	No. of cases[a]		Categories[b]	Total vitamin A [c]		Preformed vitamin A		Vit. supp. [d]	Proxies	Adjusted for
				RR	95% CI	RR	95% CI		(% cases)	
Case–control studies										
Stehr *et al.* (1985), USA	111		Two	1.7	1.02–3.1	–	–	N	100	Year of death, age, sex, race, residence
Risch *et al.* (1985), Canada	246		Per 10 000 IU	–	–	0.9	0.4–1.8	N	0	Sex, age, residence
La Vecchia *et al.* (1987a), Italy	206		Tertiles	–	–	0.8	*p*, trend = 0.4	N	0	Sex, age, residence, education
You *et al.* (1988), China	564		Quartiles	–	–	1.0	0.7–1.4	N	0	Sex, age, income
Graham *et al.* (1990b), USA	186 M		Four	–	–	3.1	1.7–5.7	N	0	Sex, age, residence
	107 F		Three			2.1	1.1–4.1			
Buiatti *et al.* (1990), Italy	1016		Quintiles	–	–	1.0	0.7–1.3	Y	0	Sex, age
Hansson *et al.* (1994), Sweden	338		Quartiles	0.8	0.5 – 1.1	0.8	0.6–1.3	N	0	Sex, age, energy intake
Gonzalez *et al.* (1994), Spain	354		Quartiles	–	–	1.5	*p*, trend = 0.1	N	0	Sex, age, residence, energy intake
La Vecchia *et al.* (1994), Italy	723		Quintiles	–	–	0.9	0.7–1.3	N	0	Age, sex, education, family history, body mass index, energy
Prospective blood-based studies	No. of cases	No. of controls				Blood retinol				
						RR	95% CI			
Nomura *et al.* (1995), USA	70	302	Three	–	–	1.2	0.6–2.2			Age

[a] Study populations include both men and women unless otherwise stated

[b] Number of categories used (if quantiles not used); otherwise number of quantiles used for categorization

[c] Relative risk for highest versus lowest category

[d] Vitamin supplement use assessed (Y) or vitamin supplement use not assessed, or unclear if it was assessed (N)

Thus, a substantial body of data suggests that components of carotenoid-rich vegetables are protective against gastric cancer, but no data suggest that preformed vitamin A has such an influence.

(d) Colon cancer

Although many studies have examined fat and fibre intake in relation to colon cancer risk, relatively few have reported data on vitamin A. McKeown-Eyssen and Bright-See (1984) reported from an international correlation study a weak positive relationship between preformed vitamin A intake and colon cancer mortality (r = 0.27), after adjustment for animal fat and cereal fibre intake; there was essentially no association with intake of vegetables and fruits (the main sources of carotenoids).

In a case–control study in Australia, Potter and McMichael (1986) did not observe a substantial protective association of preformed vitamin A or carotenoids among either men or women (Table 12). Lyon *et al.* (1987), working in Utah, United States, observed no overall relationship, although in sex-specific analyses, a modest protective association with total vitamin A intake among women was observed (adjusted for age and energy only). In a subsequent case–control study in Utah, West *et al.* (1989) observed a significant inverse association with higher intake of β-carotene after adjusting for age, obesity, crude fibre and energy intake; no significant association was observed for total vitamin A. Graham *et al.* (1988), however, found no protective association in a study performed in New York State, United States.

In a case–control study (Ferraroni *et al.*, 1994) carried out in Milan, Italy, between 1985 and 1992, high retinol intake was inversely associated with colon cancer (RR in highest versus lowest intake quintile, 0.7; 95% CI, 0.5–0.9) but not rectal cancer risk (corresponding RR, 0.8; 95% CI, 0.6–1.1).

Another large case–control study on cancer of the colon and rectum was carried out between 1992 and 1996 in six areas of Italy, using a more detailed, validated food frequency questionnaire and food composition tables (La Vecchia *et al.*, 1997). Intake level of retinol was not associated with either colon or rectal cancer.

Few prospective studies have reported data on colon cancer. Paganini-Hill *et al.* (1987) did not observe any substantial protective effect of either preformed vitamin A or provitamin A carotenoids. Heilbrun *et al.* (1989) observed a modest non-significant inverse association between higher intake of total vitamin A and both colon cancer ([RR, 0.7]; p, trend = 0.1) and rectal cancer ([RR, 0.8]; p, trend = 0.4). A similar inverse association was observed between preformed vitamin A intake for colon ([RR=0.7]; p, trend = 0.2) but not rectal (RR, 1.0; p, trend = 0.8) cancer. Interestingly, in a nested case–control study in Maryland, United States, subjects in the upper quintile of serum retinol were at reduced risk of colon cancer [RR, 0.3; 95% CI, 0.1–0.8] after up to nine years of follow-up, although this observation should not be given much weight given the limitations of serum retinol levels (Schober *et al.*, 1987). Nomura *et al.* (1985) observed higher median levels of retinol, but somewhat lower levels of β-carotene among men who subsequently developed colon cancer, compared with controls.

In summary, there is little evidence to suggest that vitamin A is protective against colon cancer. The data are sparse and inconsistent, however. As animal fat and fibre may be important determinants of colon cancer, more studies which carefully control for these are needed.

(e) Skin cancer

A few studies have investigated the relationship of vitamin A to skin cancer. Table 13 lists those concerned with non-melanocytic cancers. A mix of prospective and case–control (Middleton *et al.*, 1986; Kune *et al.*, 1992; Hunter *et al.*, 1992) studies conducted among Caucasian populations with a wide range of disease risk reported no effect of vitamin A intake: although the risk estimates in the individual studies were generally greater than unity, in every instance, the 95% confidence interval included 1.0. In addition, two prospective studies have reported on the relationship between pre-diagnostic levels of

Table 12. Studies of vitamin A intake and colon cancer

Reference, site		No. of cases[a]	Categories[b]	Total vitamin A[c]		Preformed vitamin[c]		Vit. supp.[d]	Proxies (% cases)	Adjusted for
				RR	95%	RR	95% CI			
Case–control studies										
Potter & McMichael (1986), Australia		121 M colon 99 F colon 124 M rectum 75 F rectum	Quintiles	–	–	1.4 1.6 0.7 1.3	0.8–2.4 0.7–3.5 0.4–1.4 0.6–3.0	N	0	Age
Lyon *et al.* (1987), USA		246	Four	M 1.4 F 0.7	– –	–	–	N	0	Age, county, race, energy
West *et al.* (1989), USA		112 M 119 F	Four	0.7 1.5	0.3–1.8 0.6–3.9	–	–	N	0	Age, body mass index, crude fibre, energy
Ferraroni *et al.* (1994), Italy		828 colon 498 rectum	Quintiles	–	–	0.7 0.8	0.5–0.9 0.6–1.1	N	0	Age, sex, education, family history, body mass index, energy
La Vecchia *et al.* (1997), Italy		1225 colon 728 rectum	Quintiles	–	–	1.1 1.0	1.0–1.2 0.9–1.1	N	0	Age, residence, sex, education, activity, energy, fibre
Cohort studies	Cohort size	No. of cases								
Paganini-Hill *et al.* (1987), USA	6694	52 M 58 F	Tertile	[1.3] [0.8]	*p*, trend > 0.05 *p*, trend > 0.05	[1.3] [1.0]	*p* , trend > 0.05 *p* , trend > 0.05	Y	0	Age
Heilbrun *et al.* (1989), USA	8006 M	102 colon 60 rectum	Quintiles	[0.7] [0.8]	*p*, trend = 0.1 *p*, trend = 0.4	[0.7] [1.0]	*p*, trend = 0.2 *p*, trend = 0.8	N	0	Age Age and alcohol
Prospective blood-based studies	No. of cases	No. of controls				Blood retinol[c]				
						RR	95% CI			
Schober *et al.* (1987), USA, Maryland	72	143	Quintiles	–	–	0.3	0.1–0.8			Age, sex, residence

[a] Study populations include both men and women unless otherwise stated

[b] Number of categories used (if quantiles not used); otherwise number of quantiles used for categorization

[c] Relative risk for highest versus lowest category

[d] Vitamin supplement use assessed (Y) or vitamin supplement use not assessed, or unclear if it was assessed (N)

Table 13. Studies of vitamin A intake and non-melanocytic skin cancers

Reference, site	No. of cases[a]		Categories[b]	Total vitamin A[c]		Preformed vitamin A[c]		Vit. supp.[d]	Proxies (% cases)	Adjusted for
				RR	95% CI	RR	95% CI			
Case–control studies										
Middleton *et al.* (1986), USA [SCC + BCC]	606 M 161 F		Tertiles	1.13 0.94	*p*, trend = 0.40	–	–		0	Age, smoking, alcohol
Cohort studies	Cohort size	No. of cases								
Knekt *et al.* (1990), Finland [BCC]	36 265	38 M 29 F	Quartiles	–	–	1.7	0.5–5.1		0	Smoking
Hunter *et al.* (1992), USA [BCC]	73 366 F	771		–	–	1.0	0.8 –1.2	Y	0	Age, residence, body mass index, hair colour, skin type, history of sunburn
Karagas *et al.* (1997), USA [SCC]	1805	132	Quartiles	–	–	1.4	0.8–2.6		0	Age, smoking, sex, study centre
Prospective blood-based studies	No. of cases	No. of controls				Blood retinol[c]				
						RR	95% CI			
Breslow *et al.* (1995), USA BCC SCC	32 37	32 37	Tertiles	–	–	3.3 1.8	0.9–11.6 0.6–5.8			Age, sex, race

[a] Study populations include both men and women unless otherwise stated

[b] Number of categories used (if quantiles not used); otherwise number of quantiles used for categorization

[c] Relative risk for highest versus lowest category

[d] Vitamin supplement use assessed (Y) or vitamin supplement use not assessed, or unclear if it was assessed (N)

SCC = squamous cell carcinoma, BCC = basal cell carcinoma

retinol and melanoma (Breslow *et al.*, 1995; Knekt *et al.*, 1991b), and both reported no significant association on the basis of 30 and 10 cases, respectively. This is consistent with the findings of a case–control study of melanoma and dietary intake of preformed vitamin A (Kirkpatrick *et al.*, 1994).

(f) Breast cancer

A relatively large number of studies have assessed the association between vitamin A and breast cancer (Table 14). Of the six case–control studies which have reported data for total vitamin A, all reported an inverse association between intake and risk. Four of the case–control studies that reported on the association with preformed vitamin A observed modest decreases in risk with higher intake (Katsouyanni *et al.*, 1988; Marubini *et al.*, 1988; Zaridze *et al.*, 1991; Longnecker *et al.*, 1997), while another seven studies found essentially no association (La Vecchia *et al.*, 1987b; Rohan *et al.*, 1988; Toniolo *et al.*, 1989; Ingram *et al.*, 1991; Richardson *et al.*, 1991; Yuan *et al.*, 1995; Negri *et al.*, 1996). In a meta-analysis of 12 case–control studies by Howe *et al.* (1990), the relative risk in the highest quintile for total vitamin A intake was 0.9 ($p = 0.04$), for β-carotene 0.9 ($p = 0.007$) and for preformed vitamin A 1.0 ($p = 0.52$).

In summary, the case–control data for breast cancer are compatible with a modest inverse association with higher intakes of vitamin A, and, as for lung cancer, this association is somewhat stronger for total vitamin A than for preformed vitamin A.

In a follow-up of female residents of a Californian retirement community, 123 breast cancers occurred (Paganini-Hill *et al.*, 1987). The relative risk comparing the highest tertile of total vitamin A intake with the lowest tertile was [0.8] ($p > 0.05$); for preformed vitamin A this risk was [0.7] ($p > 0.05$). In a follow-up of 89 494 nurses in the United States, Hunter *et al.* (1993) reported a relative risk of 0.8 (95% CI, 0.7–1.0) for women in the highest quintile of total vitamin A intake compared with the lowest. The comparable relative risk for preformed vitamin A was 0.8 (95% CI 0.7–1.0). The association for total vitamin A was slightly stronger among premenopausal (RR = 0.8) than postmenopausal (RR = 0.9) women. Rohan *et al.* (1993) observed suggestive evidence of an inverse association for both total vitamin A and preformed vitamin A. However, the studies of Graham *et al.* (1992), Kushi *et al.* (1996a) and Verhoeven *et al.* (1997), all conducted among postmenopausal women, observed essentially no relationship with disease risk for either total vitamin A or preformed vitamin A.

Studies of blood retinol and breast cancer risk are very limited. Knekt *et al.* (1990) reported a non-significantly lower risk associated with higher retinol levels at baseline.

(g) Prostate cancer

Graham *et al.* (1983), in a case–control study in New York State, observed a positive association between higher intakes of total vitamin A and risk of prostate cancer. In a case–control study among black men in Washington, DC, United States, Heshmat *et al.* (1985) also observed a positive association, which was statistically significant in the subgroup of men aged 30–49 years. Kolonel *et al.* (1988) reported a significantly elevated relative risk for consumption of high levels of total vitamin A but not preformed vitamin A among men 70 years or older in Hawaii, United States (the findings were essentially null for men aged < 70 years).

Most subsequent studies have not confirmed this increased risk (Table 15). In a reanalysis of the case–control study in Hawaii, the excess risk was almost entirely attributable to increased consumption of papaya (a food very high in carotenoids, not retinol) among cases. No elevation in risk was observed for β-carotene from other food sources (Le Marchand *et al.*, 1991). In Japan, Ohno *et al.* (1988) observed an inverse association for β-carotene, as did Mettlin *et al.* (1989) in New York State, Ross *et al.* (1987) in California African-Americans (the relation was null among whites) and Rohan *et al.* (1995) among Canadian men. West *et al.* (1991) observed an elevation in risk with higher intake of vitamin A for men 68 years of age or older, but not among younger men. Talamini *et al.* (1992) observed

Table 14. Studies of vitamin A intake and breast cancer

Reference, site	No. of cases[a]	Categories[b]	Total vitamin A[c]		Preformed vitamin A[c]		Vit. supp.[d]	Proxies (% cases)	Adjusted for
			RR	95% CI	RR	95% CI			
Case-control studies									
Graham *et al.* (1982), USA	2024	Four	[0.8]	p, trend < 0.05	–	–	N	0	Age
La Vecchia *et al.* (1987b), Italy	1108	Three	–	–	0.9	0.7–1.1	N	0	Age, education, family history, body mass index, reproductive factors
Katsouyanni *et al.* (1988), Greece	120	Quintiles	0.5	0.3–0.8	0.6	0.4–1.0	N	0	Age, education, residence, reproductive factors
Marubini *et al.* (1988), Italy	214	Quintiles	–	–	0.7	0.4–1.5	N	0	Age, energy, alcohol
Rohan *et al.* (1988), Australia	451	Quintiles	–	–	1.2	0.8–1.8	N	0	Age
Toniolo *et al.* (1989), Italy	250	Quartiles	–	–	1.2	p, trend > 0.05	N	0	Age, energy
Potischman *et al.* (1990), USA	83	Quartiles	[0.7]	[0.3–2.0]	–	–	Y	0	Age, family history, income, body mass index, reproductive factors
Ingram *et al.* (1991), Australia	99	Quartiles	–	–	1.0	0.6–1.7	N	0	Age, residence
Zaridze *et al.* (1991), USSR	81	Quartiles	0.2	0.0–0.8	0.5	0.1–1.7	N	0	Age, energy, education, reproductive factors
Richardson *et al.* (1991), France	409	Tertiles	–	–	1.5	1.0–2.1	N	0	Age, education, family history, benign breast disease, reproductive factors
London *et al.* (1992), USA	313	Quintiles	–	–	0.7	0.4–1.3	Y	0	Age, energy, alcohol, body mass index, family history, reproductive factors
Holmberg *et al.* (1994), Sweden	265	Quartiles	–	–	0.7	0.4–1.0	N	0	Age, residence, energy
Yuan *et al.* (1995), China	834	per 1753 IU	–	–	0.9	0.6–1.2	N	0	Age, family history, reproductive factors
Negri *et al.* (1996), Italy	2569	Quintiles	0.7	0.6–0.9	0.9	0.7–1.0	N	0	Age, centre, education, energy, alcohol, reproductive factors
Longnecker *et al.* (1997), USA	3543	Six	0.4	0.1–1.1	0.6	0.3–1.2	Y	0	Age, centre, body mass index, education, benign breast disease, family history, alcohol, reproductive factors

Table 14. (contd)

Reference, site	Cohort size	No. of cases	Categories[b]	Total vitamin A[c]		Preformed vitamin A[c]		Vit. supp.[d]	Proxies (% cases)	Adjusted for
				RR	95% CI	RR	95% CI			
Cohort studies										
Paganini-Hill *et al.* (1987), USA	[~4000]	123	Tertiles	[0.8]	*p*, trend > 0.05	[0.7]	*p*, trend > 0.05	Y	0	Age
Graham *et al.* (1992), USA	18 586	344	Quintiles	1.0	0.7–1.3	0.9	0.7–1.3	Y	0	Age, education
Hunter *et al.* (1993), USA	89 494	1439	Quintiles	0.8	0.7–1.0	0.8	0.7–1.0	Y	0	Age, energy, fat intake, family history, body mass index, alcohol, benign breast disease, reproductive factors
Rohan *et al.* (1993), Canada	56 837	519	Quintiles	0.8	0.6–1.2	0.8	0.6–1.2	Y	0	Age, energy, education, family history, benign breast disease, reproductive factors
Kushi *et al.* (1996a), USA	34 387	879	Quintiles	0.9	0.7–1.1	1.0	0.8–1.2	Y	0	Age, energy, education, family history, benign breast disease, body mass index, reproductive factors
Verhoeven *et al.* (1997), Netherlands	62 573	650	Quintiles	–	–	1.2	0.8–1.8	Y	0	Age, energy, family history, benign breast disease, alcohol, reproductive factors
Prospective blood-based studies	No. of cases	No. of controls				Blood retinol[c]				
						RR	95% CI			
Wald *et al.* (1984), Guernsey	78	39	Quintiles	–	–	0.8	*p*, trend > 0.05			Age
Knekt *et al.* (1990), Finland	93	52	Quintiles	–	–	[0.8]	[0.4–2.0]			Age, residence, smoking

[a] Study populations include both men and women unless otherwise stated

[b] Number of categories used (if quantiles not used); otherwise number of quantiles used for categorization

[c] Relative risk for highest versus lowest category

[d] Vitamin supplement use assessed (Y) or vitamin supplement use not assessed, or unclear if it was assessed (N)

Table 15. Studies of vitamin A intake and prostate cancer

Reference, site	No. of cases[a]	Categories[b]	Total vitamin A[c]		Preformed vitamin A[c]		Vit. supp.[d]	Proxies (% cases)	Adjusted for
			RR	95% CI	RR	95% CI			
Case–control studies									
Graham *et al.* (1983), USA	262	Quartiles	1.8	p, trend < 0.01	–	–	N	0	Age
Ross *et al.* (1987), USA	142 Blacks 142 Whites	Tertiles	0.8 1.0	$p > 0.05$ $p > 0.05$	– –	– –	–	0	Age, residence, race
Ohno *et al.* (1988), Japan	100	Quartiles	[0.4]	[0.2–0.8]	–	–	N	0	Age
Kolonel *et al.* (1988), USA	189 (< 70 y) 263 (> 70 y)	Quartiles	0.8 2.0	p, trend = 0.16 p, trend <0.01	0.9 1.4	p, trend = 0.82 p, trend = 0.10	Y	0	Age, ethnicity
West *et al.* (1991), USA	179 (<68 y) 179 (≥68 y)	Quartiles	1.0 1.6	0.6–1.7 0.9–2.7	– –	– –	Y	0	Age, residence
Rohan *et al.* (1995), Canada	207	Quartiles	0.8	p, trend = 0.1	0.6	p, trend = 0.02	Y	0	Age, energy
Ghadirian *et al.* (1996), Canada	232	Quartiles	0.9	p, trend = 0.87	0.8	p, trend = 0.15	N	0	Age, energy, family history
Talamini *et al.* (1992), Italy	157 (< 70 y) 114 (≥ 70 y)	Tertiles	–	–	0.8 2.2	0.5–1.3 1.1–4.2	N	0	Age, residence, education, body mass index
Andersson *et al.* (1996), Sweden	526	Quartiles	1.3	p, trend = 0.43	1.3	p, trend = 0.10	N	0	Age, energy

Table 15 (contd)

Reference, site	Cohort size	No. of cases [a]	Categories[b]	Total vitamin A[c]		Preformed vitamin A		Vit. supp. [d]	Proxies (% cases)	Adjusted for
				RR	95% CI	RR	95% CI			
Cohort studies										
Paganini-Hill *et al.* (1987), USA		93	Tertiles	1.4	$p > 0.05$	[1.1]	*p*, trend > 0.05	Y	0	Age
Hsing *et al.* (1990a), USA	17 633	78 (< 75 y) 71 (>75 y)	Quartiles	2.8 0.4	*p*, trend < 0.05 *p*, trend = 0.01	1.7 0.9	*p*, trend > 0.05 *p*, trend = 0.05	N	0	Age, smoking
Giovannucci *et al.* (1995), USA	47 894	773	Quintiles	1.1	*p*, trend = 0.47	1.3	*p*, trend = 0.004	Y	0	Age, tomato-related products, vasectomy, race
Prospective blood-based studies	No. of cases	No. of controls				Blood retinol[c]				
						RR	95% CI			
Hsing *et al.* (1990b), USA	48 (< 70 y) 55 (> 70 y)	48 55	Quartiles	–	–	0.3 0.4	*p*, trend = 0.08 *p*, trend = 0.19			Age, race
Reichman *et al.* (1990), USA	84	2356		–	–	[0.4]	[0.2–0.8]			Age
Knekt *et al.* (1990), Finland	32	59	Quintiles	–	–	[1.4]	[0.5–5.0]			Age, residence, smoking
Nomura *et al.* (1997b), USA	142	142	Quartiles	–	–	0.8	0.4–1.5			Age

[a] Study populations include both men and women unless otherwise stated

[b] Number of categories used (if quantiles not used); otherwise number of quantiles used for categorization

[c] Relative risk for highest versus lowest category

[d] Vitamin supplement use assessed (Y) or vitamin supplement use not assessed, or unclear if it was assessed (N)

no association of preformed vitamin A intake with cancer risk in northern Italy (RR in highest versus lowest tertile = 1.1, 95% CI, 0.8–1.6), but a direct association emerged for men aged 70 years or more (RR, 2.2, 95% CI, 1.1–4.2). Andersson *et al.* (1996) observed a weak positive association between retinol intake and prostate cancer. Rohan *et al.* (1995) observed a significant trend of decreasing risk of prostate cancer with increasing intake of preformed vitamin A.

Prospective data are sparse. Paganini-Hill *et al.* (1987) reported an elevation in risk for men in the highest tertile of total vitamin A, mainly attributable to increased supplemental vitamin A. In a 20-year follow-up of 17 633 white men, no overall association was observed between vitamin A intake and risk of prostate cancer (Hsing *et al.,* 1990a). An elevation in risk was apparent for men aged less than 75 years, balanced by an inverse association for men 75 years or older. Giovannucci *et al.* (1995) observed a significant positive association with retinol intake, which was stronger for men over 70 years of age.

In summary, there is no consistent evidence that dietary vitamin A protects against prostate cancer. Although initial studies suggesting an adverse effect have not been consistently confirmed, the possibility that higher intakes may increase risk requires further investigation. As most preformed vitamin A is derived from foods of animal origin, the possibility exists that other factors in animal foods may be associated with increased risk of prostate cancer, or there may be other confounding factors associated with incidence or ascertainment of prostate disease.

(h) Bladder cancer

There have been several observational epidemiological studies on the relationship between vitamin A intake and bladder cancer (see Table 16). A large hospital-based case–control study indicated lower risk associated with higher levels of total vitamin A intake (Mettlin & Graham, 1979), but the measure of vitamin A included both plant and animal sources. Subsequently, four population-based case–control studies have looked more specifically at dietary preformed vitamin A. Studies conducted in Spain (Riboli *et al.*, 1991), Hawaii (Nomura *et al.*, 1991) and Canada (Risch *et al.*, 1988) all showed no association with preformed vitamin A, but a study in the Seattle area of the United States (Bruemmer *et al.*, 1996) showed lower risk for those in the highest quintile of preformed vitamin A intake.

Taken together, the observational studies do not support the hypothesis of an association between dietary preformed vitamin A intake and the risk of bladder cancer.

(i) Cervical cancer

In a large case–control study, Marshall *et al.* (1983) observed no relation between cervical cancer risk and vitamin A derived from meats and milk (presumably mainly preformed vitamin A). In the studies of Brock *et al.* (1988), Verreault *et al.* (1989) and Herrero *et al.* (1991), little association was seen between preformed vitamin A intake and cervical cancer risk. In Milan, Italy, an index of retinol intake was not associated with invasive cervical cancer risk (La Vecchia *et al.*, 1988a). In the studies of Slattery *et al.* (1990) and Ziegler *et al.* (1990, 1991), the point estimates for high versus low consumption of total vitamin A were less than unity, but the effect was relatively small (10–20% reduction) and not statistically significant.

Potischman *et al.* (1991) analysed serum levels in the study for which Herrero *et al.* (1991) reported dietary data. A weak positive relation for serum retinol and a weak inverse relationship with β-carotene were apparent.

Overall, the available data (Table 17) suggest no relation between preformed vitamin A intake and risk of cervical cancer.

4.1.2 Intervention trials with cancer as an endpoint

4.1.2.1 Primary prevention trials

In an intervention study, each subject is allocated to one of two or more groups whose exposure is determined by the investigators. From a scientific point of view, the most reliable intervention study is one in which the allocation of exposure is carried out by randomization. Interventions which involve

Table 16. Studies of vitamin A intake and bladder cancer

Reference, site	No. of cases[a]		Categories[b]	Total vitamin A[c]		Preformed vitamin A[c]		Vit. supp.[d]	Proxies (% cases)	Adjusted for
				RR	95% CI	RR	95% CI			
Case–control studies										
Risch *et al.* (1988), Canada	826		Interquartile range	1.0	0.8 –1.2	1.0	0.9–1.2	N	0	Age, smoking, diabetes
Nomura *et al.* (1991), USA	66 F 195 M			1.1 1.0	0.4–2.6 0.6 –1.7	1.0 1.6	0.4–2.8 0.9–2.7	Y	0	Age, smoking
Bruemmer *et al.* (1996), USA	262		Quartiles	0.5	*p*, trend = 0.04	0.6	*p*, trend = 0.006	Y	0	Age, sex, county, smoking, calories
Riboli *et al.* (1991), Spain	432 M		Quartiles	–	–	1.3	*p*, trend = 0.30	N	0	Age, calories
Michalek *et al.* (1987), USA	102		Dichotomy	1.3	0.5–3.3		–	N	0	Age
Mettlin & Graham (1979), USA	112 F 377 M		Seven	[0.3] [0.5]	[0.1 –1.1] [0.3 –1.0]		–	N	0	Age
La Vecchia *et al.* (1989), Italy	163		Tertiles	–	–	0.4	*p*, trend < 0.01	N	0	Age, sex, area of residence, social class, smoking
Prospective blood-based studies	No. of cases	No. of controls				Blood retinol[c]				
						RR	95% CI			
Helzlsouer *et al.* (1989), USA	35	70	Dichotomy	–	–	[1.3]	[0.3–5.6]			Age, smoking
Knekt *et al.* (1991b), Finland	15	29	Per S.D.	–	–	0.6	*p*, trend = 0.14			Age

[a] Study populations include both men and women unless otherwise stated

[b] Number of categories used (if quantiles not used); otherwise number of quantiles used for categorization

[c] Relative risk for highest versus lowest category

[d] Vitamin supplement use assessed (Y) or vitamin supplement use not assessed, or unclear if it was assessed (N)

Table 17. Case–control studies of vitamin A intake and invasive cervical cancer

Reference, site	No. of cases[a]	Categories[b]	Total vitamin A[c]		Preformed vitamin A[c]		Vit. supp.[d]	% Proxies (cases)	Adjusted for
			RR	95% CI	RR	95% CI			
Marshall *et al.* (1983), USA	513	Seven	–	–	1.0	*p*, trend > 0.05	N	0	Age
La Vecchia *et al.* (1988a), Italy	392	Three	–	–	1.2	0.8–1.9	N	0	Age, education, parity, body mass index, smoking, sexual behaviour, contraceptive and hormone use
Verreault *et al.* (1989), USA	189	Quartiles	–	–	1.1	*p*, trend = 0.52	Y	0	Age, education, Pap smear, energy, sexual behaviour, contraceptive use
Slattery *et al.* (1990), USA	266	Quartiles	0.9	0.5–1.6	–	–	N	0	Age, education, smoking, church attendance, sexual behaviour
Ziegler *et al.* (1990), USA	271	Quartiles	0.9	*p*, trend = 0.5	–	–	Y	0	Age, centre, Pap smears, smoking, sexual behaviour, contraceptive use, vaginal infections
Herrero *et al.* (1991), Colombia, Costa Rica, Mexico, Panama	748	Quartile	–	–	1.1	0.8–1.5	N	0	Age, centre, Pap smears, sexual behaviour, pregnancies, socioeconomc status, human papillomavirus infection

[a] Study populations include both men and women unless otherwise stated

[b] Number of categories used (if quantiles not used); otherwise number of quantiles used for categorization

[c] Relative risk for highest versus lowest category

[d] Vitamin supplement use assessed (Y) or vitamin supplement use not assessed, or unclear if it was assessed (N)

substantial dietary changes are difficult to implement, due to problems of compliance. Moreover, the possibility of bias is increased if subjects in the intervention and control groups (and also the investigators) cannot easily be kept blind to their allocation. Interventions using micronutrients, such as certain retinoids, may be easier to perform if the active treatment can be packaged in the form of an anonymous dietary supplement. However, interventions of this kind may not reflect accurately the effects of micronutrients when presented in the form of complex mixtures within foods. Issues such as optimal dosage, minimal duration, latency and adverse effects cannot always be resolved in an intervention study. A single dose is usually used to maximize study power, and the trial may have to be stopped prematurely if early advantageous or adverse effects are observed. For various reasons (such as costs, patients' compliance, disclosure of early findings, emergence of new hypotheses), most intervention trials are restricted to a few years of treatment and/or observation, thus hampering the evaluation of potential long-term benefits. On the other hand, only in an intervention trial can the effects of synthetic compounds such as synthetic retinoids be assessed.

(a) Linxian trials

Two randomized chemoprevention studies were carried out in four Linxian communes, north-central China, an area with one of the world's highest rates of oesophageal cancer (Blot *et al.*, 1993, 1995; Li *et al.*, 1993). Among several dietary deficiencies common in Linxian, riboflavin deficiency seemed the most severe.

In the first study, a total of 29 584 healthy subjects (55% females) aged 40–69 years were recruited in 1985. Using a complex factorial design, the participants were randomly assigned to seven intervention groups, which were based on four combinations of nutrients: (*a*) retinyl palmitate (5000 IU/day) and zinc; (*b*) riboflavin and niacin; (*c*) vitamin C and molybdenum; (*d*) β-carotene (15 mg/day), vitamin E and selenium, and one placebo group. Supplemented doses ranged from one to two times the United States recommended daily allowance (RDA). Participant compliance (as measured by pill disappearance and quarterly blood measurements on a random sample) was very good (>90%) and treatment groups were highly comparable in terms of sex, age, smoking, alcohol drinking and diet. The study had 90% power to detect a 23% reduction in cancer mortality during the 5.25-year supplementation period. Incident cancers and deaths were identified by several methods.

A total of 2127 deaths occurred during the intervention period (March 1986 to May 1991). Cancer was the leading cause of death, with 32% of the total mortality due to oesophageal (360 deaths) and stomach (331 deaths) cancers. Relative risks (RRs) of death and 95% confidence intervals (CI) in participants given retinol and zinc compared with non-users were 1.0 (95% CI, 0.9–1.1) for all cancers, 0.9 (95% CI, 0.8–1.2) for oesophageal cancer, and 1.0 (95% CI, 0.8–1.3) for stomach cancer (Table 18). Some protection was seen, however, for stomach cancer other than cardia (78 observed deaths, RR, 0.6; 95% CI, 0.4–0.9). RRs for cancer incidence (1298 new cancer diagnoses, RR for all cancers, 1.0; 95% CI, 0.9–1.1) were similar to the RRs for cancer deaths. Among different intervention groups, significantly lower cancer mortality (RR, 0.9; 95% CI, 0.8–1.0) occurred only among participants receiving supplementation with the combination of β-carotene, vitamin E and selenium. Blot *et al.* (1995) also reported age- and sex-specific RRs that were not significantly heterogeneous, although RRs for all cancer mortality for the retinol and zinc intervention group were lower in females than in males (0.86 and 1.07, respectively) and in participants aged <55 years than in those aged ≥55 years (0.84 and 1.03, respectively).

[The Working Group noted that the supplemental dose of retinol was relatively low (i.e., one fifth of that in most other intervention studies) and that the study design makes it impossible to distinguish the effect of retinol from that of zinc. The failure of the trial to find a significant reduction in cancer mortality among those given supplements of retinol and other compounds could be related to the shortness of the intervention and follow-up. In general, the applicability of the results to populations with adequate nutritional status and for

Table 18. Randomized chemoprevention trials including vitamin A or retinyl esters

Reference and country	Participants No.	Participants Type	Intervention(s)	Average follow-up (years)	All cancer No. deaths or new cases	All cancer RR (95%CI)	Specific cancers Site	Specific cancers RR (95% CI)	Comments
Blot *et al.* (1993), China	29 584 (55% fem.)	Healthy adults (40–69 yrs)	Factorial, including group on retinol (5000 IU/d) and zinc	5.25	792 cancer deaths	1.9 (0.9–1.1)	Oesophagus	0.9 (0.8–1.2)	The combination of β-carotene, vitamin E and selenium reduced cancer risk
							Stomach	1.0 (0.8–1.3)	
Li *et al.* (1993), China	3318 (56% fem.)	Oesophageal dysplasia (40–69 yrs)	Multivitamin, including retinol (10 000 IU/d) versus placebo	6.0	221 new cases	1.0 (0.8–1.2)	Oesophagus	0.9 (0.7–1.2)	Decrease of cerebrovascular deaths in men
							Stomach	1.2 (0.9–1.6)	
Omenn *et al.* (1996a,b), USA	4060	Asbestos workers	Retinol (25 000 IU/d) and β-carotene (30 mg/d) versus placebo	4.0	1446 new cases	1.2 (1.0–1.3)	Lung (new cases)	1.3 (1.0–1.6)	Leukaemia RR, 2.2 (95% CI 1.0–5.0) No difference in mesotheliomas (14 in active treatment; 9 in placebo groups)
	14 254 (44% fem.)	Heavy smokers (mean age = 58)							
de Klerk *et al.* (1998), Western Australia	1024 (8% fem.)	Asbestos workers (median age = 57)	Retinol (25 000 IU/d) versus β-carotene (30 mg/d)	5.0	58 deaths (cancer and non-cancer)	0.6 (0.3–1.0)	Mesothelioma (3 in retinol-treated; 13 in β-carotene-treated	0.2 (0.0–0.9)	Mesothelioma rate in the retinol group was lower than among historical controls
							Lung	0.7 (0.2–2.3)	
Moon *et al.* (1997), USA	2297 (30% fem.)	Adults with ≥10 actinic keratosis (median age = 63)	Retinol (25 000 IU/d) versus placebo	3.8	115 deaths (cancer and non-cancer) 526 new skin cancers	1.1 (0.8–1.5)	Cutaneous SCC	0.7 (0.6–1.0)	50% protection in individuals with ≥8 moles and freckles
							BCC	1.1 (0.9–1.3)	
Levine *et al.* (1997), USA	525 (29% fem.)	Adults with ≥ 4 previous skin cancers (mean age = 66)	Retinol (25 000 IU/d) or isotretinoin (5–10 mg/d), or placebo	3.8	444 new skin cancers	–	Cutaneous SCC	[~1.0]	Hazard ratios and confidence intervals were not provided in detail
							BCC	[~1.0]	

RR, relative risk; CI, confidence interval; SCC, squamous cell carcinoma; BCC, basal cell carcinoma.

cancer sites other than oesophageal and stomach may be limited.]

The other intervention trial in Linxian was carried out from May 1985 through May 1991, and included 3318 persons (56% females) aged 40–69 years, who had shown cytological evidence of oesophageal dysplasia (Li *et al.*, 1993). These diagnoses were derived primarily from population-based, oesophageal balloon cytology examinations conducted in November and December 1983. Participants were randomly assigned to supplements (one β-carotene capsule (15 mg) and two 13-vitamin, 12-mineral tablets, including retinyl acetate, 10 000 IU) or a matching placebo in a two-group design. Doses were kept at less than or equal to three times the United States RDA. Good compliance (>90%) was confirmed as in the general population trial (Blot *et al.*, 1993). Cancers were identified not only through routine surveillance, but also by special cytology and endoscopy screenings after 2.5 years and 6 years. Nearly half of all cancers were diagnosed during cytological and endoscopic screening. There were no significant differences between the randomized groups at baseline with respect to any of the subject characteristics examined (e.g., smoking, alcohol drinking and selected dietary habits), but individuals assigned to supplements had a 3% higher prevalence of grade 2 dysplasia.

No significant difference was observed for all cancer mortality (87 observed deaths in the supplement group and 89 in the placebo group, RR, 1.0; 95% CI, 0.7–1.3), oesophageal cancer (38 and 44 deaths, respectively, RR, 0.8; 95% CI, 0.5–1.3) and stomach cancer (42 and 35 deaths, respectively, RR, 1.2, 95% CI, 0.8–1.9) (Table 18). In contrast with the results reported by Blot *et al.* (1993), retinol-containing supplements were not associated with decreased mortality from non-cardia stomach cancer. Total cancer incidence was similar in the treatment and placebo groups (RR, 1.0; 95% CI, 0.8–1.2), as was incidence for oesophageal/gastric cardia cancer (RR, 1.0; 95% CI, 0.8–1.2) (Table 18). RRs of death did not vary by sex and age group (Blot *et al.*, 1995). [The Working Group noted that negative findings, according to the authors (Li *et al.*, 1993), may have been due to the shortness of intervention and follow-up and/or to supplementation delay if dysplastic lesions were no longer amenable to a benefit from nutrient supplementation. Retinol was only one of 26 vitamins and microelements supplemented in the treatment group. Furthermore, it was administered at a relatively low dose (i.e., less than half of that in other intervention trials). Finally, both studies were carried out in a period when substantial improvements were taking place in the general nutritional status of the Chinese population. This may have led to concurrent increases in the intake of vitamins and microelements in the placebo group, reducing the power of the trials to identify an effect of supplementation.]

(b) CARET

Pilot studies of the Beta-Carotene and Retinol Efficacy Trial (CARET), in the United States between 1985 and 1988, investigated 816 men with substantial occupational exposure to asbestos who received a combination of 15 mg β-carotene and 25 000 IU retinol (as palmitate) daily or placebo (1:1) and 1029 men and women with extensive cigarette-smoking histories who received 30 mg β-carotene, 25 000 IU retinol, both, or neither (2 x 2 factorial design) (Omenn *et al.*, 1996a,b). In 1988, all pilot study participants in active treatment groups were converted to the CARET efficacy regimen of 30 mg β-carotene plus 25 000 IU retinol taken daily, and the project was expanded 10-fold, including six study centres around the country during the following three years (additional randomization 1:1 active/placebo). A 2 x 2 factorial design for the efficacy trial was rejected under the hypothesis that retinol and β-carotene might have a favourable effect through complementary molecular actions (Omenn *et al.*, 1994a).

The 14 254 smokers (56% men) had a mean age of 58 years and a mean of 49 pack-years of cigarette smoking, 66% were current smokers upon recruitment (mean of 24 cigarettes per day and 48 pack-years), and 34% were former smokers (mean of three years since quitting, after smoking 28 cigarettes per day and 52 pack-years). The 4060 asbestos-exposed male workers had a mean age of 57 years; 3% were never-smokers (from the pilot study), 58% were former smokers and 38% were current smokers, with a mean of 43 pack-years of smoking history (40 pack-years for former smokers and 47 pack-years for current smokers) and a mean of 10 years since quitting among the former smokers. They had means of 35 years since first asbestos exposure and 27-year duration of asbestos exposure on the job; approximately two thirds had positive chest X-ray results for asbestos-related disease. A net smoking cessation rate of 5% per year was achieved among study participants during the follow-up.

Up to December 1995, CARET received and validated reports of 2420 end-points, including 1446 cancers (in 1353 participants) and 974 deaths, with a median of 3.7 years and a mean of 4.0 years of follow-up after randomization for all CARET participants. Histological, immunohistochemical and ultrastructural criteria were used to diagnose the histological type of lung neoplasms. 746 additional cancer reports, which were not CARET end-points, were excluded (i.e., 500 basal cell and squamous cell skin cancers, eight cancers diagnosed before randomization, and 238 recurrences, metastatic presentations or non-cancers).

Based on a two-sided test for the primary analysis, CARET had 80% power, if carried to completion, to detect a 22% observed reduction or 24% observed increase in lung cancer incidence. The 73 135 person-years (median, 3.7) of follow-up accrued, however, corresponded to 66% of the total of 110 000 person-years projected, due to discontinuation of the trial 21 months earlier than planned.

The two randomized groups were well matched and withdrawal percentages were virtually the same in participants assigned to active treatment and those assigned to placebo (15% and 14% respectively among asbestos workers, and 20% and 19% among heavy smokers). After five years of supplementation, serum retinol levels were about 10% higher and serum β-carotene levels more than 12-fold higher in the active-treatment group than in the placebo group. There were no major side-effects attributable to the intervention regimen. The incidence of lung cancer was the primary end-point. Statistical analysis was based on stratified, weighted log-rank statistics with relative risks estimated by Cox regression models (Omenn *et al.*, 1994a).

Up to December 1995, 388 participants (2%) were reported as new cases of lung cancer (286 centrally reviewed, 254 fatal). The RR for lung cancer in the active-treatment group was 1.3 (95% CI, 1.0–1.6), with RRs of 1.4 (95% CI, 1.0–2.1) for asbestos workers, 1.4 (95% CI, 1.1–1.9) for heavy smokers who were smoking at the time of randomization, and 0.8 (95% CI, 0.5–1.3) for former heavy smokers (Table 18). Active treatment had no significant effect on the risk of mesothelioma (14 cases in the active-treatment group and 9 in the placebo group (RR, 1.5; 95% CI, 0.7–3.5) and non-lung cancer (1076 new cases, 300 of which were prostate cancers). None of several other common cancer types showed a significant difference in incidence (urinary bladder: RR, 1.1; 95% CI, 0.7–1.7; breast: RR, 0.8; 95% CI, 0.6–1.1; colorectal: RR, 1.0; 95% CI, 0.7–1.5; head and neck: RR, 1.3; 95% CI, 0.7–2.2; lymphoma: RR, 0.9; 95% CI, 0.4–2.0; prostate: RR, 1.0; 95% CI, 0.8–1.3), but a borderline elevated RR was found for leukaemia in the active-treatment group (26 observed, 2.2; 95% CI, 1.0–5.0; $p<0.06$). The RR of death from any cause in the active-treatment group was 1.2 (95% CI, 1.0–3.3) (Omenn *et al.*, 1996b).

There were suggestions that the excess lung cancer risk was associated with the highest quartile of alcohol intake (RR, 2.0; 95% CI, 1.3–3.1) and large-cell histology (RR, 1.9; 95% CI, 1.1–3.3) (Omenn *et al.*, 1996b).

[The Working Group noted that the CARET trial was based on the hypothesis that a favourable effect would come from the combination of retinyl palmitate and β-carotene. It was, therefore, unable to distinguish the individual effects of the two agents. Early discontinuation was influenced by the unexpected unfavourable effect of β-carotene in the Alpha-Tocopherol, Beta-Carotene Cancer Prevention Study (ATBC) in Finland (Cancer Prevention Study Group, 1994).]

(c) Wittenoom trial

A randomized, partially single-blind chemoprevention trial was carried out between June 1990 and May 1995 in Perth, Western Australia, among workers who had been occupationally exposed to blue asbestos (crocidolite) between 1943 and 1966 in a mine at Wittenoom Gorge (Musk *et al.*, 1998). Median duration of asbestos exposure was short (about one year). The base population for the study consisted of the 2695 members of the Wittenoom workers' cohort who have been followed for the health effects of asbestos since 1979 (de Klerk *et al.*, 1998). Out of the 1677 subjects who indicated interest, 1203 joined the study and 1024 (8% females) were randomly assigned to receive either retinyl palmitate (25 000 IU/day, n = 512) or β-carotene (30 mg/day, n = 512) (de Klerk *et al.*, 1998). The 996 members of the cohort not participating in the active intervention programme, but living within the catchment area of the death and cancer registries, formed a passive reference group.

Pill-counting and measurement of plasma β-carotene levels were performed in order to assess compliance. Deaths and incident cases of cancer were documented from the Western Australian Cancer Registry and death certificates. Follow-up was complete up to May 1995. All subjects attended the Perth Chest Clinic at least once and 48% had four annual follow-up visits. The two treatment groups were closely comparable at baseline by age (median 56 and 57 years), sex, cigarette smoking (21% current smokers, 52% ex-smokers), dietary intake and plasma levels of β-carotene (mean 6 mg, 0.5 μmol/L) and retinol (mean 0.7 mg, 2.6 μmol/L), and asbestos exposures (median 190 days of exposure, 30 years from first exposures). Comparison between groups was conducted by means of Cox regression and Fisher's exact tests in both intention-to-treat analyses and efficacy analyses (i.e., based on treatment actually taken).

Mesothelioma was the most common cause of death. After a median follow-up of 232 weeks (4 1/2 years), the RR with retinol compared to β-carotene for mesothelioma was 0.2 (95% CI, 0.1–0.9; 15 new cases, 11 deaths) (de Klerk *et al.*, 1998). The RR from efficacy analyses was 0.1 (95% CI, 0.0–0.8) for retinol. There was no significant difference between the groups in lung cancer incidence (RR, 0.7; 95% CI, 0.2–2.3) or other cancer mortality (RR, 1.0; 95% CI, 0.2–3.9). Total mortality was significantly lower in the retinol group (21 deaths) than in the β-carotene group (37 deaths) (RR, 0.6; 95% CI, 0.3–1.0). Compared with the passive reference group, trial participants had significantly lower mortality (RR, 0.6; 95% CI, 0.5–0.9), but the rates converged with time. The incidence of both mesothelioma (RR, 0.8; 95% CI, 0.4–1.6) and lung cancer (RR, 0.7; 95% CI, 0.3–1.4) was non-significantly lower among active participants (Musk *et al.*, 1998).

The investigators concluded that there is a possibility that retinol exerts some protective effect on mesothelioma at late stages, whereas it is clear that there was no benefit from β-carotene. Since the mesothelioma rates in the retinol-treated group were only lower than rates before the start of the study among 'historical controls', the apparent benefit should not be due to a risk increase in the β-carotene-treated group (de Klerk *et al.*, 1998).

(d) Southwest Skin Cancer Prevention Studies

Two randomized, double-blind, controlled trials to examine the efficacy of retinol supplementation on the incidence of first new non-melanoma skin cancer were conducted in Arizona, United States (Moon *et al.*, 1997; Levine *et al.*, 1997).

The first included 2297 subjects (30% females), aged 21–84 years (median 63) identified through media announcements and referral to dermatologists in 1984–88. They were considered to have a moderate skin cancer risk (having a history of more than 10 actinic keratosis and at most two cutaneous squamous cell carcinomas (SCCs) or basal cell carcinomas (BCCs)) (Moon *et al.*, 1997).

All subjects were willing to limit the intake of non-study vitamin A to no more than 10 000 IU/day and were scheduled for clinic visits one month after randomization and then every six months. After a single-blind three-month placebo run-in period, the subjects were randomly allocated to receive either oral retinol (25 000 IU/day; n = 1157) or placebo (n = 1140). The groups were fully comparable according to the baseline characteristics, including an estimate of weekly sun exposure. Capsule-count adherence and serum measurements were used to evaluate compliance. Adverse symptoms were rare (1%), but cholesterol and liver enzyme values rose for some subjects on retinol.

The study was interrupted earlier than planned for funding reasons. There were a total of 4332 study years of ascertainment period for the active treatment group and 4317 for the placebo group. Analyses of primary outcome measures were based on the Cox proportional hazards model, with adjustment for skin characteristics.

During a median follow-up time of 3.8 years, 526 subjects had a new skin cancer, 96% histologically confirmed. The active treatment group showed an RR of 0.7 (95% CI, 0.6–1.0) for cutaneous SCC (249 observed new cancers) and 1.1 (95% CI, 0.9–1.3) for BCC (417 observed new cancers), compared with the placebo group. The effect of retinol on SCC risk was consistent in different strata by age, sex, history of sun exposure and sunburn. An especially low RR, however, was found in individuals with a higher number of moles and freckles (RR, 0.5; 95% CI, 0.3–0.8). A differential (possibly lower) metabolism of retinol by basal cells compared to keratinocytes was suggested to explain the lack of benefit in terms of BCC risk (Moon *et al.*, 1997).

The second randomized, double-blind controlled trial (Levine *et al.*, 1997) included high-risk subjects (i.e., those with a history of four or more BCC or cutaneous SCC) and involved three arms: oral retinol (25 000 IU; n = 173), isotretinoin (5–10 mg according to weight; n = 178) or placebo (n = 174) daily for three years. Methods were similar to those of Moon *et al.* (1997). Out of 719 original participants, 525 (28% females, aged 21–85 years, median age 66 years) completed the run-in period and were randomized. Baseline characteristics, including an estimate of weekly sun exposure, and compliance were similar in the three groups. Toxicity was generally modest, but side-effects were greatest in the isotretinoin-treated group. A total of 125 SCCs and 319 BCCs were diagnosed clinically and confirmed pathologically. There were no differences between those who received the placebo and those who were given either isotretinoin or retinol with regard to time to the first occurrence of either BCC or SCC. In the retinol-treated group, the cumulative probability of cutaneous SCC at 36 months was about 5% in the study of Moon *et al.* (1997), but 28% in that of Levine *et al.* (1997). [The Working Group noted that relative risks were not reported, but similar curves of cumulative incidence were provided. However, the cumulative proportion of participants with a first new SCC seemed slightly higher in the retinol group than in the placebo groups, although not significantly so. The lack of benefit of retinol in terms of cutaneous SCC onset in high-risk individuals contrasted with findings from Moon *et al.* (1997) in moderate-risk individuals. The effects of retinoids may be more pronounced in the early stages of cancer promotion than later. Still, the lack of beneficial effect of retinol, compared with placebo, among high-risk individuals is inconsistent with the encouraging results in the companion study on moderate-risk individuals].

(e) Conclusions from the six primary prevention trials

Overall, there is no consistent evidence that four- to six-year supplementation of retinol reduces the risk of any type of cancer. In the CARET study, the risk of carcinoma of the lung was significantly elevated in the group supplemented with retinol and β-carotene compared with the placebo group, except for subjects who had stopped smoking. Among asbestos miners in the Wittenoom trial, lung cancer was less common in the retinol group than in the β-carotene group, but the difference was not statistically significant. Thus it remains possible that retinol may be less harmful than β-carotene or have no effect.

Mesothelioma, a rare neoplasm attributable to asbestos exposure, was studied in the CARET subcohort of asbestos-exposed workers and in the Wittenoom trial. In crocidolite-exposed workers in Australia, retinol intervention appeared to lead to a reduction in incidence of mesothelioma, whereas in the CARET study, where retinol was given in combination with β-carotene, no such reduction was seen. The apparent prevention of mesotheliomas in the only trial using retinol as such suggests that further studies on the effects of retinol on mesothelioma development are warranted. The two trials in Linxian (China) allowed evaluation of the effect of retinol, in combination with either zinc or 25 additional vitamins and microelements versus placebo, especially in the prevention of cancers of the stomach and oesophagus. Cancers at these sites were extremely frequent in the study population. The two Linxian trials did not support a benefit of retinol, even in a population where nutritional deficiencies may well have existed.

Two intervention studies from the United States agreed in ruling out a benefit with respect to basal cell carcinoma of the skin. For squamous cell carcinoma, a more threatening disease than basal cell carcinoma, a risk reduction of about 25% in moderate-risk individuals is difficult to reconcile with the lack of benefit in high-risk individuals. However, the details of the end-points of the latter study have not been published.

It is worth bearing in mind that some weaknesses are largely shared by all the six trials above, making it difficult to draw firm conclusions. All studies were large, well designed and carefully conducted. However, the complexity and heavy responsibilities entailed by investigations of this size and cost led to compromises. For example, different potentially promising agents were combined in most studies, including the CARET study, and in the Wittenoom trial it was not possible to include a placebo group. All trials, except the two Linxian trials, were interrupted or modified earlier than initially planned. Intervention duration therefore never exceeded six years, a period which leaves open the issue of potential longer-term benefits of retinol were it active on relatively early stages of carcinogenesis. Finally, the choice of specific high-risk populations, though needed in order to have sufficient study power, is not without undesirable consequences with respect to the applicability of the trial results to the general population. The spectrum of cancer sites and types, for instance, was obviously heavily distorted, in all trials, to the type(s) specifically increased in the study populations. Thus, the results were largely uninformative with respect to several important cancer sites (e.g., female cancers) and shed little light on the effects of vitamin A on overall cancer mortality, particularly in women.

4.1.2.2 Prevention of second primary cancers

After epidemiological studies of vitamin A and cancer began to emerge in the 1970s, several clinical trials tested the efficacy of various types of retinoids and, less frequently, vitamin A as adjuvant therapy in patients in relation to different malignancies (Mayne & Lippman, 1997).

In a few investigations, the distinction between second primary cancers and recurrences was not made or was problematic. Both end-points are therefore shown in certain instances.

Pastorino *et al.* (1993) tested the adjuvant effect of high-dose vitamin A on 307 patients (25 females) with stage I non-small-cell lung cancer in Milan, Italy. After curative surgery, patients were randomized between 1985 and 1989 to either oral retinyl palmitate (300 000 IU orally daily for a minimum of 12 months; $n = 150$) or no treatment ($n = 157$) [no placebo was used]. After a median follow-up of 46 months, the number of patients with either recurrence or new primary tumours was 56 (37%) in the treated group and 75 (48%) in the untreated group (Table 19). Eighteen patients in the treated group developed a second primary tumour, whereas 29 patients in the control group developed 33 second primary tumours. Onset of second primaries was significantly delayed in the treated group ($p = 0.045$, log-rank test). No significant difference in overall survival emerged. In view of the only modest side-effects, it was suggested that aqueous emulsified retinyl palmitate may be less toxic than other forms of retinol. [The Working Group noted that doses of 300 000 IU per day showed limited toxicity, although daily supplements as low as 25 000 IU in other studies have produced adverse effects.]

A chemoprevention study in curatively treated patients with oral cancer, laryngeal cancer and lung cancer was started in June 1988 in Europe (EUROSCAN; de Vries *et al.*, 1991, 1993). Treatments used were aqueous emulsified retinyl palmitate (300 000 IU per day during one year and half this dose during a second year), *N*-acetylcysteine (600 mg during two years) or both drugs or neither were used, in a 2 x 2 factorial design. The last patients were entered in 1994, and the intervention period thus

Table 19. Randomized controlled cancer trials including vitamin A or retinyl esters

Reference and country	Cancer patients		Treatment	Recurrence and/or new primary tumours		Deaths		Comments
	No.	Type		Active treatment	Controls	Active treatment	Controls	
Pastorino *et al.* (1993), Italy	307 (8% female)	Stage I lung cancer	Retinol (300 000 IU/d) versus nothing	56/150 Significant delay in new primaries	75/157	55/150	64/157	Median follow-up 46 months
Lamm *et al.* (1994), USA	65	Bladder cancer (17% fem.)	High-versus low-dose multivitamin (retinol RDA versus 40 000 IU/d)	14/35 (p<0.01)	24/30	74%	76%	At 12-month follow-up
Meyskens *et al.* (1994), USA	248 (38% female)	Malignant melanoma ≥0.75 mm	Retinol (100 000 versus nothing)	Survival RR = 1.1 (95% CI, 0.7–1.7) Disease-free survival RR = 1.2 (95% CI, 1.8–1.8)				Median follow-up > 8 years
Jyothirmayi *et al.* (1996), India	106 (31% female)	Head and neck cancer	Retinol (28 500 IU/d)	11/56	7/50	Not given		Median follow-up 3 years

RDA, recommended dietary allowance.

ended in 1996. In total, 2595 patients have been included, from 81 institutes in 14 different countries. Of these, 1566 (60.4%) patients had a head and neck cancer, while the other 1029 patients had been treated for lung cancer (van Zandwijk *et al.*, 1997). Of the patients receiving retinyl palmitate, 10% interrupted the treatment because of side-effects (mainly dryness and itching of the skin), but no major complication was observed. Analysis is in progress and a first report of results is expected to appear in 1998.

Lamm *et al.* (1994) compared the efficacy of two multiple vitamin regimens (i.e., RDA doses versus high doses) in diminishing recurrences of transitional cell carcinoma of the bladder in West Virginia, United States. Between 1985 and 1992, 65 such patients (11 females) were thus randomized to receive, in addition to other vitamins (B_1, B_2, B_3, B_5, B_6, B_{12}, C, D_3, E, folic acid) and zinc, either 5000 (n = 30) or 40 000 IU (n = 35) of retinyl acetate daily. After 12 months of treatment, there were 11 recurrences (37%) in the RDA group compared with 3 (9%) in the high-dose group (p = 0.008, Fisher's exact test). Overall recurrence rates were 80% (24/30) and 40% (14/35), respectively, but survival rates were similar (75% in RDA and 76% in the high-dose group) (Table 19). Due to the trial design, benefits from individual high-dose vitamins could not be distinguished (Lamm *et al.*, 1994).

A national cooperative group trial was conducted in the United States in patients with early-stage cutaneous malignant melanoma thicker than 0.75 mm, to determine if vitamin A (100 000 IU orally daily for 18 months) can increase disease-free or overall survival (Meyskens *et al.*, 1994). A total of 248 patients were randomized to vitamin A (n = 119) or observation (n = 121), with eight late exclusions. Median follow-up exceeded eight years. No differences emerged between the two groups (RR, 1.1, p = 0.71 for survival; and 1.2, p = 0.41, for disease-free survival) (Table 19). This held true for subset analyses by sex, type of other therapy, and Breslow's thickness. Overall, 12% of patients who received vitamin A experienced severe toxicity.

In Trivandrum, India, Jyothirmayi *et al.* (1996) evaluated in 1992–93 the effectiveness of vitamin A (retinyl palmitate, 28 500 IU per day orally for one year) in the prevention of local relapses and second primaries of head and neck cancer. Randomization to either vitamin A or placebo included 106 patients. Compliance was good, and no major side-effect was reported. Eleven of 56 patients [19.6%] in the vitamin A group had loco-regional recurrence compared with 5/50 [10%] in the placebo group (non-significant difference). No second primaries were observed in the vitamin A group as opposed to two in the placebo group (Table 19). The number of deaths was not reported.

One nested case–control study (Day *et al.*, 1994) in the United States investigated the possible relationship between dietary retinol intake and risk of second primary tumours in a cohort of 1090 oral and pharyngeal cancer patients. Individuals in the highest-intake quartile showed an RR of 1.6 of developing a second primary compared with individuals in the lowest quartile (p value of chi square for trend, 0.09).

In summary, of four randomized studies, only the investigation of Pastorino *et al.* (1993) showed a significant benefit from supplementation (i.e., a significant delay in new primary cancer after resection of lung cancer).

4.1.3 Preneoplastic lesions and intermediate end-points

4.1.3.1 Oral premalignancy

Stich *et al.* performed several studies on the frequency of micronuclei in cells scraped from the inside of the human cheek as a measure of chromosomal breakage (Stich *et al.*, 1982, 1984a,b, 1985, 1988a,b, 1991a,b; Stich & Rosin, 1984). Supplementation for three months in 40 Filipino betel-quid chewers with retinol (100 000 IU per week) and β-carotene (300 000 IU per week) was associated with a three-fold decrease in the mean proportion of cells with micronuclei. The frequency of micronucleated buccal mucosa cells decreased from an average of 4.2% to 1.4% (Stich *et al.*, 1984a,b; Stich & Rosin, 1984). [The Working Group noted that the study was neither randomized, blinded, nor placebo-controlled. The results were based on comparisons made in the supplemented group before and after the supplementation and not between supplemented and placebo groups.]

Stich *et al.* (1988a) later randomized fisherman from Kerala (betel-quid chewers) to placebo, β-carotene (180 mg per week) or vitamin A 100 000 IU per week and β-carotene during six months. After three months, the frequency of micronucleated cells in the group receiving vitamin A and β-carotene (n = 51) was significantly reduced from 4.0% to 1.2% in areas of leukoplakia and from 4.2% to 1.2% in normal mucosa. [The Working Group noted that the blindness of the treatment group assignment was compromised by yellowing of the oral mucosa of those participants receiving β-carotene. The results were based on comparisons made in the supplemented group before and after the supplementation and not between supplemented and placebo groups.]

In another study (Stich *et al.*, 1988b, 1991a,b), the same population participants received 200 000 IU vitamin A per week (n = 21) or placebo (n = 33) during six months. Markers under study were the number of layers of spinous cells (decrease in 85% of the participants), loss of polarity of basal cells (reduced from 72% to 22%) and subepidermal lymphocytic infiltration (diminished from 66% to 5%); nuclei with condensed chromatin disappeared from the epidermal layer (72% to 0%). The protective effect of the original treatment could be maintained for at least eight additional months by administration of lower doses of vitamin A or β-carotene. [The Working Group noted that the blindness of the study during follow-up and end-point assessment was not mentioned in the reports.]

Prasad *et al.* (1995) performed a study in reverse smokers of chutta (rolled tobacco) (n = 298). 150 subjects were randomized to receive vitamin A (10 000–25 000 twice a week for a year), riboflavin, zinc and selenium; 148 received placebo. Micronuclei and DNA adducts in the exfoliated cells of the buccal mucosa were used as markers. After 12 months, the frequency of micronuclei and the concentration of DNA adducts among those with lesions at baseline decreased significantly ($p < 0.001$) in the supplemented group compared with the placebo group. [The Working Group noted that the blindness of the study during follow-up and end-point assessment was not mentioned in the reports. Many of the reported results were based on comparisons made in the supplemented group before and after the supplementation and not between supplemented and placebo groups. In addition, micronuclei can only be regarded as a measure of DNA damage.]

Ramaswamy *et al.* (1996) studied serum levels of vitamin A in 50 patients with oral leukoplakias and 50 normal controls, 25 betel-quid chewers and 25 non-chewers, in India. A significant decrease in the serum level of vitamin A in the patients with oral leukoplakia was found, compared with the controls.

Copper *et al.* (1998) found no differences in plasma levels of the major retinoids, retinol, all-*trans*-retinoic acid, 13-*cis*-retinoic acid and 13-*cis*-4-oxoretinoic acid in 25 head and neck cancer patients from those in controls without cancer. In addition, in 10 patients from the EUROSCAN chemoprevention trial, the effect on retinoid levels of retinyl palmitate (300 000 IU/day intake during one month) was measured. The medication caused significant elevation in plasma levels of retinol (1.2-fold), all-*trans*-retinoic acid (2.2-fold), 13-*cis*-retinoic acid (5.8-fold) and 13-*cis*-4-oxoretinoic acid (8.9-fold). 13-*cis*-4-Oxoretinoic acid seems a good candidate to serve as marker to monitor compliance in future chemoprevention trials with retinol.

4.1.3.2 Reversal of oral premalignancy

Head and neck cancer (oral cancer in particular, laryngeal cancer to a lesser extent) is preceded by precancerous lesions in a considerable proportion of cases. Oral leukoplakia has been regarded as a good model to study the value of chemopreventive interventions, since the effect is directly visible and material for analysis is easily obtainable from the site of the disease. Reversal of premalignant lesions is regarded as an intermediate end-point. In many studies and chemoprevention trials, the efficacy of chemopreventive agents (retinoids, retinol and/or β-carotene) in reversing oral leukoplakia has been demonstrated (Silverman *et al.*, 1963; Raque *et al.*, 1975; Koch, 1978, 1981; Stich *et al.*, 1982, 1984a,b, 1985, 1988a,b; Shah *et al.*,

1983; Hong *et al.*, 1986; Garewal *et al.*, 1990; Toma *et al.*, 1992; Chiesa *et al.*, 1992, 1993; Lippman *et al.*, 1993; Prasad *et al.*, 1995; Sankaranarayanan *et al.*, 1997), but only in a minority was retinol the chemopreventive drug under study (Silverman *et al.*, 1963; Stich *et al.*, 1984a,b, 1988a,b; Prasad *et al.*, 1995; Sankaranarayanan *et al.*, 1997).

Silverman *et al.* (1963) were the first to administer topical vitamin A to oral leukoplakia patients, in doses of 300 000 to 900 000 IU for 1–15 weeks, with positive responses in 43%. All patients had relapses after cessation of treatment. The lower dose (300 000 IU) was as effective as the dose of 900 000 IU. [The Working Group noted the uncontrolled, open design of the study.]

Stich and co-workers have conducted a number of studies in India with betel-quid chewers, who have a high incidence of leukoplakia, using vitamin A alone or vitamin A and β-carotene together. In one study, 130 patients were randomized to placebo (n = 35), β-carotene 180 mg per week (n = 35), and β-carotene 180 mg per week with vitamin A 100 000 IU per week (n = 60) (Stich *et al.*, 1988a). At six months, complete responses were 3, 15 and 28%, respectively. New lesions were better suppressed in the combined treatment group (8%) than in the β-carotene (15%) and placebo (21%) groups. [The Working Group noted that the blindness of the treatment group assignment was compromised by yellowing of the skin of those participants receiving β-carotene.]

In a second randomized trial (Stich *et al.*,1988b), patients received placebo (n = 33) or 200 000 IU vitamin A per week (n = 21) during six months. A 57% complete remission rate and complete suppression of new lesions occurred in the treatment group, compared with a 3% remission and 21% new lesions in the placebo arm. This study population was different from that in other trials (a vitamin A deficiency cannot be excluded) and the lesions may have been caused by tobacco and betel-quid chewing. [The Working Group noted that the blindness of the study during follow-up and end-point assessment was not mentioned in the reports.]

In the study of Prasad *et al.* (1995) described in Section 4.1.3.1, complete regression of leukoplakia occurred in 57% of subjects on supplementation and 8% on placebo. [The Working Group noted that the blindness of the study during follow-up and end-point assessment was not mentioned in the reports. The reported results were based on comparisons made in the supplemented group before and after the supplementation and not between supplemented and placebo groups.]

Sankaranarayanan *et al.* (1997) conducted a double-blind placebo-controlled trial to evaluate the chemopreventive potential of either retinol alone or β-carotene alone in subjects with oral leukoplakia in Kerala, India. Fishermen and women with oral precancerous lesions (n = 160) were randomized to receive oral vitamin A (retinyl acetate 300 000 IU per week, n = 50), or β-carotene (360 mg per week, n = 55) or placebo (n = 55) for 12 months. The results were based on 43 compliant subjects on placebo, 42 on vitamin A and 46 on β-carotene. The complete regression rates were: [7%] in the placebo arm, 52% with vitamin A ($p < 0.0001$) and [33%] with β-carotene ($p < 0.05$). Half of the responders with β-carotene and two thirds of those with vitamin A relapsed after treatment. [The Working Group noted the use of only 'compliant' participants and the rejection of the intention-to-treat principle.]

In conclusion, retinol seems to be active in oral leukoplakia. Recurrences occur after treatment. The meaning of these findings remains unclear, in particular as to how far these results can be extrapolated to overt oral cancer.

4.1.3.3 Larynx

Issing *et al.* (1997) performed a study of laryngeal squamous cell hyperplasia using retinyl palmitate in a induction-phase dose of 300 000 IU daily, increasing in case of resistant lesions and with a later maintenance phase of 150 000 IU/day. Fifteen out of 20 cases showed complete response, while in the other five patients partial remission was seen.

4.1.3.4 Oesophagus and stomach

A randomized double-blind intervention trial was carried out in Huixian, China, to determine whether combined treatment with retinol, riboflavin and zinc could lower the prevalence of precancerous lesions of the oesophagus. Subjects received either retinol (50 000 IU), 200 mg riboflavin and 50 mg zinc once a week (n = 305) or placebo (n = 305) (Muñoz *et al.*, 1985, 1987a). The intervention did not affect the prevalence of oesophageal lesions; after one year, the prevalence of oesophagitis with or without atrophy or dysplasia was 45.3% in the placebo group and 48.9% in the vitamin/zinc group. Significant site-specific suppression of micronuclei (oesophageal but not buccal) was observed in treated subjects. However, the plasma retinol levels increased substantially in both treatment and placebo groups (Thurnham *et al.*, 1988). This may have been due to social changes taking place in China at that time, although there was no change in riboflavin status in the placebo group. The data were therefore re-analysed using logistic regression analysis in which all data were combined and the prevalence of oesophageal lesions was shown to be significantly lower in those whose retinol increased over the years (Wahrendorf *et al.*, 1988). Thus, improvement in vitamin A status may have reduced the inflammatory lesions in the oesophagus.

Wang *et al.* (1994) reported on a randomized intervention trial among 29 504 residents of Linxian, China [Linxian General Population Study, see also Section 4.1.2.1(*a*) and Blot *et al.* (1993)]. A fractional factorial study design allowed evaluation of four different combinations of nutrients: (*a*) retinol and zinc, (*b*) riboflavin and niacin, (*c*) vitamin C and molybdenum, and (*d*) β-carotene, vitamin E and selenium, in seven groups including placebo. At the end of the 5.25-year intervention, endoscopy was performed on 391 individuals. A reduction in risk (RR, 0.38, p = 0.09) was seen for the effect of retinol and zinc on the prevalence of gastric cancer. Oesophageal biopsy results showed no convincing evidence that any of the supplement combinations decreased the prevalence of oesophageal dysplasia.

In a cross-sectional study of serum micronutrient levels and prevalent dysplasia, subjects with dysplasia had lower carotene levels, but equivalent retinol levels, to controls (Haenszel *et al.*, 1985). In a similar study in China, serum levels of β-carotene were lower among subjects with intestinal metaplasia or dysplasia than among controls; retinol levels were equivalent (Zhang *et al.*, 1994).

4.1.3.5 Colorectum

Nearly all colorectal cancers arise from adenomas which are polypoid neoplasms usually present for years before progression to invasive cancer. Several epidemiological studies have examined nutritional factors in colorectal adenomas (see Potter, 1996, for review). Two case–control studies have presented results for vitamin A. A study in Denmark found lower risk with higher intake of dietary vitamin A (RR, 0.7; 95% CI, 0.4–1.1 for highest tertile) (Olsen *et al.*, 1994). However, a study in Spain found a similar association with total vitamin A (RR, 0.5 for highest quartile, p, trend < 0.05), but no association with retinol (RR, 1.0 for highest quartile, p, trend > 0.05) (Benito *et al.*, 1993). This limited evidence would support a protective role for pre-vitamin A compounds in fruits and vegetables, but not any association specific to retinol in colorectal adenomas.

4.1.3.6 Lung

A randomized, placebo-controlled clinical trial of β-carotene and retinol was conducted among 755 former asbestos workers in Texas, United States (McLarty *et al.*, 1995). The targeted endpoint for the intervention study was a reduction in the incidence and prevalence of sputum atypia. The dosage of 50 mg β-carotene per day and 25 000 IU retinol per day on alternate days resulted in significant increases in serum concentrations of both agents with no significant clinical toxicity. No significant reduction in sputum atypia was observed after treatment compared with placebo.

4.1.3.7 Cervical dysplasia

Lambert *et al.* (1981) compared serum levels of vitamin A and carotene in 14 patients with cervical intraepithelial neoplasia (CIN) with those in 10 controls, in order to study a possible vitamin A deficiency as a causative factor in malignant transformation of cervical metaplasia. No significant vitamin A deficiency was found in these patients.

Brock *et al.* (1988a) investigated blood and dietary measures of vitamin A status in 117 patients with *in situ* cervical cancer and 196 matched controls. Neither retinol from food nor plasma retinol was related to cancer risk.

La Vecchia *et al.* (1988a) analysed 392 cases of invasive cervical cancer compared with 392 age-matched controls, and 247 cases of CIN compared with 247 controls with normal smears. No association emerged between any of the food items containing vitamin A and CIN.

Cuzick *et al.* (1990) investigated serum vitamin A and vitamin E levels in women aged 16–40 years, in a case–control study of CIN. The findings showed no association between serum vitamin A levels and cervical neoplasia.

Ziegler *et al.* (1991) performed a case–control study of 229 women with *in situ* cervical cancer and 502 controls. Vitamin A intake was unrelated to the risk of *in situ* cervical cancer.

De Vet *et al.* (1991) performed a case–control study of the effects of β-carotene and several other dietary factors on the risk of cervical dysplasia. Cases (n = 257) were the participants in a randomized trial assessing the effect of β-carotene on cervical dysplasia, and controls (n = 705) were sampled from the general population. An increased risk of cervical dysplasia was observed for women with a high intake of β-carotene, but no association was found with the intake of retinol.

Liu *et al.* (1995) evaluated the effect of human papillomavirus type 16 (HPV-16) infection and nutritional status on the course of cervical dysplasia in 206 women. HPV-16 infection was found to be related to the progression of cervical dysplasia, with a relative risk of 1.2. High plasma levels of retinol were related to the regression of cervical dysplasia, especially in HPV-16-positive women. Compared with women having plasma retinol levels below 0.45 μg/mL, the relative risk was 0.7 for those with retinol levels of 0.45–0.61 μg/mL, and 0.7 for those with retinol levels above 0.61 μg/mL.

Buckley *et al.* (1992) found no difference in retinol intake between American Indian women with cervical dysplasia (n = 42) and women with normal cervical cytology (n = 58).

Palan *et al.* (1996) investigated plasma levels of β-carotene, lycopene, canthaxanthin, retinol, and α- and τ-tocopherol. The target population of 235 included women with histopathological diagnosis of CIN or cervical cancer and a control group. The mean plasma level of carotenoids as well as that of α-tocopherol were significantly lower in women with CIN and cervical cancer. The mean level of τ-tocopherol was higher among patients with CIN, while the mean plasma levels of retinol were similar among the groups.

4.1.3.8 Systemic biomarkers

The relationships between plasma levels or dietary intake of retinol and levels of carcinogen–DNA adducts have been investigated. Mooney *et al.* (1997) evaluated DNA adducts with polycyclic aromatic hydrocarbons by competitive ELISA with fluorescence detection in leukocytes of 159 heavy smokers, and found an inverse association with their plasma levels of retinol. Wiencke *et al.* (1995) measured smoke-related DNA adducts by ^{32}P-postlabelling analysis in blood mononuclear cells and lung tissue obtained at surgery from 31 lung cancer patients. DNA adducts in both blood and lung were inversely related to the dietary intake of retinol.

Urinary excretion of aflatoxin B_1–DNA adducts in healthy Taiwanese males was positively associated with plasma levels of α- and β-carotene, but no association of the adducts levels with plasma levels of retinol was found (Yu *et al.*, 1997).

The incidence of chromosomal aberrations in cultured lymphocytes of 109 styrene-, formaldehyde- and phenol-exposed workers was compared with that of 64 controls. There was a marked increase in the incidence of the structural chromosomal aberrations in the first mitotic division metaphases of the occupationally exposed workers. 22 occupationally exposed workers were selected for a trial including one month's administration of capsules with retinyl palmitate 100 000 IU plus 0.1 mg α-tocopherol acetate dissolved in 0.2 mL of oil at a dose of 1–2 capsules for five days per week. The drug combination caused a significant decrease in occupationally induced chromosomal damage in lymphocytes (Mierauskienè *et al.*, 1993).

4.1.3.9 Summary

In conclusion, studies using biomarkers as intermediate end-points have been performed in relation to oral leukoplakia and oesophageal dysplasia. Although changes in expression were found in some instances, their relevance remains to be established.

Of the premalignant lesions, oral leukoplakia is the best studied. Studies performed in developing countries have shown positive results, but it remains unclear how far these results can be extrapolated to other populations.

4.2 Experimental models

4.2.1 Tumour induction

In the following section, studies evaluating effects of retinol and retinyl esters on experimental carcinogenesis are described. Several tumour models have been used to study the effects of vitamin A and its analogues on the development of cancers. These have largely used chemical carcinogens for induction of target organ-specific cancers. For example, 7,12-dimethylbenz[*a*]anthracene (DMBA) and *N*-methyl-*N*-nitrosourea (MNU) were used for induction of breast cancer, whereas *N*-[4-(5-nitro-2-furyl)-2-thiazolyl]formamide (FANFT) was used for induction of urinary bladder cancer. It should be noted that the majority of carcinogenesis studies are carried out at a high carcinogen concentration and the modulatory chemopreventive agents are used as pharmacological doses rather than physiological concentrations. This poses problems in correlating the results with those derived from clinical trials. Secondly, the mammary carcinogenesis studies were conducted with young animals and therefore may not model closely the effects of vitamin A on breast cancer in post-menopausal women.

Several further studies have been reported evaluating effects of vitamin A and esters, but were inadequately designed. Such studies were not included in this section. Effects of vitamin A and esters on the development of spontaneous tumours are described in Section 6.

4.2.1.1 Lung (Table 20)

(a) Rat

Over 230 Fischer 344 rats (males and females; 15–22 rats per subgroup [not further specified]) were placed on a semisynthetic vitamin A-free diet (TD-69389, General Biochemicals) at three weeks of age. One week thereafter, they were divided into three groups which received retinyl acetate twice weekly by gavage amounting to weekly doses of 17.4, 174 or 1740 mg retinyl acetate per rat. Five weeks later, the animals were treated with two intratracheal instillations (on consecutive days) of 3-methylcholanthrene (MCA); the total dose amounted to 1.25, 2.5, 5 or 10 mg of carcinogen, providing four groups of rats for each level of retinyl acetate. The animals were killed when moribund or at 180 weeks after carcinogen treatment. Pulmonary squamous-cell cancer incidence was higher among rats at a low dose of retinyl acetate (17.4 mg/week/rat) in comparison with rats given the highest retinyl acetate supplement. This phenomenon was observed at all four dose levels of carcinogen: 10 mg (93% versus 66%), 5 mg (65% versus 20%), 2.5 mg (27% versus 9%) and 1.25 mg (23% versus 10%) (Nettesheim *et al.*, 1979).

(b) Hamster

Two groups of 36 male and 36 female Syrian golden hamsters, 12 weeks of age, were given intratracheal instillations of benzo[*a*]pyrene (BP) adsorbed onto ferric oxide particles (3 mg BP + 3 mg ferric oxide in 0.2 mL saline) once a week for 10 weeks. Group 1 received no further treatment. Group 2 received retinyl palmitate (5000 IU in 0.1 mL corn oil) by stomach tube twice weekly for life starting seven days after the last intratracheal instillation. The incidence of respiratory tract tumours (tracheal and bronchial squamous-cell papillomas and carcinomas combined) was 11/53 in the BP-only group versus 1/46 in the group given BP plus retinyl palmitate. It was suggested that retinyl palmitate has a systemic inhibitory effect on the development of metaplastic and benign and malignant neoplastic lesions in the respiratory tract of BP-treated hamsters (Saffiotti *et al.*, 1967). [The Working Group noted that this was a pilot study without statistical evaluation of the data.]

In a similar experiment, the effects of intragastrically administered retinyl acetate on lung tumour development in hamsters induced by

Table 20. Effects of vitamin A and retinyl esters on lung tumorigenesis

Species, strain, sex, age	No. of animals	Carcinogen (dose/route)	Retinoid (dose/route)	Treatment relative to carcinogen	Preventive efficacy[a]	Reference
Rat, Fischer 344, male and female, 3 weeks old	230 rats (15–22 rats/group)	3-MCA, intratracheally 0.5 dose × 2 times (total dose, 1.3, 2.5, 5 or 12 mg/rat)	Retinyl acetate, 17.4, 174 or 1740 µg/rat/week given by stomach tube; 0.5 dose 2 times/week for up to 180 weeks	Before and during	Effective at all doses of carcinogen	Nettesheim *et al.* (1979)
Hamster, Syrian golden, male and female, 12 weeks old	36 males and 36 females per group	BP (3 mg) + ferric oxide (3 mg), intratracheal instillation weekly for 10 weeks	5000 IU retinyl palmitate in 0.1 mL corn oil twice weekly, intragastrically for life	After	Effective	Saffiotti *et al.* (1967)
Hamster, Syrian golden, male, 12 weeks old	83 74 73	12 × 3 mg BP 12 × 3 mg BP 12 × 3 mg BP	Retinyl acetate 100 µg/week 1600 µg/week 2400 µg/week, intragastrically for life	After	Ineffective	Smith *et al.* (1975a)
Hamster, Syrian golden, male, 12 weeks old	109 111 107	12 × 3 mg BP 12 × 3 mg BP 12 × 3 mg BP	Retinyl acetate 100 µg/week 1600 µg/week 2400 µg/week for life	After	Ineffective	Smith *et al.* (1975b)

Abbreviations: BP, benzo[*a*]pyrene; MCA, 3-methylcholanthrene

[a] Effective implies a statistically significant inhibition

BP adsorbed onto ferric oxide particles (12 weekly intratracheal instillations) were studied. One week after the last carcinogen administration, the hamsters, which were fed a commercial diet, were divided into three groups receiving either 100 μg (Group 1), 1600 μg (Group 2) or 3300 μg (Group 3; later reduced to 2400 μg) retinyl acetate intragastrically in cotton seed oil for life [a control group not receiving retinyl acetate was not included]. In Group 1, 48/83 animals (58%) had benign and malignant respiratory tract tumours combined (72 tumours total); in Group 2, 52/74 animals (70%) had respiratory tract tumours (70 tumours in total); in Group 3, 59/73 animals (81%) had respiratory tract tumours (84 tumours in total). The increase in the tumour incidence in Group 3 versus Group 1 was statistically significant ($p < 0.01$). However, the incidence of squamous-cell carcinomas and adenocarcinomas in the respiratory tract was similar in all three groups (Smith *et al.*, 1975a).

Similar results were obtained by Smith *et al.* (1975b). Hamsters were exposed to the same BP/ferric oxide mixture and treated with the same retinyl acetate doses and were maintained on a semi-synthetic diet and kept in conventional housing or in laminar flow units (to reduce respiratory infections). The incidence of respiratory tract tumours was not statistically significantly different between the low- and high-dose retinyl acetate groups. It was noted, however, that the proportions of hamsters with stomach papillomas were significantly reduced ($p < 0.005$) in the two high-dose retinyl acetate groups (1600 μg and 2400 μg retinyl acetate, respectively) compared with the low-dose retinyl acetate group (100 μg retinyl acetate), namely 25% and 26% with papillomas, respectively, compared with 50%.

4.2.1.2 Mammary gland *(Table 21)*

All of the following studies were conducted in young adult animals.

(a) Mouse

Groups of 20–30 female C3H/A mice were fed retinyl acetate in the diet starting either at conception, as weanlings or at three months of age. The groups received retinyl acetate at concentrations of either 21, 41, 83, 166 or 333 mg/kg of diet in the form of gelatin beadlets. No significant difference in the incidence of mammary carcinomas was found between controls and retinyl acetate-fed mice. The incidence in experimental groups of mice varied from 80 to 92%. The number of tumours per mouse and the tumour latency period were also not influenced by retinyl acetate in the diet (Maiorana & Gullino, 1980).

Forty-day-old GR/A female mice were treated with estrone (0.5 mg/L in the drinking-water) and progesterone (50 mg subcutaneous pellet made with 10 mg cholesterol). Animals were fed either basal diet (not specified) or diet containing retinyl acetate at a concentration of 82 mg/kg of diet in the form of beadlets for 13–14 weeks, at which time the study was terminated. The incidence of mammary tumours [not examined histologically] was 22/65 (34%) in controls compared with 37/65 (57%) ($p < 0.05$) in retinyl acetate-treated mice. This enhancement of tumour development was recorded for both nulliparous and multiparous mice (Welsch *et al.*, 1981).

(b) Rat

Groups of 50 female Sprague–Dawley rats were treated with a single intragastric dose of either 2.5, 5 or 15 mg DMBA in 1 mL sesame oil. Retinyl acetate treatment (1 or 2.5 mg/rat per day in the form of gelatin beadlets mixed in the diet) was initiated seven days after carcinogen treatment for 211 days. All animals were maintained on conventional diets. There was only 8% incidence of histopathologically confirmed mammary carcinomas in the 2.5 mg DMBA control group of rats. At 5 and 15 mg DMBA, the incidence of mammary carcinomas was 46 and 75%, respectively. Retinyl acetate was ineffective at the 1 mg dose regardless of DMBA dose; however, at 2.5 mg retinyl acetate dose, there was a significant ($p < 0.05$) decrease in the incidence of adenocarcinomas (11/50 compared with 23/50 in controls) and of adenomas (30/50 compared with 43/50 in controls) (Moon *et al.*, 1976).

Groups of 30 female Sprague-Dawley rats, 50 days of age, were injected twice intravenously

Table 21. Effects of vitamin A and retinyl esters on breast tumorigenesis

Species, strain, sex, age	No. of animals	Carcinogen (dose/route)	Retinoid (dose/route)	Treatment relative to carcinogen	Preventive efficacy	Reference
Mouse, C3H/A, female, 3 weeks old	Control 102, experimental 20–30/group	Murine mammary tumour virus positive	Retinyl acetate, 21, 41, 83, 166 or 333 mg/kg of diet	From conception, from weanling or from 3 months	Ineffective	Maiorana & Gullino (1980)
Mouse, GR/A, females, 40 days old	65/group	Estrone + progesterone	Retinyl acetate, 82 mg/kg diet for 13–14 weeks	Before, during and after	Increased tumour incidence	Welsch *et al.* (1981)
Rat, Sprague-Dawley, females, 50 days old	50/group	DMBA: 2.5, 5 or 15 mg	Retinyl acetate: 1 or 2.5 mg per day in diet for 211 days	After	Ineffective at 1 mg. Effective at 2.5 mg	Moon *et al.* (1976)
Rat, Sprague-Dawley, females, 50 days old	30/group	MNU: 12.5, 25 or 50 mg/kg bw intravenous injection × 2	Retinyl acetate: 250 ppm in the diet	Before, during and after	Effective at all doses of carcinogen	Moon *et al.* (1977)
Lewis rats, females, 50 days old	20/group	DMBA: 20 mg intragastrically at 50 days of age	Retinyl acetate: 250 mg/kg of diet	(a) Before and during (b) After, 1–30 weeks (c) After, 1–2 weeks (d) After, 12–30 weeks (e) Before, during and after	Effective Effective Effective Effective Effective	McCormick *et al.* (1980)
Rat, ACI, female 59–65 days old	24/group	17_-Ethinylestradiol pellet (1 mg/pellet)	Retinyl acetate 420 IU/g diet + 4 IU retinyl palmitate/g diet for 25 weeks	Before and during	Effective	Holtzman (1988)

Table 21 (contd)

Species, strain, sex, age	No. of animals	Carcinogen (dose/route)	Retinoid (dose/route)	Treatment relative to carcinogen	Preventive efficacy	Reference
Rat, Lew/Mai females, 50 days old	20/group	BP: 50 mg single dose intragastrically 6.25 mg/wk/8 wks	Retinyl acetate: 250 mg/kg diet for up to 90 weeks	(a) Before and during (b) After and during, up to 90 weeks (c) After and during, up to 20 weeks (d) After, 20–35 weeks –2 to +90 weeks	Effective Effective Ineffective Effective Effective Effective	McCormick *et al.* (1981)
Rat, Sprague-Dawley, females, 50 days old	25/group	DMBA: 15–20 mg single dose intragastrically	Retinyl acetate: 328 mg/kg diet for 240 days	+1 to + 17 weeks	Effective	Thompson *et al.* (1982)
Rat, Sprague-Dawley, females, 50 days old	30/group	MNU: 50 mg/kg bw single dose intravenously	Retinyl acetate: 328 mg/kg diet (duration not given)	+1 to + 17 weeks	Effective	Moon *et al.* (1983)
Rat, Sprague-Dawley, females, 50 days old	30/group	DMBA: 16 mg single dose intragastrically	Retinyl acetate: 250 mg/kg diet	Before and during After Before, during and after	Ineffective Effective Effective	McCormick *et al.* (1986)
Rat, Sprague-Dawley, females, 50 days old	30/group	DMBA: 5 mg intragastrically, 6 times	Retinyl acetate: i.p. injection once weekly at 350 mg/kg bw for 50 days; 250 mg/kg bw for 90 days; and 200 mg/kg bw for 60 days until 240 days of age	Before and during	Effective	Ramesha *et al.* (1990)
Rat, Holtzman, female, 50 days old	20/group	DMBA: 20 mg single dose intragastrically	Retinyl acetate 50 mg/kg diet	Before, during and after, up to 10 days	Ineffective	Rao *et al.* (1990)

Abbreviations: BP, benzo[*a*]pyrene; DMBA, 7,12-dimethylbenz[*a*]anthracene; MNU, *N*-methyl-*N*-nitrosourea with either 12.5, 25 or 50 mg/kg bw MNU. The injections were given one week apart. Retinyl acetate in the form of gelatin beadlets was mixed with the Purina Lab chow diet at a concentration of 0 or 250 mg/kg of diet. The treatment was started one week after initiation and continued for 175 days. Retinyl acetate inhibited tumour incidence significantly compared with groups treated with carcinogen alone. The incidence of mammary tumour-bearing (retinyl acetate-treated versus untreated) was: 15/30 versus 25/30 in the high-dose MNU group, 7/30 versus 12/29 in the mid-dose MNU group and 0/30 versus 6/30 in the low-dose MNU group. At the high dose, control rats developed 61 cancers compared with 25 cancers in the retinyl acetate-treated group (Moon *et al.*, 1977).

Groups of 20 female Lewis rats, 50 days of age, were treated with 20 mg DMBA in 1 mL sesame oil. Retinyl acetate in gelatin beadlets was mixed with Purina Lab chow at a concentration of 250 mg/kg of diet. In relation to the time of DMBA treatment, rats were given retinyl acetate during weeks –2 to +1, –2 to +30, +1 to +30, +1 to +12 or +12 to +30. The experiment was terminated at 30 weeks. The greatest inhibition of mammary tumour yield was observed in the group receiving retinyl acetate for the longest time (–2 to +30 weeks); mammary tumour multiplicity was approximately 60% of that in the controls. A similar inhibition of 60% was also reported after a shorter exposure to retinyl acetate of –2 to +1 week (McCormick *et al.*, 1980). [The Working Group noted that the mammary tumours were not examined histologically and that data were presented only as graphs.]

McCormick and Moon (1982) studied the effect of delaying retinyl acetate treatment after MNU administration. All experimental details were the same as described by Moon *et al.* (1977), except that a single injection of 25 mg/kg bw MNU was given. Treatment with retinyl acetate at a concentration of 328 mg/kg of diet was initiated 1, 4, 8, 12, 16 or 20 weeks after the carcinogen treatment. The results showed that the treatment with retinyl acetate could be delayed for as long as 12 weeks without loss of efficacy.

Groups of 20 Lew/Mai rats, 50 days of age, received either a single dose of 50 mg BP in 1 mL sesame oil intragastrically or eight weekly doses of 6.25 mg BP. Rats were given Purina Lab chow as control diet or a diet containing 250 mg/kg of diet retinyl acetate in the form of gelatin beadlets. In relation to the time of BP treatment, retinyl acetate was given during weeks –2 to +1, +1 to +90, +1 to +20 or +20 to +90. Animals were weighed monthly and killed 90 weeks after the carcinogen treatment. Rats given only the single injection of BP had a 77% incidence of mammary tumours. The incidence in the retinyl acetate-treated groups was: –2 to +1, 44% ($p < 0.01$); +1 to +90, 42% ($p < 0.01$); +1 to +20, 71%; and +20 to +90, 45% ($p < 0.01$). There was a 67% incidence of mammary tumours in animals given eight injections of BP alone; retinyl acetate given from –2 to +90 weeks reduced this to 40% ($p < 0.01$) (McCormick *et al.*, 1981). [The Working Group noted that the tumours were not evaluated histopathologically.]

Groups of 25 Sprague–Dawley rats, 50 days of age, received 20 mg DMBA intragastrically and were ovariectomized at various times in relation to carcinogen treatment. Intact and ovariectomized animals were treated with retinyl acetate at a concentration of 328 mg/kg of diet. The incidence of mammary adenocarcinomas was 10/25 in ovariectomized rats compared with 4/25 in the rats that were ovariectomized and received retinyl acetate treatment. Tumour multiplicity in this study was also reduced by retinyl acetate (Thompson *et al.*, 1982).

Four groups of 30 female Sprague–Dawley rats were treated with 50 mg/kg bw MNU by intravenous injection. Rats were either kept intact or were ovariectomized 14 days after carcinogen treatment. Both intact and ovariectomized rats either served as separate controls or received 1 mmol retinyl acetate/kg of diet [328 mg/kg of diet] in the form of gelatin beadlets. Although retinyl acetate reduced the incidence of mammary adenocarcinomas from 80% in controls to 59% in the retinyl acetate-treated group, ovariectomy reduced the incidence to 35%. The combination of ovariectomy and retinyl acetate resulted in a tumour incidence of less than 10%. This remarkable suppression of carcinogenesis was accompanied by increased latency of tumour development from 30–50 days in controls to 150 days in the combined treatment group (Moon *et al.*, 1983). [The Working Group noted that data were presented only as graphs.]

McCormick *et al.* (1986) studied the effect of combined treatment with retinyl acetate and butylated hydroxytoluene (BHT) in groups of 30 female Sprague–Dawley rats treated with 16 mg of DMBA in 1 mL sesame oil at 50 days of age. Animals were given either 250 mg retinyl acetate/kg of diet as gelatin beadlets alone or in combination with BHT at a concentration of 5 g/kg of diet. In relation to the time of DMBA treatment, retinyl acetate/BHT was given during weeks –2 to +1, +1 to + 26, or –2 to + 26 (180 days). Body weights were not affected in these studies. The multiplicity of mammary carcinomas was reduced from 7.5 tumours per rat in controls to 4.97 and 4.74 following treatment with retinyl acetate from + 1 to + 26 and from –2 to + 26 weeks, respectively (66% and 63% of controls, respectively). The combination of BHT and retinyl acetate was more effective than either treatment alone.

Two groups of 30 Sprague–Dawley rats, 40 days of age, were treated with 5 mg DMBA in sesame oil per week for six weeks (total dose, 30 mg). Retinyl acetate was injected intraperitoneally once weekly at doses of 350 mg/kg bw (40 days), 250 mg/kg bw (90 days) and 200 mg/kg bw (60 days) until the animals reached the age of 240 days. Retinyl acetate significantly reduced the numbers of of tumour-bearing animals from 28/28 in DMBA-treated controls to 13/28 ($p < 0.001$). When retinyl acetate treatment was combined with other compounds such as sodium selenite, magnesium chloride and ascorbic acid, the inhibitory effect of retinyl acetate was enhanced (Ramesha *et al.*, 1990).

Female Holtzman rats were treated with 20 mg DMBA in 0.5 mL oil. They were given either control diet or diet mixed with retinyl acetate (50 mg/kg of diet) alone or in combination with tamoxifen, tocopherol, aminoglutethimide, ergocryptine and/or selenium. The chemopreventive agent in the diet was given for 21 days beginning 10 days before carcinogen treatment and continuing to 10 days after carcinogen treatment. Rats were killed 180 days after carcinogen treatment and the tumours were examined histopathologically. Mammary adenomas developed in 10/15 DMBA-exposed rats and in 12/20 rats treated with DMBA plus retinyl acetate. When retinyl acetate was given in combination with two or more other agents, the tumour incidence was reduced from 64% to 20–30% ($p < 0.05$) (Rao *et al.*, 1990).

Two groups of female ACI rats were divided into 24 rats per group. All animals received AIN-16A semisynthetic diet with 4000 IU of retinyl palmitate. The active treatment group had its diet supplemented with 412 000 IU of retinyl acetate per kg diet. After two weeks, subcutaneous pellets of 1 mg 17α-ethinylestradiol were implanted into both groups of rats. Animals were killed 25 weeks later. Retinyl acetate treatment did not affect body weight. The incidence of mammary carcinomas was 88% (21/24) in controls rats and 70% (16/23) in the retinyl acetate-treated group ($p < 0.05$). The multiplicity was reduced from 5.6 cancers per rat in controls to 2.7 cancers per rat in the retinyl acetate-treated group ($p < 0.05$) (Holtzman, 1988).

4.2.1.3 Urinary bladder (Table 22)

(a) Rat

Three groups of 40 weanling female Sprague–Dawley rats, weighing 44 to 76 g, were fed vitamin A-deficient diets and received either (1) 100 IU retinyl palmitate via stomach tube during weeks 9 and 16; (2) 5 IU retinyl palmitate/g diet or (3) 250 IU retinyl palmitate/g diet for the first four weeks and 500 IU/g diet thereafter. After one week, 0.188% FANFT was added to these diets for 12 weeks and 0.1% for the following eight weeks. At 22 weeks, the incidences of bladder carcinomas (transitional-cell and squamous-cell) were 21/40, 17/40 and 16/40 in the three groups, respectively (Cohen *et al.*, 1976).

In a second experiment, two groups of 36 weanling female Sprague–Dawley rats, weighing 44 to 76 g, were fed a basal diet either with or without added retinyl palmitate (930 up to 2500 IU/g diet). After one week on these diets, 0.1% FANFT was added to the diet for 20 weeks, after which the rats received their respective

Table 22. Chemopreventive activity of vitamin A and retinyl esters on urinary bladder carcinogenesis

Species, strain, sex	No. of animals	Carcinogen, dose, route and duration of administration	Retinoid (dose/route)	Treatment relative to carcinogen	Preventive efficacy	Reference
Rat, Sprague-Dawley, female, 3–4 weeks old	40/group	*N*-4-(5-Nitro-2-furyl)-2-thiazolyl formamide in the diet; 0.188% for 12 weeks and 0.1% for the next 8 weeks	Retinyl palmitate, 0, 5, 250, 500 IU per g diet for 22 weeks	Before and during	Ineffective	Cohen *et al.* (1976)
Rat, Sprague-Dawley, female, 3–4 weeks old	36/group	*N*-4-(5-Nitro-2-furyl)-2-thiazolyl formamide in the diet (0.1%) for 20 weeks	Retinyl palmitate, 0, 930, 2500, 1100 IU per g diet for 35 weeks	Before, during and after	Ineffective	Cohen *et al.* (1976)
Rat, Wistar, male, weight 165 g	18/group	*N*-Butyl-*N*-(4-hydroxy-butyl)-nitrosamine via drinking water, 0, 0.01, 0.025% for 20 weeks	Retinyl acetate, 0, 100, 200 IU per g diet for 20 weeks	During	Effective at 200 IU	Miyata *et al.* (1978)

diets without FANFT. All rats alive at 35 weeks were killed. Signs of hypervitaminosis A occurred by 11 weeks in the group maintained on 2500 IU/g diet (fed in weeks 6–13). Therefore the concentration was reduced to 1100 IU/g diet after 13 weeks. The incidence of transitional-cell carcinomas (2/36 in both groups) was similar in the group fed normal vitamin A diet and in the group on the retinyl palmitate-supplemented diet (Cohen *et al.*, 1976).

Nine groups of 18 male Wistar rats, weighing approximately 165 g, were treated simultaneously with *N*-butyl-*N*-(4-hydroxybutyl)nitrosamine (BBN) in the drinking water and/or retinyl acetate in the diet for 20 weeks as follows: (1) 200 IU retinyl acetate/g diet and 0.025% BBN; (2) 100 IU retinyl acetate/g diet and 0.025% BBN; (3) 0.025% BBN; (4) 200 IU retinyl acetate/g diet and 0.01% BBN; (5) 100 IU retinyl acetate/g diet and 0.01% BBN; (6) 0.01% BBN; (7) 200 IU retinyl acetate/g diet; (8) 100 IU retinyl acetate/g diet and (9) controls, with 10 IU of retinyl acetate in basal diet. All surviving rats were killed after 20 weeks. Administration of 200 IU retinyl acetate/g diet reduced the incidence of transitional cell papillomas (1/18 vs 7/16) and carcinomas (4/16 vs 10/14) in groups receiving 0.01% and 0.025% BBN, respectively, compared to controls ($p < 0.02$) (Miyata *et al.*, 1978).

4.2.1.4 Skin *(Table 23)*

(a) Mouse

Four groups of 20 or 10 female Swiss mice, 8 weeks of age, were treated as follows: (1) MCA was applied on the shaved skin (0.1 mL/mouse as a 0.3% solution in acetone) twice weekly for the first five weeks and then once weekly during the sixth to ninth weeks (14 applications); (2) MCA as in group 1 and, during the third to fifth weeks, retinyl palmitate (6 mg/0.1 mL acetone/mouse) was applied to the same treated areas of the skin twice weekly (6 applications) and subsequently, once weekly during the sixth to ninth weeks (4 applications); (3) retinyl palmitate alone as group 2 (10 applications) and (4) acetone alone (14 applications). From the 10th week on, no further treatment was given until the end of the experiment at 23 weeks. Groups 1 and 2 comprised 20 mice per group and groups 3 and 4, 10 mice per group. The tumours were classified histopathologically. In the group treated with MCA and retinyl palmitate, the incidence of mice with papillomas (3/20) was lower than in mice treated with

Table 23. Chemopreventive activity of vitamin A and retinyl esters on skin carcinogenesis

Species, strain, sex	No. of animals/group	Carcinogen, dose, route and duration of administration	Vitamin A (dose)	Treatment relative to carcinogen	Preventive efficacy	Reference
Mouse, Swiss, female	20/group	MCA, 0.1 ml of 0.3% solution in acetone, applied to the shaved skin (14 applications)	Retinyl palmitate, 6 mg/0.1 mL in acetone applied on the skin	During	Effective (papillomas) Ineffective (carcinomas)	Abdel-Galil *et al.* (1984)
Mouse, Skh-hr1, Hairless, female 10–12 weeks old	20/group	UVR; 280–700 nm, 5 days/week for 12 weeks	Retinyl palmitate 60 IU or 300 IU, 3 times per week by stomach tube until death	Before and during	Ineffective	Kelly *et al.* (1989)
Mouse, CD-1, female	35/group	DMBA, single topical application of 150 nmol; promoted twice weekly with 8 nmol TPA for 21 weeks	Retinyl palmitate, 60, 200, 700/350 IU per g diet	During promotion with TPA	Effective (papillomas)	Gensler *et al.* (1987)
Mouse, C3H/HeN, female, 6 weeks old	20–30/group	UVB radiation, 280–320 nm, 30 min/day, 5 days/week from week 18–42	Retinyl palmitate, 0, 120 IU per g diet for 45.5 weeks	Before and during	Inconclusive	Gensler *et al.* (1990)
Mouse, Oslo/Bom inbred hairless, female (age not given)	44/group	UVB (280–320 nm) or UVAB (280–380 nm) for 18 weeks	0.3–0.6 mg retinol/kg diet or 4–6 mg/kg diet for 78 weeks	1 month before and during	Increased tumour incidence	Mikkelsen *et al.* (1998)

Abbreviations: DMBA, 7,12-dimethylbenz[*a*]anthracene; MCA, 3-methylcholanthrene; TPA, 12-*O*-tetradecanoylphorbol 13-acetate

MCA only (9/19). The incidence of mice with carcinomas was similar in both groups (4/20 versus 5/19). No skin tumour was seen in control groups (Abdel-Galil *et al.*, 1984).

Four groups of 35 female CD-1 mice, 6 weeks of age, were treated with a single topical application of 150 nmol of DMBA in 0.2 mL acetone and, starting three weeks later, 12-*O*-tetradecanoylphorbol 13-acetate (TPA) (8 nmol) was applied in 0.2 mL acetone twice weekly for 21 weeks. The control diet (AIN-76A) contained 3.9 IU retinyl palmitate/g diet. Mice were fed diets supplemented with retinyl palmitate for 21 weeks at a level of 60, 200 or 700 IU/g diet (the high dose was reduced to 350 IU per g of diet after five weeks). There were 14.3 ± 2.6, 8.2 ± 2.0 and 3.4 ± 1.2 papillomas per mouse in the groups on the low, medium and high doses of retinyl palmitate, respectively, versus 15.6 ± 2.7 in controls, corresponding to reductions of 9%, 37% ($p < 0.02$) and 65% ($p < 0.02$) (Gensler *et al.*, 1987).

Groups of 20 inbred, hairless (Skh-hr1) female mice, 10–12 weeks of age, were exposed to 280–700 nm ultraviolet light on five days per week for 12 weeks. The initial daily exposure was 0.53 J/cm^2. Subsequent exposure times were increased by 20% every two weeks. After 12 weeks, the exposure was increased to 1.60 J/cm^2 and from that time up to 25 weeks following the start of treatment was held at that level at a frequency of twice weekly. Retinyl palmitate (60 or 30 IU) was dissolved in arachis oil and administered intragastrically three times weekly beginning two weeks before the start of treatment and continuing until death. All tumours were classified histopathologically. The incidence of skin tumours (papillomas and carcinomas) in both retinyl palmitate-treated groups was similar to that in controls (Kelly *et al.*, 1989).

Groups of 20–30 female C3H/HeNCrlBR mice, six weeks of age, were fed: (1) an AIN-76A basal diet containing 4 IU retinyl palmitate/g diet; (2) basal diet supplemented with 120 IU retinyl palmitate/g diet; (3) basal diet supplemented with 1% canthaxanthin or (4) basal diet supplemented with 1% canthaxanthin plus 120 IU retinyl palmitate/g diet. The animals were maintained on their respective diets for at least 45 1/2 weeks. During weeks 18–42, the shaved dorsal skin of the animals was irradiated with ultraviolet light (280–320 nm) for 30 minutes per day on five days per week. There was no significant difference in tumour incidence in irradiated mice fed retinyl palmitate (32%), canthaxanthin (36%), retinyl palmitate plus canthaxanthin (31%) and controls (37%). Dietary supplementation with retinyl palmitate, however, significantly reduced the mean skin tumour burden at four weeks (sum of the tumour areas on each mouse) by 41% in comparison with controls ($p < 0.008$; analysis of variance of the log tumour burden). Canthaxanthin reduced the tumour burden per mouse by 45%, whereas canthaxanthin plus retinyl palmitate treatment resulted in a 68% reduction in tumour burden, indicating no interaction between retinyl palmitate and canthaxanthin (Gensler *et al.*, 1990). [The Working Group noted that the measurement of skin tumour burden was rather unusual for skin carcinogenesis studies.]

Four groups of 44 hairless female mice of the Oslo/Bom inbred strain [age not specified] were fed a standard laboratory diet containing low (0.3–0.6 mg/kg diet) or high (4–6 mg/kg diet) levels of retinol. After the mice had been fed these diets for one month, the animals were exposed daily to irradiation with ultra-violet B (280–320 nm) or B and A (280–380 nm) for 18 weeks followed by an observation period of up to 60 weeks. After one year, the incidence of skin squamous cell carcinomas was 49–63% in the high-retinol group versus 25–39% in the low-retinol group ($p < 0.003$). Two months later, these figures were 66–72% versus 50–53% for the high- and low-retinol groups, respectively ($p = 0.01$) (Mikkelsen *et al.*, 1998).

4.2.1.5 Oesophagus and forestomach (Table 24)

(a) Mouse

Three groups of 150 male ICR/Jcl mice, four weeks of age, were treated as follows: (1) no treatment with carcinogen; (2) 0.2 mg BP in 0.2 mL corn oil by gavage twice a week to a total dose of 2.0 mg and (3) 2.0 mg BP in 0.2 mL corn oil to a total dose of 20.0 mg. Each of these groups was divided into five subgroups

Table 24. Chemopreventive effects of vitamin A and retinyl esters in other organs

Species, strain, sex	No. of animals	Carcinogen (dose/route)	Vitamin A (dose/route)	Treatment relative to carcinogen	Preventive efficacy	Reference
Forestomach						
Mouse, ICR/Jcl, male, 4 weeks old	30/group	BP in corn oil by gavage; twice weekly to total dose of 2 mg or 20 mg	Retinyl palmitate: 5 IU, 50 IU or 200 IU/day in diet for 66 weeks	Before and during in one group and after in another group	Effective at low dose of BP on incidence of papillomas Ineffective at high dose of BP	Yamada *et al.* (1995)
Oesophagus						
Rat, Sprague-Dawley, sex and age unspecified	60/group	*N*-Nitroso-*N*-methyl-benzylamine, 2.5 mg/kg bw twice a week for 5 weeks, intragastrically	Retinyl acetate: 0.3 mg/kg, 2.2 mg/kg or 29.9 mg/kg in diet for 15 weeks	Before, during and after carcinogen	Ineffective	Nauss *et al.* (1987)
Large intestine						
Rat, Sprague-Dawley, male, age not given	50/group	Aflatoxin B_1 in semi-synthetic diet (0.1 mg/kg diet)	Retinyl palmitate: 5, 50 or 500 mg/day/rat in diet for 24 months	During	Colon carcinomas developed in the retinyl palmitate deficient group	Newberne & Rogers (1973)
Rat, Sprague-Dawley, male, weanling	12/group	1,2-Dimethylhydrazine, two injections 25 mg/kg bw three days apart	Retinyl palmitate: 200 IU/g diet for 12 weeks	After		Cassand *et al.* (1997)
Rat, Fischer 344, male, 6 weeks old	9 or 10/group	Azoxymethane, two intraperitoneal injections 15 mg/kg bw one week apart	Retinyl palmitate: 0.5 or 1.0 mmol/kg diet for 5 weeks	After		Zheng *et al.* (1997)
Thyroid						
Rat, Fischer 344, male	15/group	*N*-Nitroso-*N*-bis(2-hydroxy-propyl)amine, 2800 mg/kg bw, one subcutaneous injection + 0.2% thiourea in drinking-water	Retinyl acetate: 320 IU/g diet	After	Ineffective	Mitsumori *et al.* (1996)

Abbreviations: BP, benzo[*a*]pyrene

of 30 mice each, which were given dietary retinyl palmitate supplementations as follows: (A) 50 IU/day (assumed to be an adequate vitamin A intake for ICR/Jcl mice); (B) 5 IU/day; (C) 200 IU/day (retinyl palmitate supplementation was given during the initiation and post-initiation phases); (D) 5 IU/day, and (E) 200 IU/day. Groups D and E both received 50 IU retinyl palmitate/day during the initiation phase and the low (5 IU) and high (200 IU) levels during the post-initiation phase. All surviving animals were killed at 66 weeks. In animals treated with the low dose of BP, the incidence of forestomach papilloma-bearing mice of the two high retinyl palmitate groups was significantly lower ($p < 0.05$) in comparison with the group given 50 IU/day (2/27, 2/27 versus 8/28), whereas the incidence of forestomach papilloma-bearing mice in the group given 5 IU retinyl palmitate/day was significantly ($p < 0.05$) higher than in controls fed 50 IU/day (15/26 vs 8/28). Carcinomas were not induced with this low dose of BP. No effect of retinyl palmitate was seen on papillomas and carcinomas in the groups treated with a high dose of BP (Yamada *et al.*, 1995).

(b) Rat

Groups of 65 Sprague–Dawley rats (sex unspecified) were fed semipurified diets containing levels of retinyl acetate which were either adequate (2.2 mg/kg of diet), deficient (0.30 mg/kg of diet) or high (29.9 mg/kg of diet). After four weeks of adaptation to the experimental diets, 60 rats per dietary group received 2.5 mg/kg bw *N*-nitroso-*N*-methylbenzylamine (NMBA), twice a week for five weeks. NMBA was dissolved in 10% ethanol and administered by gavage. Five animals in each group received vehicle only. Fifteen weeks after the last dose of carcinogen, the animals were killed and the oesophagus was evaluated for presence of neoplasms, using routine histopathological procedures. The incidence and multiplicity of carcinomas, papillomas and preneoplastic lesions were similar in all groups, indicating that dietary retinyl acetate levels did not influence oesophageal tumour development induced by NMBA (Nauss *et al.*, 1987).

4.2.1.6 Large intestine *(Table 24)*

(a) Rat

Groups of 50 male Sprague–Dawley rats were maintained on a semi-synthetic diet containing aflatoxin B_1 at a concentration of 0.1 mg/kg diet. Retinyl palmitate was mixed into the diet to provide 5, 50 or 500 mg/day per rat based on measured food consumption. The study was carried out for 24 months. Six colon carcinomas developed in the retinyl palmitate-deficient group. No such tumours were found in any of the other groups (Newberne & Rogers, 1973).

Sprague–Dawley weanling male rats were divided into two groups of 12 animals. Rats were treated with 50 mg/kg 1,2-dimethylhydrazine hydrochloride (DMH) in two injections of 25 mg/kg three days apart. Starting one week after the last injection, rats received either semi-synthetic diet as control or diet supplemented with 200 IU/g retinyl acetate for 12 weeks. Animals were then killed and the colon was fixed and stained for aberrant crypts, considered to be precursors of colon cancers. Adenocarcinomas were also removed and microscopically identified. Retinyl acetate-treated animals exhibited 4.2 aberrant crypts per cm^2, compared with 5.7 per cm^2 in controls. The total number of adenocarcinomas per rat decreased from 364 to 252 ($p < 0.08$) (Cassand *et al.*, 1997).

Two groups of 9 or 10 male Fischer 344 rats, six weeks of age, were treated with retinyl palmitate at concentrations of 0.5 or 1.0 mmol/kg in AIN-76A basal diet (263 or 525 ppm) for five weeks after prior treatment with two weekly intraperitoneal injections of 15 mg/kg bw azoxymethane for two weeks. The numbers of preneoplastic aberrant crypt foci per rat were 51.3 $\pm$ 5.38 and 36.2 $\pm$ 6.49 at the low and high doses of retinyl acetate, respectively, whereas the control group had 65.2 $\pm$ 5.22 aberrant crypt foci per rat; this constitutes a 44.5% reduction at the highest dose ($p < 0.01$) (Zheng *et al.*, 1997).

4.2.1.7 Liver

(a) Rat

In the study of Newberne and Rogers (1973) described in Section 4.2.1.6, the number of aflatoxin B_1-induced liver tumours was unaffected by retinyl palmitate administration.

4.2.1.8 Thyroid (Table 24)

(a) Rat

Four groups of male Fischer 344 rats, four weeks of age, received a single subcutaneous injection of 2800 mg/kg bw *N*-nitroso-*N*-bis(2-hydroxypropyl)amine (DHPN). Group 1 (5 rats), received tap water; group 2 (5 rats) received 0.1% retinyl acetate in the diet; group 3 (15 rats) received 0.2% thiourea; and group 4 (15 rats) received thiourea plus retinyl acetate in the diet. Animals were killed 20 weeks after the carcinogen treatment. No thyroid tumours were found in animals receiving DHPN and either retinyl acetate alone or basal diet. In animals treated with DHPN plus thiourea, the incidence of follicular-cell tumours [exact histology not given] was similar to that in the group given DHPN + thiourea + retinyl acetate (Mitsumori *et al.*, 1996).

4.2.1.9 Other sites

(a) Mouse

Groups of 20 male CBA/J mice, six weeks of age, were fed basal diet (Teklad) for three days before experiment. They were then fed either control diet or diet supplemented with 150 mg/kg of diet retinyl palmitate throughout the experiment. All animals were inoculated with murine sarcoma virus at three concentrations. Animals were killed 20 days after virus inoculation. At a 1×10^{-3} dilution of virus (low dose), the tumour incidence [site not specified] was 37.5% in controls compared with 0% in the retinyl palmitate-treated group. At higher virus concentrations (1×10^{-2} and 1×10^{-1}), there was a 62.5% tumour incidence in controls compared with 25% and 12.5% incidence, respectively, in the retinyl palmitate-treated groups. Results showed significant suppression of virally induced sarcoma by retinyl palmitate ($p < 0.01$, *t*-test) (Seifter *et al.*, 1983).

Pregnant female albino rats [number unspecified] were given 75 mg/kg bw *N*-ethyl-*N*-nitrosourea by intravenous injection. The mothers were treated with retinyl acetate (300 IU/g diet) during the suckling phase of the offspring. The pups were given retinyl acetate in diet. Animals were allowed to live until natural death. Tumours of the nervous system and kidney developed in all offspring. Retinyl acetate did not affect the incidence of any tumour type or the average life span of the rats (Alexandrov *et al.*, 1991).

4.2.2 Intermediate biomarkers

The ability of retinol, retinal, retinoic acid and retinyl esters to modulate intermediate biomarkers was evaluated in rodents (mouse, rat, hamster) treated with a variety of genotoxic agents, including alkylating agents, polycyclic aromatic hydrocarbons, aromatic amines, mycotoxins and cytostatic agents. The investigated end-points included DNA or RNA binding, DNA damage and clastogenic damage, as assessed by determining the frequency of sister chromatid exchanges, micronuclei and chromosomal aberrations. Table 25 summarizes the outline of these studies and the results obtained.

Five studies evaluated the formation of DNA or RNA adducts under various experimental conditions. The ability of ^{14}C-labelled 2-acetylaminofluorene to bind DNA or RNA of liver cells was not affected in Sprague–Dawley rats given retinyl palmitate orally twice a week according to a dose escalation schedule from the 1st to the 12th week before intraperitoneal injection of the carcinogen (Rondahl *et al.*, 1985). The formation of DNA adducts was investigated by ^{32}P-postlabelling analysis in skin cells of CD–1 mice receiving topical applications of (7*S*,8*S*)-dihydroxy-7,8-dihydrobenzo[*a*]pyrene [(+)-BP-7,8-diol] and of TPA. TPA was administered both 24 h earlier and simultaneously with (+)-BP-7,8-diol. The topical application of retinoic acid had no effect on the formation of (–)-*syn*-BP diol epoxide adducts, whereas it significantly decreased the formation of (–)-*anti*-isomer adducts, but only when co-administered with the second TPA application (Marnett & Ji, 1994). Retinyl acetate, given by gavage for seven days, attenuated the binding of [^{3}H]benzo[*a*]pyrene, given as a single intraperitoneal injection, to the DNA of hepatocytes and stomach cells, but did not affect its binding to the DNA of lung and kidney cells (McCarthy *et al.*, 1987). Administration of retinyl acetate with the diet for two weeks decreased the formation of ^{32}P-postlabelled DNA adducts in mammary cells of Sprague–Dawley rats receiving a single treatment by gavage with 7,12-dimethylbenz[*a*]anthracene (DMBA)

Table 25. Assay of retinol, retinal, retinoic acid and retinyl esters for ability to modulate intermediate biomarkers in animal models

End-point	Code[a]	Modulator (administration schedule and tested doses)[b]	Genotoxic agent (administration schedule and tested doses)[b]	Animal strains and species, and cells	Investigated effect	Result[c]	Inhibitory dose (IDx)[d]	Reference
D	BVP	Retinyl palmitate p.o. twice a week for 12 weeks (0.9 to 7.2 mg/administration)	2-Acetylaminofluorene, single i.p. injection (0.94 mg/kg bw)	Sprague–Dawley rats, liver cells	Binding to RNA	–	NA	Rondahl *et al.* (1985)
D	BVD	Retinyl palmitate p.o. twice a week for 12 weeks (0.9 to 7.2 mg/administration)	2-Acetylaminofluorene, single i.p. injection (0.94 mg/kg bw)	Sprague–Dawley rats, liver cells	Binding to DNA	–	NA	Rondahl *et al.* (1985)
D	BVD	Retinyl acetate by gavage for 7 days (80 mg/kg bw)	[^{3}H]BP, single i.p. injection (2 mg/kg bw)	Sprague–Dawley rats, hepatocytes	Binding to DNA	(+)	80 mg/kg bw (ID27)	McCarthy *et al.* (1987)
D	BVD	Retinyl acetate by gavage for 7 days (80 mg/kg bw)	[^{3}H]BP, single i.p. injection (2 mg/kg bw)	Sprague–Dawley rats, stomach cells	Binding to DNA	(+)	80 mg/kg bw (ID32)	McCarthy *et al.* (1987)
D	BVD	Retinyl acetate by gavage for 7 days(80 mg/kg bw)	[^{3}H]BP, single i.p. injection (2 mg/kg bw)	Sprague–Dawley rats, lung cells	Binding to DNA	–	NA	McCarthy *et al.* (1987)
D	BVD	Retinyl acetate by gavage for 7 days (80 mg/kg bw)	[^{3}H]BP, single i.p. injection (2 mg/kg bw)	Sprague–Dawley rats, kidney cells	Binding to DNA	–	NA	McCarthy *et al.* (1987)
D	BVD	Retinoic acid (50 μg topical)	(7S,8S)-Dihydroxy-7,8-dihydrobenzo[*a*]pyrene, topical (200 nmol) + TPA, topical (10 nmol)	CD-1 mice, skin cells	Binding to DNA [(–) *anti*-BPDE-dG adducts]	+	50 μg (ID50)	Marnett & Ji (1994)
D	BVD	Retinoic acid (50 μg topical)	(7S,8S)-Dihydroxy-7,8-dihydrobenzo[*a*]pyrene, topical (200 nmol) + TPA, topical (10 nmol)	CD-1 mice, skin cells	Binding to DNA [(+)*syn*-BPDE-dG adducts]	–	NA	Marnett & Ji (1994)
D	BVD	Retinyl acetate p.o. for 2 weeks (328 mg/kg diet)	DMBA, single gavage administration (25 mg/kg bw)	Sprague–Dawley rats, mammary cells	Binding to DNA	(+)	328 mg/kg diet (ID30)	Amagase *et al.* (1996)

Table 25 (contd)

End-point	Code[a]	Modulator (administration schedule and tested doses)[b]	Genotoxic agent (administration schedule and tested doses)[b]	Animal strains and species, and cells	Investigated effect	Result[c]	Inhibitory dose (IDx)[d]	Reference
D	BVD	Retinol by gavage for 7 days (100 mg/kg bw/day)	Ochratoxin A single gavage administration (2 mg/kg bw)	Swiss mice, kidney cells	Binding to DNA	+	100 mg/kg bw (ID59)	Grosse *et al.* (1997)
D	DVA	Retinyl palmitate p.o. for 8 weeks (5–500 IU/g diet)	Aflatoxin B_1, single i.p. injection (1 mg/kg bw)	Sprague–Dawley rats, hepatocytes	Single-strand breaks	(+)	5 IU/g diet (ID65)	Decoudu *et al.* (1992)
D	DVA	Vitamin A [unspecified] p.o. from day 7 of pregnancy to day 10 post delivery (90 IU)	DMBA, single dose by gavage in the female offspring (80 mg/kg bw), and phenobarbital, single dose by gavage 24 hours earlier (60 mg/kg bw)	Sprague–Dawley rats, liver cells	Single-strand breaks	+	90 IU (ID66)	Bolognesi *et al.* (1992)
D	DVA	Vitamin A [unspecified] p.o. from day 7 of pregnancy to day 10 post delivery (90 IU)	DMBA, single dose by gavage in the female offspring (80 mg/kg bw)	Sprague–Dawley rats, liver cells	Single-strand breaks	(+)	90 IU (ID39)	Bolognesi *et al.* (1992)
D	DVA	Vitamin A [unspecified] p.o. from day 7 of pregnancy to day 10 post delivery (90 IU)	DMBA , single dose by gavage in the female offspring (80 mg/kg bw), and phenobarbital, single dose by gavage 24 hours earlier (60 mg/kg bw)	Sprague–Dawley rats, mammary gland cells	Single-strand breaks	+	90 IU (ID54)	Bolognesi *et al.* (1992)
D	DVA	Vitamin A [unspecified] p.o. from day 7 of pregnancy to day 10 post delivery (90 IU)	DMBA, single dose by gavage in the female offspring (80 mg/kg bw)	Sprague–Dawley rats, mammary gland cells	Single-strand breaks	+	90 IU (ID50)	Bolognesi *et al.* (1992)
D	DVA	Vitamin A [unspecified] p.o. from day 7 of pregnancy to day 10 post delivery (90 IU)	MNU, single dose by gavage in the female offspring (50 mg/kg bw), and phenobarbital, single dose by gavage 24 hours earlier (60 mg/kg bw)	Sprague–Dawley rats, liver cells	Single-strand breaks	–	NA	Bolognesi *et al.* (1992)

Table 25 (contd)

End-point	Code[a]	Modulator (administration schedule and tested doses)[b]	Genotoxic agent (administration schedule and tested doses)[b]	Animal strains and species, and cells	Investigated effect	Result[c]	Inhibitory dose (IDx)[d]	Reference
D	DVA	Vitamin A [unspecified] p.o. from day 7 of pregnancy to day 10 post delivery (90 IU)	MNU single dose by gavage in the female offspring (50 mg/kg bw), and phenobarbital, single dose by gavage 24 hours earlier (60 mg/kg bw)	Sprague–Dawley rats, mammary gland cells	Single-strand breaks	–	NA	Bolognesi *et al.* (1992)
D	DVA	Retinyl palmitate p.o. for 2 weeks after 9 weeks on a vitamin A deficient diet (50-100 IU/day)	Aflatoxin B_1, single i.p. injection (7 mg/kg bw)	Wistar rats, hepatocytes	Single-strand breaks	(+)	100 IU/day (ID15)	Webster *et al.* (1996)
D	DVA	Retinyl palmitate p.o. for 2 weeks (50–100 IU/day)	*N*-Nitrosodimethylamine single i.p. injection (10 mg/kg bw)	Wistar rats, hepatocytes	Single-strand breaks	(+)	100 IU/day (ID20)	Webster *et al.* (1996)
S	SVA	Retinyl acetate p.o. for 10 weeks (20 mg/kg diet)	Aflatoxin B_1 single s.c. injection (16–32 mg/kg bw)	C57BL/6J mice, bone marrow cells	Sister chromatid exchanges	+	20 mg/kg diet (ID70)	Qin & Huang (1986)
S	SVA	Retinyl acetate p.o. for 10 weeks (20 mg/kg diet)	BP single i.p. injection (200–400 mg/kg bw)	C57BL/6J mice, bone marrow cells	Sister chromatid exchanges	-	NA	Qin & Huang (1986)
S	SVA	Retinyl acetate p.o. for 10 weeks (20 mg/kg diet)	Cyclophosphamide single i.p. injection (8–16 mg/kg bw)	C57BL/6J mice, bone marrow cells	Sister chromatid exchanges	–	NA	Qin & Huang (1986)
M	MVM	Retinyl palmitate by gavage, twice a week for 7 weeks (32 mg/kg bw)	Cyclophosphamide single i.p. injection (10–50 mg/kg bw)	NMRI mice, bone marrow cells	Micronuclei	–	NA	Busk *et al.* (1984)
M	MVM	Vitamin A [unspecified], single oral administration (150 IU)	BP, single oral administration (75 mg/kg bw) 1 hour before vitamin A	Swiss albino mice, bone marrow cells	Micronuclei	+	150 IU (ID100)	Rao *et al.* (1986)
M	MVM	Retinyl palmitate by gavage for 14 weeks (132 IU/kg bw/day)	Aflatoxin B_1 by gavage for 14 weeks (0.05 µg/kg bw/day)	Swiss albino mice, erythrocytes from bone marrow	Micronuclei	+	132 IU/kg bw/day (ID66)	Sinha & Kumari (1994)

Table 25 (contd)

End-point	Code[a]	Modulator (administration schedule and tested doses)[b]	Genotoxic agent (administration schedule and tested doses)[b]	Animal strains and species, and cells	Investigated effect	Result[c]	Inhibitory dose (IDx)[d]	Reference
M	MVR	Retinyl palmitate p.o. for 5 weeks (20 000 U/kg diet)	4-(Methylnitrosamino)-1-(3-pyridyl)-1-butanone, single i.p. injection (25–100 mg/kg bw), followed by partial hepatectomy	Fischer rats, hepatocytes	Micronuclei	+	20,000 U/kg diet (ID95)	Alaoui–Jamali *et al.* (1991b)
C	CBA	Retinol, single gavage administration (1–25 mg/kg bw)	Busulfan (myleran), single gavage administration (50 mg/kg bw)	Chinese hamsters, bone marrow cells	Chromosomal aberrations	–	NA	Renner (1985)
C	CBA	Retinol, single gavage administration (1–25 mg/kg bw)	Cyclophosphamide, single gavage administration (20 mg/kg bw)	Chinese hamsters, bone marrow cells	Chromosomal aberrations	–	NA	Renner (1985)
C	CBA	Retinol, single gavage administration (1–25 mg/kg bw)	Thio-TEPA, single gavage administration (10 mg/kg bw)	Chinese hamsters, bone marrow cells	Chromosomal aberrations	–	NA	Renner (1985)
C	CBA	Retinol, single gavage administration (1–25 mg/kg bw)	Methyl methanesulfonate, single gavage administration (40 mg/kg bw)	Chinese hamsters, bone marrow cells	Chromosomal aberrations	–	NA	Renner (1985)
C	CBA	Retinyl palmitate by gavage for 14 weeks (132 IU/kg bw/day)	Aflatoxin B_1 by gavage for 14 weeks (0.05 μg/kg bw/day)	Swiss albino mice, bone marrow cells	Chromosomal aberrations	+	132 IU/kg bw/day (ID73)	Sinha & Kumari (1994)
C	CBA	Retinyl palmitate by gavage for 14 days (132 IU/kg bw/day)	Ochratoxin by gavage for 14 days (1 μg/kg bw)	Swiss albino mice, bone marrow cells	Chromosomal aberrations	+	132 IU/kg bw/day (ID68)	Kumari & Sinha (1994)
C	CCC	Retinyl palmitate by gavage for 14 weeks (132 IU/kg bw/day)	Aflatoxin B_1 by gavage for 14 weeks (0.05 μg/kg bw/day)	Swiss albino mice, primary spermatocytes	Chromosomal aberrations	+	132 IU/kg bw/day (ID85)	Sinha & Kumari (1994)
C	CCC	Retinyl palmitate by gavage for 14 days (132 IU/kg bw/day)	Ochratoxin by gavage for 14 days (1 μg/kg bw)	Swiss albino mice, primary spermatocytes	Chromosomal aberrations	+	132 IU/kg bw/day (ID67)	Kumari & Sinha (1994)

[a] See Appendix 2.

[b] Doses of compounds are as reported by the authors

[c] +, inhibition of the investigated end-point (≥ID50) ; *(+), weak inhibition of the investigated end-point ≤ID50); –, no inhibition of the investigated end-point*

[d] IDx, dose inhibiting the x % of the investigated end-point; NA, not applicable.

Abbreviations: BP, benzo[*a*]pyrene; BPDE, benzo[*a*]pyrene diol epoxide; DMBA, 7,12-dimethylbenz[*a*]anthracene; MNU, *N*-methylnitrosourea; TPA, 12-*O*-tetradecanoylphorbol 13-acetate

24 h before killing. The levels of DNA adducts, most of which were identified as the *anti*-dG adduct, were significantly decreased in rats receiving the retinyl acetate-supplemented diet compared with rats fed the basal diet. Moreover, a further significant decrease in DNA adducts was observed following combined treatment with retinyl acetate and either garlic (20 g/kg diet) or garlic plus selenite (0.5 mg/kg diet) (Amagase *et al.*, 1996). A single administration by gavage of the mycotoxin ochratoxin resulted in the formation of 13 distinct DNA adducts in kidney cells of Swiss mice, as detected by ^{32}P-postlabelling. Pretreatment of mice with retinol by gavage for seven days caused a significant decrease in total adduct levels. In particular, seven adducts were markedly decreased and five adducts were no longer detectable, the major adduct being the only one which was unaffected in retinol-pretreated mice (Grosse *et al.*, 1997).

In a rat liver bioassay with initiation by *N*-nitrosodiethylamine (DEN) and promotion by polybrominated biphenyls, feeding 200 IU retinyl acetate/g of diet from day 7 to day 180 (end of study) decreased the number and volume of γ-glutamyltranspeptidase-positive foci, compared with the group given a low dose (2 IU/g of diet). Only the difference in percentage of volume occupied by foci between the high- and low-dose groups was significant (Rezabek *et al.*, 1989).

In a rat liver assay for foci of hepatocellular alterations with DEN initiation and 2-acetylaminofluorene promotion, retinyl acetate given as an intragastric dose of 10 mg/kg bw every other day throughout the study did not decrease the number and mean size of γ-glutamyltranspeptidase-positive foci compared with controls (Moreno *et al.*, 1995).

Two groups of 20 male weanling albino Wistar rats (Cpb/WU) were given intraperitoneal injections of 30 mg/kg bw azaserine at 19 days of age. Twelve days after initiation, the animals were fed a semisynthetic diet (AIN-based) high in saturated fat (20% lard) without (controls) or with 100 IU of retinyl acetate and retinyl palmitate (50:50 ratio). Four months after initiation, all animals were killed and the number and size of acidophilic foci were determined. The area as % of pancreas occupied by acidophilic focus tissue was significantly lower ($p < 0.05$) in the group maintained on the diet supplemented with retinyl acetate/retinyl palmitate (Woutersen & van-Garderen-Hoetmer, 1988).

Administration of retinyl palmitate in the diet significantly attenuated the induction of DNA single-strand breaks, as assessed by alkaline elution assay, in hepatocytes of Sprague-Dawley rats receiving a single intraperitoneal injection of aflatoxin B_1 (Decoudu *et al.*, 1992) and in hepatocytes of Wistar rats receiving single intraperitoneal injections of aflatoxin B_1 and *N*-nitrosodimethylamine (Webster *et al.*, 1996). Using the same technique, vitamin A [unspecified], given to Sprague-Dawley rats during embryonal and fetal life, gave protection against the induction of DNA single-strand breaks in liver and mammary gland cells of the female progeny treated by gavage with a single dose of DMBA. However, no protective effect was observed in rats treated with MNU (Bolognesi *et al.*, 1992).

Qin and Huang (1986) compared the ability of retinyl acetate, given in the diet for 10 weeks, to decrease the frequency of sister chromatid exchanges in bone marrow cells of C57BL/6J mice treated with either aflatoxin B_1, BP or cyclophosphamide by intraperitoneal injection. Administration of retinyl acetate yielded a concentration of 274 μg vitamin A per g liver, versus 38 μg/g in control mice. A protective effect was only observed towards aflatoxin B_1 (Busk *et al.*, 1984). A lack of modulation of sister chromatid exchanges induced by cyclophosphamide was also observed in bone marrow cells of NMRI mice receiving retinyl palmitate by gavage, twice a week for seven weeks, before the intraperitoneal injection of this cytostatic drug (Busk *et al.*, 1984). Conversely, oral retinyl palmitate produced a significant decrease in micronuclei in peripheral blood erythrocytes of Swiss albino mice co-treated by gavage with aflatoxin B_1 (Sinha & Kumari, 1994) in bone marrow cells of Swiss albino mice receiving BP orally (Rao *et al.*, 1986), and in hepatocytes of Fischer rats receiving an intraperitoneal injection of 4-(*N*-nitrosomethylamino)-1-(3-pyridyl)-1-butanone

(NNK), followed by partial hepatectomy (Alaoui-Jamali *et al.*, 1991b).

In Chinese hamsters, a single administration of retinol by gavage did not significantly affect the increased frequency of chromosomal aberrations induced in bone marrow cells either by the simultaneous administration by gavage of busulfan or cyclophosphamide, or administration by gavage of aziridine 1,1′,1″-phosphinothioylidynetris (thiotepa) 2 h later, or intraperitoneal injection of methyl methanesulfonate 6 h later (Renner, 1985). Retinyl palmitate decreased the induction of chromosomal aberrations in bone marrow cells and spermatocytes of Swiss albino mice co-treated by gavage with either ochratoxin for 14 days (Kumari & Sinha, 1994) or aflatoxin B_1 for 14 weeks (Sinha & Kumari, 1994). In both studies, retinyl palmitate also decreased the frequency of spermatozoa showing abnormal head morphology due to treatment with these mycotoxins.

4.2.3 In-vitro models

4.2.3.1 Modulation of cell proliferation and differentiation

Most studies of cell proliferation and differentiation have been carried out with malignant cells and few with normal cells or immortalized cells. None of these cell systems is an optimal representative of premalignant cells. Therefore, the findings cannot be related directly to cellular processes that are modulated during carcinogenesis or during chemoprevention. Nonetheless, the findings point to possible mechanisms that might mediate effects on chemoprevention *in vivo*.

Vitamin A (retinol) can be converted to several classes of active metabolites: retinoic acids (all-*trans*-retinoic acid, that can be isomerized to 9-*cis*-retinoic acid and 13-*cis*-retinoic acid), 4-oxoretinol, and two retro-retinoids, anhydroretinol and 14-hydroxy-4,14-retro-retinol (14-HRR). All of these metabolites exert distinct effects on the growth, differentiation and apoptosis of various normal and malignant cells in culture.

Lotan and Nicolson (1977) described the ability of retinyl acetate and retinoic acid, both at 10 μmol/L, to inhibit the proliferation of a large number types of untransformed, transformed and malignant rodent and human cells in culture. The susceptible cell lines represented many different histological tumour types such as neuroblastoma, sarcoma, melanoma, mammary carcinoma, lymphoma, myeloma and lymphosarcoma. The sensitivity to the retinoids was independent of the type of transforming agent used to derive some of the rodent cell lines, including chemical carcinogens such as BP, MCA, DMBA, mineral oil, polyoma virus, Abelson leukaemia virus, or spontaneous transformation. Retinyl acetate was usually less potent than retinoic acid. Subsequent studies with selected cell lines demonstrated that the growth-inhibitory effects were dose- and time-dependent and were reversible upon removal of the retinoid from the medium (Lotan *et al.*, 1978). Because initial studies demonstrated that retinyl acetate was less potent in inhibition of cell growth than retinoic acid, most subsequent studies have employed the acid metabolite. However, this section describes only studies with retinol and retinyl esters, typically at pharmacological doses. The cells that have been analysed for response to retinol addition or removal from the growth medium include primary cultures (e.g., epidermal keratinocytes), immortalized cells (e.g., keratinocytes transfected with human papillomavirus E6 or SV40 T antigen) and malignant cells (e.g., established tumour cell lines). The type of effects that retinol exerted on the cells included modulation of cell proliferation and differentiation.

(a) Epidermal keratinocytes and squamous carcinoma cells

Exposure of primary cultures of mouse epidermal keratinocytes to retinyl acetate inhibits cell proliferation and suppresses squamous cell differentiation. The differentiation of cells treated with 40 μmol/L retinyl acetate was suppressed. Treated cells exhibited prolonged survival despite the inhibition of proliferation, due to a reduced rate of cell death. Such death normally follows squamous cell differentiation in culture (Yuspa *et al.*, 1977). Similarly, retinol inhibited calcium-induced stratification and terminal differentiation with keratinization in confluent culture of cutaneous keratinocytes from the newborn rat. The addition of retinol to the medium enhanced features characteristic of the secretory epithelium, such as formation of an extensive endoplasmic reticulum, enlargement of the Golgi zone and an increase in the number of vacuoles. Thus, retinol redirected epithelial differentiation from a stratifying and keratinizing epithelium towards a secretory epithelium (Brown *et al.*, 1985).

Treatment of mouse epidermal keratinocytes with retinyl acetate affected several parameters presumed to be important in chemical carcinogenesis (Yuspa *et al.*, 1977). Whereas the activity of constitutive aryl hydrocarbon hydroxylase (AHH) was not significantly affected after exposure to retinyl acetate, the level of AHH induced by BP was reduced to 20% of that in controls. Further, in the presence of retinyl acetate, binding of DMBA to epidermal cell DNA was markedly decreased.

Retinyl acetate stimulated the outgrowth of human epidermal keratinocytes in primary skin cultures. Treated cultures exhibited higher mitotic index, higher labelling index and a larger growth fraction than control cultures. In addition, the number of keratohyaline granules in treated cultures decreased, indicating an effect on the differentiation process, although there was no evidence of mucous metaplasia (Chopra & Flaxman, 1975). The effects of retinol on the differentiation of various keratinocytes were defined in cellular and molecular terms by the studies of Fuchs and Green (1981) and Green and Watt (1982), who established that endogenous retinol present in the serum, when added to the growth medium, affects the differentiation of cultured keratinocytes derived from skin and from other stratified squamous epithelia. The removal of retinol from serum causes a reduction in cell motility, an increase in cell adhesiveness and inhibition of pattern formation. Further, removal of vitamin A leads to synthesis of a 67 kDa keratin characteristic of terminally differentiating epidermis and to much reduced synthesis of the 52 kDa and 40 kDa keratins typical of conjunctiva. The addition of retinyl acetate to the medium restored cell motility and pattern formation and enhanced the detachment of the most mature cells from the surface of the stratified epithelium. In addition, the production of the 67 kDa keratin was prevented and the synthesis of the 40 and 52 kDa keratins was stimulated. The formation of cross-linked envelopes, which occurs during the last stage of terminal differentiation, was inhibited by the addition of retinyl acetate.

Whereas the above studies used normal keratinocytes in short-term culture, a few studies have used immortalized keratinocytes as a model for premalignant cells *in vitro*. Two approaches have been successful for the immortalization technique, one using a recombinant retrovirus encoding the simian virus 40 (SV40) large T-antigen (Agarwal & Eckert 1990) and the other involving transfection of various normal human keratinocyte cell strains with human papillomavirus type 16 (HPV-16) DNA (Pirisi *et al.*, 1992). The SV40-T-immortalized human keratinocyte cells (cell line KER-1) do not form colonies in soft agar and are non-tumorigenic. The pattern of keratin gene expression in non-immortalized and KER-1 cells is similar, except that KER-1 cells express keratin 7 (K7), which is not expressed by non-immortalized keratinocytes. Incubation with retinol (0.2 or 2 µmol/L) results in a 40-fold increase in K7 expression in KER-1 cells. The formation of cross-linked cornified envelopes is reduced by retinol in both non-immortalized keratinocytes and KER-1 cells, without affecting the level of the envelope precursor, involucrin (Agarwal & Eckert 1990). Thus, the response of 'premalignant' keratinocytes to retinol is similar to that of normal cells in terms of modulation of differentiation.

Comparison of normal human foreskin keratinocytes (HKc) and four HPV16-immortalized HKc lines revealed that all the immortalized lines were 10- to 100-fold more sensitive than normal HKc to growth inhibition by retinol in both clonal and mass culture growth assays. In addition, the immortalized cell lines were more sensitive to modulation of keratin expression by retinol, despite a similar rate of uptake of [^{3}H]retinol by normal and immortalized cells. Retinoic acid, which can be formed from retinol in skin keratinocytes (Siegenthaler, 1990), also inhibited the growth of immortalized cells preferentially and, further, was found to reduce the expression of the HPV-16 open reading frames of E2, E5, E6 and E7 two- to four-fold. These results suggest that the increased sensitivity of the immortalized cell lines to growth control by retinol and retinoic acid may be mediated by inhibition of the expression of HPV-16 oncogene products which are required for the maintenance of continuous growth (Pirisi *et al.*, 1992; Creek *et al.*, 1994). Retinoic acid treatment (1 nmol/L) of normal HKc, during or immediately following transfection with HPV-16 DNA, inhibited immortalization by about 95%. Overall, these results point to a possible biochemical basis for a role of dietary retinoids in chemoprevention of HPV-induced cancers (Creek *et al.*, 1994).

The antiproliferative and differentiation-suppressing effects of retinyl acetate have also been demonstrated in fully malignant epidermal keratinocyte cell lines (e.g., SCC-13), derived from human squamous cell carcinomas (Cline & Rice, 1983). The competence to form cross-linked envelopes in confluent SCC-13 cell cultures, which was about 50% in medium without retinyl acetate supplementation, was reduced to 10% after addition of retinyl acetate. A similar reduction was observed in the levels of involucrin. The results suggest that some potential differentiated character of malignant keratinocytes may be suppressed by vitamin A. During carcinogenesis, there is a loss of differentiation potential, which is apparent after the removal of vitamin A from the medium, as the maximal degree of differentiation attained by SCC cells is lower than that of normal keratinocytes (Kim *et al.*, 1984). Still, the SCC cells respond to changes in vitamin A levels in the medium, as shown by the altered expression of 67-kDa and 40-kDa keratins in SCCs from tongue and epidermis. When the vitamin A concentration in the medium was raised, the expression of the 40-kDa keratin increased. Conversely, a reduction in the amount of vitamin A led to increased expression of the 67-kDa keratin and the cells underwent stratification and terminal differentiation (Kim *et al.*, 1984).

(b) Normal and malignant airway epithelial cells

Extensive studies have been carried out with organ cultures and with normal bronchial epithelial cells derived from rat, rabbit, hamster, monkey and human trachea. These have demonstrated that vitamin A is required for the maintenance of proper differentiation *in vitro*. For example, the expression of a normal mucocilary epithelium in explants of rat trachea required supplementation with retinyl acetate. The explants secreted mucous glycoproteins into the medium and the production of the mucins was dependent upon the vitamin A status of the explant. In the absence of vitamin A (serum-free medium), the explants underwent a metaplastic change to a keratinizing squamous epithelium. The addition of 0.1, 2 or 10 μg retinyl acetate per mL of medium stimulated mucin synthesis within 24 hours which continued throughout the 21-day exposure period in a concentration-dependent fashion. The keratinizing squamous epithelium began to revert to a mucus-secreting tissue as early as 24 hours after addition of 10 μg retinyl acetate to the medium. The response was slower with the lower vitamin concentrations (Clark & Marchok 1979; Clark *et al.*, 1980). Studies with two carcinoma cell lines (T8 and 100 WT), derived from a mucus-secreting adenocarcinoma and a keratinizing squamous cell carcinoma, respectively, revealed that retinyl acetate added to medium at 6.6 and 33 μmol/L inhibited cell growth by 25 and 50%, respectively. Retinyl acetate also induced characteristics of secretory cells in the 100 WT squamous cells and enhanced these features in the T8 cells. This effect was evidenced by an increase in the synthesis and secretion of mucins and reduction of cell stratification (Marchok *et al.*, 1981).

Organ cultures of tracheas from hamsters fed a vitamin A-deficient diet underwent squamous metaplasia and keratinization. Retinyl acetate reversed these metaplastic changes (Clamon *et al.*, 1974; Newton *et al.*, 1980). This organ culture was used to screen numerous retinoids for reversal of keratinization. The concentration required for 50% effectiveness (ED_{50}) was 0.7 nmol/L for retinol and 1 nmol/L for retinyl acetate. In contrast, retinoic acid and some synthetic retinoids had greater potency than retinol (e.g., ED_{50} < 0.03 nmol/L) (Newton *et al.*, 1980). Cigarette smoke condensate increased cell proliferation in hamster tracheal organ culture, whereas retinol suppressed this hyperplastic effect (Rutten *et al.*, 1988a).

Not only organ culture but also primary epithelial cells derived from hamster trachea have been studied for the effects of vitamin A and found to respond to vitamin A deficiency and supplementation in a similar fashion as in organ culture and *in vivo*. Thus, hamster tracheal epithelial cells maintained in primary culture in serum-free medium (vitamin A-deficient state) appeared squamous-like and stratified and produced a more complex keratin pattern (keratins 5–7, 8, 14, and 17–19) than cells cultured in vitamin A-supplemented medium, which formed a simple cuboidal epithelium and produced only four simple epithelial keratins (7, 8, 18 and 19) (Edmondson *et al.*, 1990). Further studies in this cell system have shown that hamster tracheal epithelial cells maintained in vitamin A-deficient medium had decreased expression of differentiation-related keratins (5, 6, 14 and 17) after exposure to the carcinogen BP. In contrast, cells maintained in medium containing 1 μmol/L retinol showed no effect of BP on the keratin expression pattern, indicating a protective effect of vitamin A (Edmondson & Mossman, 1991). Studies with primary hamster tracheal epithelial cells in serum-free, hormone-supplemented medium showed that cigarette smoke condensate inhibited dye-coupled intercellular communication between the epithelial cells, whereas retinol given to the cells at pharmacological concentrations concurrently with the condensate counteracted the inhibitory effect of cigarette smoke condensate on intercellular communication (Rutten *et al.*, 1988b). This observation suggests that maintenance of gap junctional communication by retinol may contribute to chemopreventive activity.

Wu and his colleagues investigated the effects of vitamin A on human and non-human primate tracheobronchial epithelium. They found that vitamin A inhibited the synthesis of keratins 5, 6, 14, 16 and 17 and stimulated keratins 7, 8, 10, 13, 15, 18 and 19 (Huang *et al.*, 1994) and also increased the production of hyaluronate (Wu & Wu, 1986). Optimal conditions for the expression of mucociliary function (ciliogenesis or mucin secretion) were achieved when early-passage human tracheobronchial cells were transplanted onto tracheal grafts, not onto plastic plates. Although cell attachment and proliferation were stimulated when tissue culture plates were coated with collagen gel, the expression of mucous cell function in culture occurred only when retinol was present in the medium (Wu *et al.*, 1990).

Different mechanisms mediate the effects of retinol on the levels of differentiation markers. Whereas the expression of a squamous cell marker, namely small proline-rich protein gene (*spr1*) (An *et al.*, 1993) and several keratins (Huang *et al.*, 1994) was down-regulated post-transcriptionally by retinol, the expression of mucin 2 (*MUC2*) gene was suppressed at the level of transcription (An *et al.*, 1994). The effects of retinol on the growth of human tracheobronchial epithelial cells in serum-free medium were variable, depending on the presence or absence of epidermal growth factor (EGF). In the absence of EGF, retinol caused a dose-dependent inhibition of growth, whereas in the presence of EGF, retinol was slightly growth-stimulatory (Miller *et al.*, 1993). Further studies suggested that the cells secreted a transforming growth factor (TGF)-α-like mitogen in the absence of retinol and that retinol suppressed the production of this factor (Miller *et al.*, 1993). Retinol also suppressed the growth of a cell line derived from human fetal lung in collagen gel culture (Emura *et al.*, 1988).

Only a few studies have analysed the effects of vitamin A on distal airway epithelial cells. These cells exhibit extensive proliferative capacity and have the potential to differentiate into mucociliary or epidermoid phenotype. Small amounts of serum induce undifferentiated cells to become ciliated and non-ciliated secretory cells, whereas they differentiate into epidermoid cells in retinol-free or serum-free medium (Kitamura *et al.*, 1990). Shibagaki and co-workers (1994) found that retinol enhanced the outgrowth of epithelial cells from explants of human peripheral lung tissue at 0.01 and 0.1 μmol/L, whereas 10 μmol/L retinol inhibited the growth. However, long-term growth on a plastic surface was suppressed by retinol even at 0.1 μmol/L. The efficiency of colony formation by these epithelial cells on a fibroblast feeder layer was reduced by retinol at both 0.1 and 10 μmol/L. DNA synthesis was also inhibited by retinol. These findings highlight the role of retinol in regulating the proliferation and differentiation of tracheobronchial and distal lung epithelial cells, which may be the basis for the chemopreventive effects of retinyl palmitate *in vivo* in animal models (Saffiotti *et al.*, 1967) and human patients (Pastorino *et al.*, 1993).

Most lung cancer cell lines examined are resistant to growth inhibition by retinoids (Geradts *et al.*, 1993). However, a two-day pretreatment with retinyl acetate inhibited the migration and invasion of A549 human lung carcinoma cells *in vitro* through a human amnion basement membrane and the degradation of proline-labelled basement membrane components by 50% at non-cytotoxic concentrations of 0.09 and 3 μg/mL, respectively. This effect was accompanied by a significant decrease in type IV collagenase activity without a change in tissue transglutaminase activity. These findings suggest that retinol may suppress the expression of invasive phenotype in carcinoma *in situ* and thereby might prevent the development of a malignant lesion from a premalignant one (Fazely *et al.*, 1988).

Effects of vitamin A on normal and malignant oral cavity epithelial cells have not been investigated extensively, although animal studies have demonstrated chemopreventive effects of retinoids (Shklar *et al.*, 1980; Inoue *et al.*, 1993) and clinical trials have demonstrated that premalignant lesions and second primary tumours in the head and neck regions are prevented by 13-*cis*-retinoic acid (Hong *et al.*, 1995). Nonetheless, retinyl acetate caused a 50% reduction in the survival rate of a human tongue cancer cell line (Inoue *et al.*, 1995) and a maxillary cancer cell line (Yamamoto *et al.*, 1996) in a colony-forming assay in monolayer cell cultures at concentrations of 60 and 28 μg/mL, respectively. Cell cycle analysis demonstrated an increase in G_0/G_1 phase in the presence of vitamin A, which indicated that growth inhibition may be the result of suppression of DNA synthesis. Effects on squamous differentiation were noted in head and neck squamous carcinoma cell line 1483. Cells grown in delipidized serum depleted of endogenous retinoids expressed keratins with molecular weights of 67, 56, 54, 52, 48, 46 and 40 kDa (Poddar *et al.*, 1991). In contrast, cells grown in medium with 10% fetal bovine serum, which contained about 0.06 μmol/L retinol, expressed much less 67 kDa keratin, whereas the levels of keratins of molecular weight 46 and 48 kDa were lower and the amounts of the 52 and the 40 kDa keratins were higher than those expressed in cells grown in delipidized serum. Thus, vitamin A present in serum modulated the expression of several keratins in the 1483 cells (Poddar *et al.*, 1991).

(c) Normal and malignant leukocytes

Retinol or retinyl acetate modulate the proliferation and differentiation of normal and malignant haematopoietic cells. Retinyl acetate (3 μmol/L) stimulated clonal growth of committed myeloid stem cells from normal human bone marrow to form colonies of granulocytes and/or macrophages in soft agar in the presence but not in the absence of colony-stimulating activity factor (CSF). These retinoids potentiated the response of the stem cells to the growth factor CSF. Interestingly, at 30 μmol/L all these retinoids inhibited colony formation (Douer & Koeffler, 1982).

B-cells deprived of retinol in cell culture die within days by a process that is neither classical apoptosis nor the result of cell cycle arrest. The cells can be rescued by physiological concentrations of retinol and retinal, but not by retinoic acid. Retinol is not metabolized to retinoic acid in these cells. However, it is converted into several metabolites, one of which has the ability to sustain B-cell growth in the absence of an external source of retinol (Buck *et al.*, 1990, 1991b). The active metabolite of retinol in B-lymphocytes and other cell lines is 14-HRR and it mediates the effect of retinol on cell growth (Buck *et al.*, 1991a). Thus, a distinct retinoid signalling pathway may regulate the growth of some cells. In addition to being an essential cofactor for growth of B-lymphocytes in culture, retinol is also required for activation of T-lymphocytes by antigen receptor-mediated signals. 14-HRR has been implicated as the intracellular mediator of this effect. Anhydroretinol, a retinol metabolite derivative with a retro-structure produced in activated human B-lymphocytes, reversibly inhibits retinol- and 14-HRR-dependent effects and blocks B-lymphocyte proliferation as well as activation of resting T-lymphocytes (Buck *et al.*, 1993). Anhydroretinol given to T-cells in the absence of 14-HRR induces rapid cell death which does not require messenger RNA and protein synthesis. The data suggest that retro-retinoids act in the cytoplasm as second messengers like diacyl glycerol or ceramide and do not require modulation of gene expression by nuclear retinoid receptors (O'Connell *et al.*, 1996).

Breitman and his collaborators have demonstrated that retinoic acid (1 μmol/L, 6 days) can induce the differentiation of >90% of HL-60 myeloid leukaemia cells into granulocytes. Retinol and retinyl acetate at the same concentration caused <20% of HL-60 cells to differentiate. In contrast, 0.1 μmol/L of retinoic acid induced the differentiation of 50% of the cells (Breitman *et al.*, 1980). In HL-60 myeloid leukaemia cells, retinol is metabolized to 14-HRR, anhydroretinol, retinoic acid and retinyl esters. Exogenous application of the retinol metabolites in retinol-depleted serum-free cultures of HL-60 allowed the identification of unique cellular functions for each metabolite: 14-HRR is a growth factor for HL-60; anhydroretinol is a functional antagonist of 14-HRR with growth-inhibiting activity, and retinoic acid is a potent inducer of granulocyte differentiation accompanied by growth arrest (Eppinger *et al.*, 1993).

Retinol–RBP and chylomicron remnant retinyl esters in concentrations normally found in human plasma inhibit growth of normal human B-lymphocytes. Physiological concentrations of retinoic acid (about 30 nmol/L) were less active than physiological concentrations of retinol (about 3 μmol/L). Pharmacological concentrations of retinol and retinoic acid were more active than the concentrations normally found in plasma. Retinol (3 μmol/L) inhibited anti-IgM-mediated DNA synthesis by 78%. Furthermore, cells were blocked in the mid-G_1 phase of the cell cycle. The late activation markers (transferrin receptor expression and actinomycin D staining at 48 hours of stimulation) were markedly inhibited. After 48 h, retinol also reduced the interleukin-6 production that was induced either by anti-IgM or by interleukin-4. Retinoids reduced the formation of plaque-forming cells (i.e., Ig synthesis) (Blomhoff *et al.*, 1992).

(d) Untransformed and transformed fibroblasts

The anchorage-independent growth of human fibroblasts induced by platelet-derived growth factor (PDGF) or by basic fibroblast growth factor (bFGF) was inhibited by physiological concentrations of either retinol (0.5 μmol/L) or retinoic acid (1.0 nmol/L), but not by anhydroretinol (0.5 μmol/L). Retinol also reduced the frequency of anchorage-independent growth of the human fibrosarcoma-derived cell line, HT1080, which formed colonies in semi-solid medium without added growth factors. These results suggest that physiologically active retinoids suppress properties associated with transformation (Palmer *et al.*, 1989).

Treatment of postconfluent cultures of C3H 10T1/2 mouse fibroblasts with certain carcinogens has been shown to cause transformation to focus-forming cells. The development of this in-vitro cell transformation system has enabled investigators to examine the ability of vitamin A to intervene in such transformation. Retinyl acetate was found to be highly active in inhibition of MCA-induced neoplastic transformation of C3H 10T1/2 cells. When MCA-treated cultures were treated continuously with retinyl acetate (0.1 μg/mL), or for 24 hours with 2.5 μg/mL starting seven days after MCA exposure, or after delaying retinyl acetate treatment up to three weeks after MCA exposure, neoplastic transformation was inhibited by 100%, 70% and 80% respectively (Merriman & Bertram, 1979). The efficacy of retinol and retinal in this system was similar to that of retinyl acetate. The ability of retinyl acetate to inhibit transformation even when added one week after the carcinogen excluded an effect on carcinogen metabolism, on the initiation phase of carcinogenesis or on the fixation of the carcinogenic damage. The effect of retinyl acetate on transformation was reversible, as transformed foci began to appear after the retinoid was removed for three to five weeks, suggesting that, when present, retinyl acetate suppressed the progression of preneoplastic cells to fully neoplastic cells. Further, fully transformed cell lines derived from cultures exposed to MCA appeared to be resistant to growth inhibition by retinyl acetate (0.1 μg/mL) when cultured on confluent monolayers of 10T1/2 cells, suggesting that the effect of retinyl acetate in this system was limited to preneoplastic cells (Merriman & Bertram, 1979; Mordan *et al.*, 1982). Subsequent studies have demonstrated that retinyl acetate increased the degree of adhesion of C3H 10T1/2 cells to a plastic substrate (Bertram, 1980) and that their ability to communicate via gap junctions, which was reduced by exposure to MCA, was enhanced by retinyl acetate at the same concentrations that inhibited neoplastic transformation (Hossain *et al.*, 1989). More recently, it was found that retinoids induce the gap junctional protein connexin 43 (Rogers *et al.*, 1990). These observations suggest that the chemopreventive effects of retinoids may be explained partially by enhanced gap junctional communication.

Cultured C3H 10T1/2 cells transfected with the plasmid pdPBV-1 harbouring bovine papillomavirus (BPV) DNA were used for assessing *in vitro* the tumour-promoting and chemopreventive activities of various agents. The exposure of such cells to extracts of areca nut (used in betel quid), which have been linked to the high incidence of precancerous oral lesions and oral cancers in India, enhanced the formation of BPV DNA-induced transformed foci approximately tenfold. The addition of retinol to the areca nut extract inhibited its tumour-promoting effect in a dose-dependent manner, completely abolishing the promoting activity at a dose of 1 μmol/L. This effect was proposed to be one of the mechanisms by which vitamin A intake could reduce oral cancer incidence among chewers of areca nut/tobacco mixtures and of the chemopreventive effect of vitamin A administered to betel quid chewers (Stich & Tsang, 1989).

The transformation of C3H 10T1/2 mouse fibroblasts was shown to be induced in density-arrested initiated cells by PDGFs in serum and was correlated with the mitogenic response of the preneoplastic cells to PDGF or EGF. The stimulation of DNA synthesis and cell division in normal and carcinogen-treated C3H 10T1/2 fibroblasts by serum after density-dependent growth arrest was inhibited by retinyl acetate to the same extent that neoplastic transformation was inhibited by this retinoid. On the basis of these data, Mordan (1989) suggested that the inhibition of neoplastic transformation by retinol is the result of blocking the G_0 to G_1 transition in the mitotic response of initiated cells to platelet growth factors which act as autocrine or endogenous promoters of transformation.

(e) Mammary cancer cell lines

Several studies have demonstrated that vitamin A can modulate the proliferation and differentiation of rat and human mammary cancer cells. In a rat mammary cancer stem-like cell line (Rama 25), differentiation to alveolar-like cells is evidenced by the increase in production of domes (hemispheric blisters) in the cell monolayer and the appearance of immunoreactive casein in the tissue culture medium. This differentiation was enhanced by retinol and retinyl acetate (0.04 to 4 μmol/L) in the presence of the hormones prolactin, hydrocortisone, insulin and 17β-estradiol. These retinoids also caused a reduction in the rate of DNA synthesis. Pretreatment of the Rama 25 cells with retinyl acetate before injection into immunocompromised young female nu/nu (nude) mice decreased the incidence of tumours compared with injections of untreated cells. The findings suggest that the ability of retinoids to suppress rat mammary gland carcinogenesis may be due to their differentiation-inducing properties and their ability to suppress DNA synthesis (Rudland *et al.*, 1983). Indeed, Mehta and Moon (1980) observed suppression of DNA synthesis in mammary cells from rats exposed to DMBA or MNU and placed on a diet supplemented with retinyl acetate, as compared to cells from rats exposed to the carcinogens but fed a diet without retinyl acetate supplement. There was no effect of retinyl acetate on DNA synthesis in cells from rats that were not exposed to carcinogens, suggesting a selective effect on initiated or transformed cells.

Inhibition of the growth of human breast cancer cell lines by retinol has been reported by several groups. Ueda *et al.* (1980) observed a good correlation between the ability of retinol to inhibit cell proliferation and the synthesis of DNA (thymidine incorporation) in MCF-7 mammary carcinoma cells in culture, suggesting that suppression of DNA synthesis is the primary cause of cell growth inhibition. Other studies have shown that retinol inhibited the anchorage-dependent and anchorage-independent growth of the human mammary carcinoma cell line MDA-MB-231. Clones resistant to growth inhibition by retinol were isolated from this cell line in soft agar. Because the clones were still susceptible to growth inhibition by all-*trans*- and 13-*cis*-retinoic acid, it is possible that metabolism of retinol to all-*trans*-retinoic acid was absent in these cells (Halter *et al.*, 1990).

Although in many cell systems, retinol is metabolized to retinoic acid, which is presumed to be the ultimate mediator of the effects of retinol on gene expression and the changes in cell growth and differentiation that these lead to, there are cell types that do not metabolize retinol to retinoic acid. For example, retinoic acid inhibits the growth of 'normal' human breast epithelial cell strains AD074 and MCF10A and the estrogen receptor-positive (ER+) breast cancer cell lines MCF-7 and T47D. However, these cells do not metabolize retinol to retinoic acid, but instead form 4-oxoretinol. Interestingly, exogenous 4-oxoretinol inhibits the growth of these cells. Further, 4-oxoretinol also inhibits the growth of the ER– breast cancer lines MDA-MB-231, MDA-MB-468 and BT20, although these cells do not metabolize retinol to 4-oxoretinol (Chen *et al.*, 1997b). Because 4-oxoretinol has been shown to activate nuclear retinoic acid receptors to mediate gene transcription, it is possible that the growth inhibitory effects of both retinol and 4-oxoretinol are mediated by alterations in gene expression (Achkar *et al.*, 1996).

Some additional clues on the mechanism of breast cancer growth suppression by retinol have come from studies that showed that pretreatment of two human mammary carcinoma cell lines (retinoid-sensitive T47D and retinoid-resistant MDA-MB-468) for 48 hours with retinol resulted in inhibition of TGFα stimulation of growth. In the T47D cell line, the mechanism appeared to be loss of TGFα-induced stimulation of the EGF receptor substrate, phospholipase C-g 1. Alteration of phospholipase C-g 1 activity was not responsible for the inhibition of cell growth seen in the presence of retinol in the absence of TGFα stimulation. In the MDA-MB-468 cell line, pretreatment with retinol resulted in a decrease in tyrosine phosphorylation of the EGF receptor (Halter *et al.*, 1993). Thus, retinol may interfere with EGF receptor-mediated mitogenic signalling.

(f) Prostate cells

Mouse prostate gland exposed to MCA or maintained in organ culture in vitamin A-deficient medium undergoes hyperplasia and squamous metaplasia. These changes are reversed after addition of retinol to the medium and prevented in organ cultures exposed to both carcinogen and vitamin A (Lasnitzki, 1955, 1962; Lasnitzki & Goodman, 1974).

Retinoic acid was more effective in this organ culture system than retinol. In tissues, most of the endogenous retinoic acid is formed from retinol and could mediate the effects of vitamin A. Support for this conclusion comes from studies that demonstrated the ability of liarozole, an inhibitor of cytochrome P450 enzymes, to suppress keratinization of a rat prostate carcinoma. Further, *in vivo*, therapy with liarozole increases plasma and tissue levels of retinoic acid, which may be a contributing factor in its retinoid-mimetic effects. In the rat Dunning prostate cancer models, liarozole inhibited the growth of androgen-independent as well as androgen-dependent carcinomas relapsing after castration. Concurrently, changes in the pattern of cytokeratins characteristic of increased differentiation were observed (De Coster *et al.*, 1996). More importantly, liarozole inhibited *in vitro* the secretion of type IV collagenase and invasion through Matrigel in a Boyden chamber by the androgen-independent PC-3ML-B2 human prostatic carcinoma clone without inhibiting cell proliferation and cell attachment. *In vivo*, liarozole treatment increased the retinoic acid levels in tumours that developed in severe-combined immunodeficient (SCID) mice, blocked type IV collagenase production in established subcutaneous tumours and reduced the growth of bone metastases of the PC-3ML-B2 cells (Stearns *et al.*, 1993). All of these effects are presumed to be caused by the accumulation of retinoic acid derived from endogenous intracellular stores of vitamin A.

(g) Bladder cancer cells

Vitamin A deficiency in the rat has been reported to lead to rapid growth and keratinization *in vivo* and in organ culture, suggesting a role for vitamin A in the control of differentiation of bladder epithelial cells. Indeed, retinol increased the level of alkaline phosphatase, which is decreased in serum-depleted medium, but did not suppress hyperplasia (Reese & Politano, 1981). The rat Nara Bladder Tumor No. 2 (NBT II) cell line, established from a urinary bladder carcinoma in the Wistar rat, underwent squamous differentiation including the formation of keratin pearls when cultured as multicellular aggregates. Supplements of vitamin A in the form of retinyl palmitate (1 to 10 IU/mL) to the medium prevented keratinization but did not inhibit aggregate formation. Vitamin A also enhanced the number of cells engaged in DNA synthesis. The inhibition of keratinization was reversible; after vitamin A was removed from the medium, the cells in the aggregates resumed the process of keratinization (Toyoshima & Leighton, 1975; Tchao, 1980). The ability of retinol to prevent keratinization in six transformed rat bladder cell lines was related to the expression of cellular RBP (Kawamura & Hashimoto, 1980).

(h) Colon cancer cells

Retinyl palmitate at concentrations of 0.1 μmol/L and above decreased by about 80% DNA synthesis measured by thymidine incorporation after one day of treatment of a rat Prob colonic tumour cell line. The treatment also induced intestinal-type alkaline phosphatase expression, and increased slightly the proportion of floating apoptotic cells as indicated by DNA ladder formation and chromatin condensation (Maziere *et al.*, 1997).

Retinol added to freshly passaged cultures of FHC, a human colonic epithelial cell line, inhibited proliferation in dose-dependent fashion. Polyamine content, specifically the spermidine content and the spermidine/spermine ratio, decreased in response to culture with retinol, suggesting that ornithine decarboxylase (ODC) was inhibited (Higuchi & Wang, 1995). The same investigators also found that physiological concentrations of retinol stimulated the induction of NAD(P)H:quinone reductase, a phase II detoxifying enzyme, in human Colo205 colon carcinoma cell line (Wang & Higuchi, 1995). These findings suggest that anticarcinogenic effects of retinol in colon epithelium may be mediated by induction of detoxifying enzymes, decreased cell proliferation, enhanced differentiation and apoptosis.

(i) Transformed ovarian cells

Studies with Chinese hamster ovary cells have demonstrated that retinol blocks cell cycle progression in the G_1 phase of the cell cycle, and that there is a concentration-dependent inhibition of ODC induction. Retinol inhibited the induction of ODC activity only when added in the first 2–3 h of G_1 progression. Because polyamines required for normal cellular growth are produced by ODC, it was postulated that the antiproliferative properties of retinoids are related to their ability to inhibit ODC expression by inhibition of ODC mRNA synthesis (Russell & Haddox, 1981). This finding may be relevant also to suppression of carcinogenesis, because ODC is increased by tumour-promoting agents and suppressed by retinoids in mouse skin (Verma *et al.*, 1979) and in rat liver (Van Rooijen *et al.*, 1984).

(j) Embryonal teratocarcinoma cells

Retinol induced the differentiation of several mouse embryonal teratocarcinoma cell lines (certain F9, OC15S1 and Nulli-SCC1) in culture, albeit with a lower potency than retinoic acid (Eglitis & Sherman, 1983). However, its physiological concentration is also much higher than that of retinoic acid and therefore retinol may have an important function in modulating differentiation *in vivo*. Recently, it was found that F9 cells metabolize retinol to 4-oxoretinol and that the latter can activate nuclear retinoic acid receptors to enhance transcription of specific genes and thereby cause cell differentiation. This constitutes a novel pathway for signalling by retinol without metabolism to all-*trans*- or 9-*cis*-retinoic acid (Achkar *et al.*, 1996).

(k) Miscellaneous normal and tumour cells

Previous studies have demonstrated that retinoic acid can induce the expression of TGFβ *in vivo* in vitamin A-deficient rat tissues (Glick *et al.*, 1991). This finding suggested indirectly that retinol may be involved in normal regulation of TGFβ expression in certain tissues. However, it was reported recently that retinol can activate a latent form of TGFβ in isolated avian osteoclasts (Bonewald *et al.*, 1997). The effect of retinol was restricted to mature osteoclasts and was not observed in osteoclast precursors. The mechanism of activation is not known, but it appears to be independent of the plasmin–plasminogen activator pathway. Because TGFβ is a multifunctional cytokine, which is found in many tissues in a latent form, its activation by retinol may be an important effect if reproduced in other cell types, especially in view of the growth inhibitory effect of TGFβ on many epithelial cancer cells.

Retinol inhibited the growth of three cell lines derived from a single Shope carcinoma and differing in their degree of differentiation. The growth-retarding effect was reversible in the undifferentiated subline upon removal of retinol from medium, but the two differentiated sublines did not revert. A seven-day pretreatment of the differentiated sublines with retinol decreased the tumorigenic potential of the differentiated sublines, whereas the potential of the undifferentiated subline was only slightly reduced. These results suggest that retinol may be effective against differentiated squamous cell carcinomas, but not against undifferentiated tumours (Isono & Seto, 1991).

Vitamin A added to the culture medium at a 50 μmol/L concentration caused a 60% inhibition of DNA synthesis in melanoma (SK Mel 28) and cervical carcinoma (HeLa) cell lines; the inhibition was reversible and this treatment did not select for retinol-resistant clones (Ferrari *et al.*, 1983). The inhibitory effect of retinol on HeLa cells was correlated with inhibition of plasma membrane NADH oxidase activity, an activity which has been implicated in the progress of cell proliferation (Dai *et al.*, 1997).

(l) Molecular mechanisms of gene regulation by retinol

There is ample evidence that the major mechanism by which retinoids, including retinol, exert their various effects on cell growth and differentiation is via modulation of gene expression (DeLuca, 1991; Gudas *et al.*, 1994). Nuclear retinoic acid receptors, which are members of the steroid hormone receptor superfamily, function as ligand-activated trans-acting transcription modulating factors and have been implicated as the proximal mediators of the effects of retinoids on gene expression (Chambon, 1996; Mangelsdorf & Evans, 1995; Mangelsdorf *et al.*, 1994).

Retinol can regulate the transcription of genes by serving as a precursor for metabolites that activate nuclear retinoid receptors. There are at least two ways by which retinol can do this. One pathway requires the formation of all *trans*- and 9-*cis*-retinoic acid. Both isomers can bind to nuclear retinoic acid receptors (RAR) α, β and γ, whereas 9-*cis*-retinoic acid can also bind to retinoid X receptors (RXR) α, β and γ (Chambon, 1996; Mangelsdorf & Evans, 1995; Mangelsdorf *et al.*, 1994).

Evidence to support the above pathway is described below. Studies with cultured human keratinocytes have demonstrated that the biological activity of retinol in activation of gene expression (determined as reduction of type I transglutaminase and stimulation of a β-retinoic acid response element $(RARE)_3$-driven reporter gene activity) requires receptors, because dominant-negative mutant receptor cotransfection eliminated the effects of retinol. Further, inhibition by citral of metabolism of all-*trans*-retinol to all-*trans*-retinoic acid reduced β $RARE_3$-tk-CAT activity by 98%. These data indicate that retinol-induced responses in human keratinocytes are mediated by its metabolite retinoic acid, which functions as a ligand to activate nuclear retinoic acid receptors (Kurlandsky *et al.*, 1994). Cope and Wille (1989) reported that treatment of human malignant keratinocytes with 30 µmol/L antisense oligodeoxynucleotides corresponding to human nuclear RAR-α blocked the induction of alkaline phosphatase by retinol in these cells. It is noteworthy that there is no simple relationship between the expression of nuclear retinoid receptors and response of cells to growth-inhibitory effects of retinol.

Another pathway is based on the reported ability of the retinol metabolite 4-oxoretinol at low doses (0.1 and 1 nmol/L) to activate the transcription of a reporter gene driven by RARE via RARs (Achkar *et al.*, 1996).

A nuclear receptor-independent mechanism has also been suggested to account for the activity of the retinol metabolite anhydroretinol, which acts without requiring synthesis of either mRNA or protein and appears to be able to affect cell growth and differentiation by a still unknown process (O'Connell *et al.*, 1996).

It is of interest to note that vitamin A deficiency (Haq *et al.*, 1991; Verma *et al.*, 1992), treatment with tumour promoters (Kumar *et al.*, 1994) and the development of premalignant and malignant lesions *in vivo* (Darwiche *et al.*, 1995; Lotan *et al.*, 1995; Xu *et al.*, 1994, 1997) are all associated with decreased expression of certain nuclear retinoid receptors *in vivo*. The expression of these receptors can be restored to normal levels by supplementation with retinoic acid (Haq *et al.*, 1991; Lotan *et al.*, 1995).

4.2.3.2 In-vitro inhibition of genetic and related effects

Many studies have dealt with the antimutagenic effects of retinol, retinal, retinoic acid and retinyl esters in short-term tests using prokaryotes or eukaryotes under in-vitro conditions. Reviews (Odin, 1997) and antimutagenicity profiles have been published in recent years (Brockman *et al.*, 1992; Waters *et al.*, 1990, 1996a, b). Such profiles are presented in Figures 6–8.

The results of studies using *Salmonella typhimurium* strains as targets of genotoxicity are summarized in Table 26. One study (Okai *et al.*, 1996) evaluated inhibition of mutagen-induced *umu* C gene expression in strain TA1535/- pSK 1002. Retinol, retinyl acetate, retinyl palmitate and retinoic acid inhibited the induction of *umu* C gene expression by the heterocyclic amine 3-amino-3,4-dimethyl-5*H*-pyrido[4,3-*b*]indole (Trp-P-1). In contrast, retinol, retinyl acetate and retinoic acid were ineffective when *umu* C gene expression was induced by the direct-acting mutagens adriamycin and mitomycin C.

A number of studies were performed with the Ames *Salmonella*/microsome test. Neither retinol nor retinoic acid affected the mutagenicity of hydrogen peroxide in strain TA104 (Han, 1992). Retinyl acetate decreased the mutagenicity of cysteine, occurring at high, non-physiological concentrations in strain TA102 (Stark *et al.*, 1994).

Vitamin A and its derivatives failed to inhibit the mutagenicity of certain direct-acting mutagens, as shown, for example, by the inactivity of retinyl palmitate and retinoic acid towards 4-nitroquinoline 1-oxide mutagenicity in TA100 (Camoirano *et al.*, 1994), and of retinol towards that of either adriamycin in TA98 (Baird & Birnbaum, 1979), mitomycin C in TA102, irrespective of the presence of rat liver S9 fractions (Qin & Huang, 1985), diepoxybutane in TA1535 (Busk & Ahlborg, 1980), photoactivated 2-azido-9-fluorenone oxime in TA1538 (White & Rock, 1981) and 4-nitro-*o*-phenylenediamine in TA98 (Balbinder *et al.*, 1983). The mutagenic potency of the last compound was decreased in the presence of S9 mix, and the effect was not influenced by retinol (Balbinder *et al.*, 1983). In the case of *N*-methyl-*N*'-nitro-*N*-nitrosoguanidine (MNNG), retinol and retinal displayed antimutagenic activity in strain TA100, which contrasted with the lack of activity of retinoic acid, retinyl acetate and retinyl palmitate (Shetty *et al.*, 1988). On the other hand, the direct mutagenicity of nitro compounds (2-nitrofluorene, 1-nitropyrene and 3-nitrofluoranthene) in TA98 was decreased by retinol and retinoic acid and, with greater potency, by retinal and retinyl palmitate (Tang & Edenharder, 1997). Moreover, retinol significantly inhibited the direct mutagenicity in TA100 of methylazoxymethanol, a metabolite of 1,2-dimethylhydrazine, but the effect was not dose-

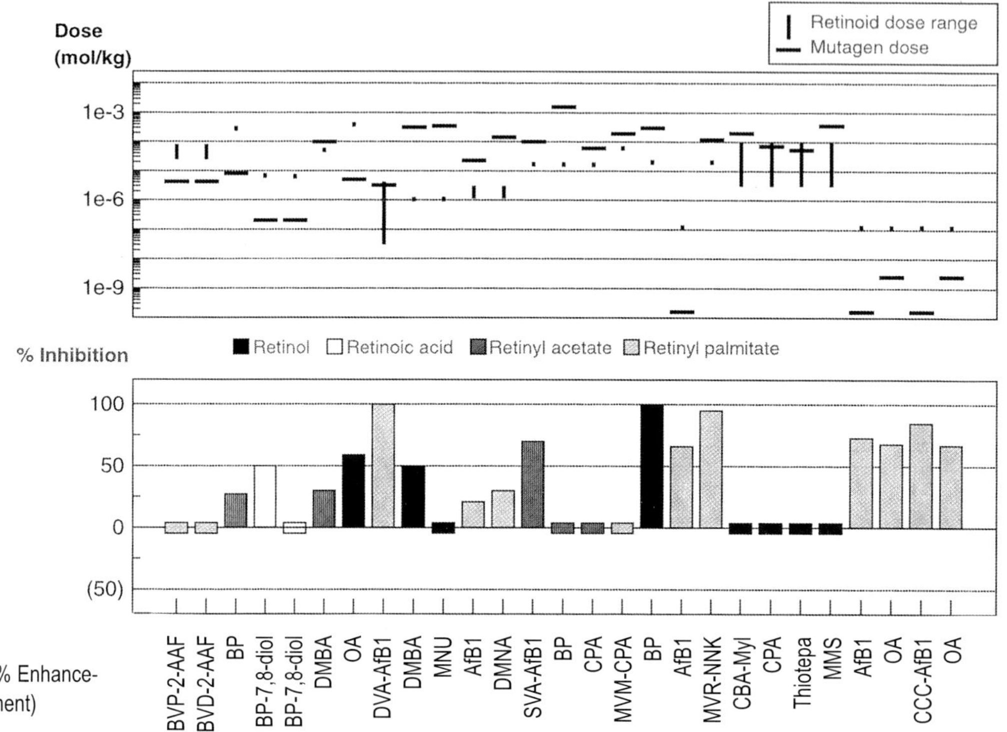

Figure 6. The antimutagenicity profile shows the performance of retinol, retinoic acid and retinyl esters to modulate genotoxin-induced effects in mammals *in vivo*.
The profile is organized using the test codes and chemical abbreviations to identify each item across the profile, and only the first occurrence of each test code is given. In the upper panel, doses from the data in Table 25 are plotted in molar units for the genotoxins and the retinoids. In the lower panel positive values are the maximum percent inhibition of the genotoxin-induced effects, negative values are the maximum percent enhancement of the effects, and values equal to zero indicate that no significant difference was observed relative to the induced effects. A brief description of the antimutagenicity profile methodology and test code definitions are given in the appendices. Abbreviations: 2-acetylaminofluorene, 2-AAF; aflatoxin B_1, AfB1; benzo[*a*]pyrene, BP; (7S,8S)-dihydroxy-7,8-dihydrobenzo[*a*]pyrene, BP-7,8-diol; cyclophosphamide, CPA; 7,12-dimethylbenz[*a*]anthracene, 7,12-DMBA; dimethylnitrosamine, DMNA; methyl methanesulfonate, MMS; *N*-methylnitrosourea, MNU; busulfan (myleran), Myl; 4-(*N*-nitrosomethylamino)-1-(3-pyridyl)-1-butanone, NNK; ochratoxin A, OA.

dependent (Tavan *et al.*, 1997). Retinol weakly inhibited the direct mutagenicity in TA98 of complex mixtures, including coal dust, diesel emission particles, tobacco snuff and airborne particles, as well as the S9-mediated mutagenicity of fried beef extracts (Ong *et al.*, 1989).

Retinol, retinal, retinoic acid, retinyl acetate and retinyl palmitate were consistently effective in inhibiting the S9-mediated mutagenicity of aflatoxin B_1 in TA98 and TA100 (Busk & Ahlborg, 1980; Raina & Gurtoo, 1985; Qin & Huang, 1985; Bhattacharya *et al.*, 1987). Only in one study (Raina & Gurtoo, 1985) did retinoic acid fail to inhibit aflatoxin B_1 mutagenicity in TA100, although it was antimutagenic in TA98. Retinol, retinoic acid and retinyl acetate were approximately equipotent in a comparative study (Qin & Huang, 1985), whereas in another study (Bhattacharya *et al.*, 1987) the potency to decrease aflatoxin B_1

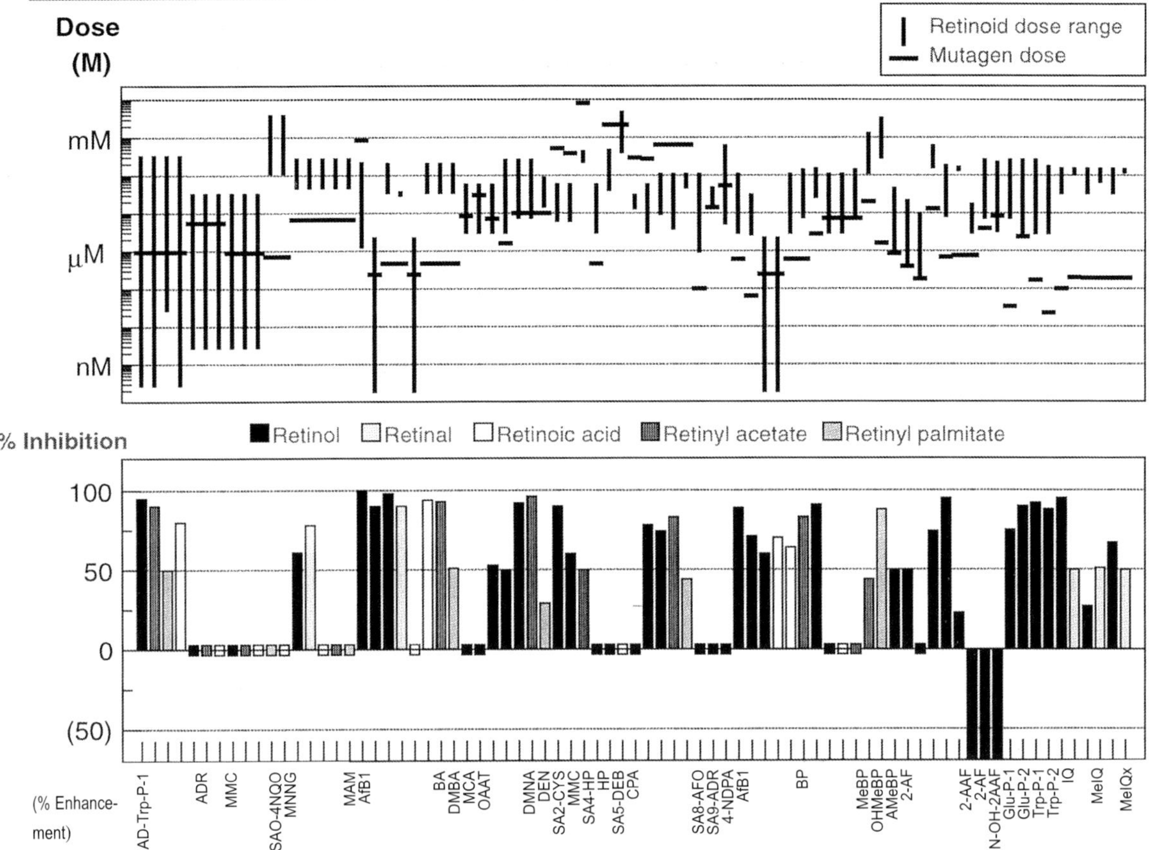

Figure 7. The antimutagenicity profile displays the performance of retinol, retinal, retinoic acid, and retinyl esters to modulate mutagen-induced effects in *Salmonella typhimurium* strains.

The profile is organized using the test codes and chemical abbreviations to identify each item across the profile, and only the first occurrence of each test code and/or mutagen is given. In the upper panel, doses from the data in Table 26 are plotted in molar units for both the mutagens and the retinoids. In the lower panel positive values are the maximum percent inhibition of the mutagen-induced effects, negative values are the maximum percent enhancement of the effects, and values equal to zero indicate that no significant difference was observed relative to the mutagen-induced effects. A brief description of the antimutagenicity profile methodology and test code definitions are given in the appendices. Abbreviations: 2-acetylaminofluorene, 2-AAF; 2-aminofluorene, 2-AF; adriamycin, ADR; aflatoxin B_1, AfB1; 2-azido-9-fluorenone; AFO; 6-acetoxymethylbenzo[*a*]pyrene, AMeBP; benz[*a*]anthracene; BA; benzo-[*a*]pyrene, BP, cyclophosphamide, CPA; cysteine, CYS; diepoxybutane, DEB; *N*-nitrosodiethylamine, DEN; 7,12-dimethyl-benz[a]-anthracene, DMBA, *N*-nitrosodimethylamine; DMNA; 2-amino-6-methylpyrido[1,2-*a*:3'2'-*d*]imidazole, Glu-P-1; 2-amino-dipyrido[1,2,-*a*:3',2'-*d*]imidazole, Glu-P-2; hydrogen peroxide, HP; 2-amino-3-methylimidazo[4,5-*f*]quinoline, IQ; methylazoxy-methanol, MAM; 3-methylcholanthrene, MCA; 6-methylbenzo[*a*]pyrene, MeBP; 2-amino-3,4-dimethylimidazo[4,5-*f*]quinoline, MeIQ; 2-amino-3,8-dimethylimidazo[4,5-*f*]quinoxaline, MeIQx; mitomycin C, MMC; *N*-methyl-*N'*-nitro-*N*-nitrosoguanidine, MNNG; *N*-hydroxy-2-acetoaminofluorene, N-OH-2AAF; 4-nitro-*o*-phenylenediamine; 4NPDA; 4-nitroquinoline 1-oxide, 4-NQO; *o*-aminoazotoluene, OAAT; 6-hydroxybenzo[*a*]pyrene, OHMeBP; 3-amino-1,4-dimethyl-5*H*-pyrido[4,3-*b*]indole, Trp-P-1; 3-amino-1-methyl-5*H*-pyrido[4,3-*b*]indole, Trp-P-2.

mutagenicity ranked as follows: retinal > retinol and retinoic acid > retinyl acetate > retinyl palmitate. The antimutagenic effect was more evident when retinoic acid was added at the start of the metabolic activation reaction than when it was added after the reaction was terminated by menadione, suggesting an effect of retinoic acid on aflatoxin B_1 metabolism (Raina & Gurtoo, 1985). Inhibition of the metabolic activation of aflatoxin B_1 to mutagenic

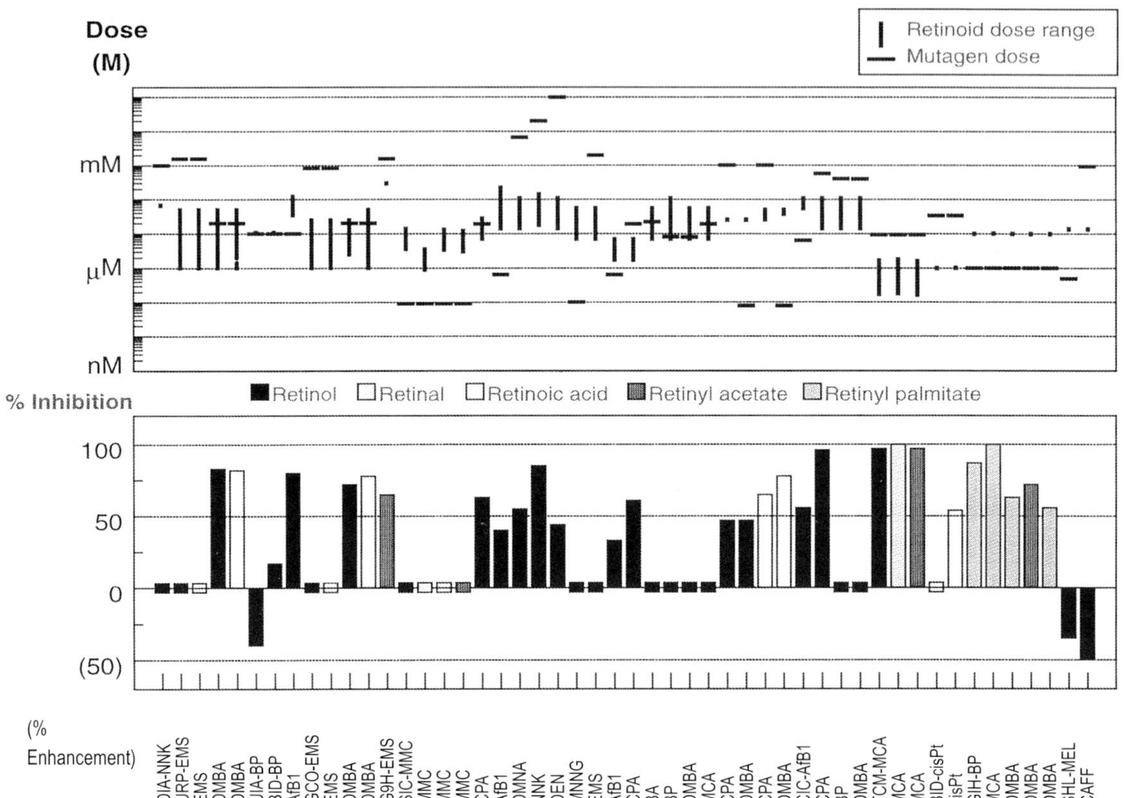

Figure 8. The antimutagenicity profile shows the performance of retinol, retinal, retinoic acid and retinyl esters to modulate genotoxin-induced effects in mammalian cells *in vitro*.
The profile is organized using test codes and chemical abbreviations to identify each item across the profile with only the initial occurrence of each test code given. In the upper panel doses from the data in Table 27 are plotted in molar units for both the genotoxins and retinoids. In the lower panel positive values are the maximum percent inhibition of the genotoxin-induced effects, negative values are the maximum percent enhancement of the effects, and values equal to zero indicate that no significant differences were observed relative to the induced effects. A brief description of the antimutagenicity profile methodology and test code definitions are given in the appendices. Abbreviations: aflatoxin B_1, AfB1; benz[*a*]anthracene, BA; benzo[*a*]pyrene, BP; caffeine, CAFF; cisplatin, cisPt; cyclophosphamide, CPA; *N*-nitrosodiethylamine, DEN; 7,12-dimethylbenz[*a*]anthracene, DMBA; *N*-nitrosodimethylamine, DMNA; ethyl methanesulfonate, EMS; 3-methylcholanthrene, MCA; melphalan, MEL; mitomycin C, MMC; *N*-methyl-*N'*-nitro-*N*-nitrosoguanidine, MNNG; 4-(*N*-nitrosomethlyamino)-1-(3-pyridyl)-1-butanone, NNK.

metabolites was also observed when liver S9 fractions from mice maintained on a diet supplemented with either retinyl acetate (Qin & Huang, 1986) or retinyl palmitate (Decoudu *et al.*, 1992) were used, as compared to liver S9 fractions from mice maintained on a vitamin A-deficient diet.

Vitamin A and its derivatives were less consistently effective in decreasing the S9-mediated mutagenicity of polycyclic aromatic hydrocarbons. Thus, in a single comparative study in strain TA98 (Qin & Huang, 1985), retinol, retinoic acid and retinyl acetate failed to decrease the mutagenicity of BP, and retinol was also ineffective towards benz[*a*]anthracene and DMBA. A protective effect of retinol in this study was observed only towards MCA. There was no difference in the activation of BP to mutagenic metabolites in TA98 when liver S9 fractions from mice maintained on a vitamin

Table 26. Assay of retinol, retinal, retinoic acid and retinyl esters for the ability to inhibit standard mutagens in in-vitro systems using *Salmonella typhimurium* strains

End-point [a]	Code [a]	Modulator (tested doses) [b]	Mutagen (tested doses) [b]	*S. typhimurium* strain	S9 mix	Result [c]	Inhibitory dose (IDx) [d]	Reference
D	SAD	Retinol (0.0003–300 μM)	Trp-P-1 (0.2 μg/mL)	TA1535/ pSK1002	+	+	0.12 μM (ID50)	Okai *et al.* (1996)
D	SAD	Retinyl acetate (0.0003–300 μM)	Trp-P-1 (0.2 μg/mL)	TA1535/ pSK1002	+	+	0.3 μM (ID50)	Okai *et al.* (1996)
D	SAD	Retinyl palmitate (0.0003–300 μM)	Trp-P-1) (0.2 μg/mL)	TA1535/ pSK1002	+	+	60 μM (ID50)	Okai *et al.* (1996)
D	SAD	Retinoic acid (0.0003–300 μM)	Trp-P-1) (0.2 μg/mL)	TA1535/ pSK1002	+	+	0.54 μM (ID50)	Okai *et al.* (1996)
D	SAD	Retinol (0.003–30 μM)	Adriamycin (3 μg/mL)	TA1535/ pSK1002	–	–	NA	Okai *et al.* (1996)
D	SAD	Retinyl acetate (0.003–30 μM)	Adriamycin (3 μg/mL)	TA1535/ pSK1002	–	–	NA	Okai *et al.* (1996)
D	SAD	Retinoic acid (0.003–30 μM)	Adriamycin (3 μg/mL)	TA1535/ pSK1002	–	–	NA	Okai *et al.* (1996)
D	SAD	Retinol (0.003–30 μM)	Mitomycin C (0.3 μg/mL)	TA1535/ pSK1002	–	–	NA	Okai *et al.* (1996)
D	SAD	Retinol acetate (0.003–30 μM)	Mitomycin C (0.3 μg/mL)	TA1535/ pSK1002	–	–	NA	Okai *et al.* (1996)
D	SAD	Retinoic acid (0.003–30 μM)	Mitomycin C (0.3 μg/mL)	TA1535/ pSK1002	–	–	NA	Okai *et al.* (1996)
G	SA4	Retinol (0.1–1 μmol/plate)	Hydrogen peroxide (5 μmol/plate)	TA104	–	–	NA	Han (1992)
G	SA4	Retinoic acid (1–10 μmol/plate)	Hydrogen peroxide (5 μmol/plate)	TA104	–	–	NA	Han (1992)
G	SA2	Retinyl acetate (0.2–1 μmol/plate)	Cysteine (20 μmol/plate)	TA102	–	+	1 μmol/plate (ID50)	Stark *et al.* (1994)
G	SA9	Retinol (10–25 μg/plate)	Adriamycin (5–15 μg/plate)	TA98	–	–	NA	Baird & Birnbaum (1979)
G	SA0	Retinyl palmitate (0.33–10 μmol/plate)	4-Nitroquinoline 1–oxide (2 nmol/plate)	TA100	–	–	NA	Camoirano *et al.* (1994)

Table 26 (contd)

End-point [a]	Code [a]	Modulator (tested doses) [b]	Mutagen (tested doses) [b]	*S. typhimurium* strain	S9 mix	Result [c]	Inhibitory dose (IDx) [d]	Reference
G	SA0	Retinoic acid (0.33–10 μmol/plate)	4-Nitroquinoline 1-oxide (2 nmol/plate)	TA100	–	–	NA	Camoirano *et al.* (1994)
G	SA2	Retinol (2.5–40 μg/plate)	Mitomycin C (0.4 μg/plate)	TA102	–	–	NA	Qin & Huang (1985)
G	SA2	Retinol (2.5–40 μg/plate)	Mitomycin C (0.4 μg/plate)	TA102	+	–	NA	Qin & Huang (1985)
G	SA5	Retinol (8–16 μg/plate)	Diepoxybutane (10–50 μg/plate)	TA1535	–	–	NA	Busk & Ahlborg (1980)
G	SA8	Retinol (1–100 μM)	Photoactivated 2-azido-9-fluorenone oxime (0.1 μM)	TA1538	–	–	NA	White & Rock (1981)
G	SA9	Retinol (5–500 μg/plate)	4-Nitro-*o*-phenylendiamine (5–25 μg/plate)	TA98	–	–	NA	Balbinder *et al.* (1983)
G	SA0	Retinoic acid (0.1–0.5 μmol/plate)	MNNG (13.6 nmol/plate)	TA100	–	+	0.35 μmol/plate (ID50)	Shetty *et al.* (1988)
G	SA0	Retinyl acetate (0.1–0.5 μmol/plate)	MNNG (13.6 nmol/plate)	TA100	–	+	NA	Shetty *et al.* (1988)
G	SA0	Retinol (0.1–0.5 μmol/plate)	MNNG (13.6 nmol/plate)	TA100	–	+	0.35 μmol/plate (ID50)	Shetty *et al.* (1988)
G	SA0	Retinal (0.1–0.5 μmol/plate)	MNNG (13.6 nmol/plate)	TA100	–	+	0.14 μmol/plate (ID50)	Shetty *et al.* (1988)
G	SA0	Retinyl palmitate (0.1–0.5 μmol/plate)	MNNG (13.6 nmol/plate)	TA100	–	–	NA	Shetty *et al.* (1988)
G	SA9	Retinol (up to 1 μmol/plate)	2-Nitrofluorene (unspecified dose)	TA98	–	(+)	1 μmol/plate (ID43)	Tang & Edenharder (1997)
G	SA9	Retinal (up to 2 μmol/plate)	2-Nitrofluorene (unspecified dose)	TA98	–	+	0.2 μmol/plate (ID50)	Tang & Edenharder (1997)
G	SA9	Retinoic acid (up to 1 μmol/plate)	2-Nitropyrene (unspecified dose)	TA98	–	(+)	1 μmol/plate (ID33)	Tang & Edenharder (1997)

Table 26 (contd)

End-point [a]	Code [a]	Modulator (tested doses) [b]	Mutagen (tested doses) [b]	*S. typhimurium* strain	S9 mix	Result [c]	Inhibitory dose (IDx) [d]	Reference
G	SA9	Retinyl palmitate (up to 2 µmol/plate)	2-Nitropyrene (unspecified dose)	TA98	–	+	0.3 µmol/plate (ID50)	Tang & Edenharder (1997)
G	SA9	Retinoic acid (up to 1 µmol/plate)	1-Nitropyrene (unspecified dose)	TA98	–	(+)	1 µmol/plate (ID45)	Tang & Edenharder (1997)
G	SA9	Retinoic acid (up to 2 µmol/plate)	1-Nitropyrene (unspecified dose)	TA98	–	+	0.06 µmol/plate (ID50)	Tang & Edenharder (1997)
G	SA9	Retinoic acid (up to 1 µmol/plate)	1-Nitropyrene (unspecified dose)	TA98	–	+	1 µmol/plate (ID50)	Tang & Edenharder (1997)
G	SA9	Retinyl palmitate (up to 2 µmol/plate)	1-Nitropyrene (unspecified dose)	TA98	–	+	0.06 µmol/plate (ID50)	Tang & Edenharder (1997)
G	SA9	Retinol (up to 1 µmol/plate)	3-Nitrofluoranthene (unspecified dose)	TA98	–	+	0.1 µmol/plate (ID50)	Tang & Edenharder (1997)
G	SA9	Retinal (up to 2 µmol/plate)	3-Nitrofluoranthene (unspecified dose)	TA98	–	+	0.05 µmol/plate (ID50)	Tang & Edenharder (1997)
G	SA9	Retinoic acid (up to 1 µmol/plate)	3-Nitrofluoranthene (unspecified dose)	TA98	–	+	0.6 µmol/plate (ID50)	Tang & Edenharder (1997)
G	SA9	Retinyl palmitate (up to 2 µmol/plate)	3-Nitrofluoranthene (unspecified dose)	TA98	–	+	0.07 µmol/plate (ID50)	Tang & Edenharder (1997)
G	SA0	Retinol (1–150 µg/plate)	Methylazoxymethanol (200 µg/plate)	TA100	–	+	5 µg/plate (ID62)	Tavan *et al.* (1997)
G	SA9	Retinol (0.21–1.72 µmol/plate)	Coal dust extract (75 mg/plate)	TA98	–	(+)	1.72 µmol/plate (ID29)	Ong *et al.* (1989)
G	SA9	Retinol (0.21–1.72 µmol/plate)	Diesel emission particles extract (2 mg/plate)	TA98	–	(+)	1.72 µmol/plate (ID31)	Ong *et al.* (1989)
G	SA9	Retinol (0.21–1.72 µmol/plate)	Tobacco snuff extract (85 mg/plate)	TA98	–	(+)	1.72 µmol/plate (ID29)	Ong *et al.* (1989)

Table 26 (contd)

End-point [a]	Code [a]	Modulator (tested doses) [b]	Mutagen (tested doses) [b]	*S. typhimurium* strain	S9 mix	Result [c]	Inhibitory dose (IDx) [d]	Reference
G	SA9	Retinol (0.21–1.72 μmol/plate)	Airborne particles extract (4 mg/plate)	TA98	–	(+)	3.45 μmol/plate (ID45)	Ong *et al.* (1989)
G	SA9	Retinol (0.21–1.72 μmol/plate)	Fried beef extract (750 mg/plate)	TA98	+	(+)	1.72 μmol/plate (ID48)	Ong *et al.* (1989)
G	SA9	Retinol (1.6–16 μg/plate)	Aflatoxin B_1 (0.04 μg/plate)	TA98	+	+	16 μg/plate (ID70)	Busk & Ahlborg (1980)
G	SA9	Retinol (0.0002–2 μM)	Aflatoxin B_1 (0.2 μg/plate)	TA98	+	+	0.0006 μM (ID55)	Raina & Gurtoo (1985)
G	SA0	Retinol (0.0002–2 μM)	Aflatoxin B_1 (0.2 μg/plate)	TA100	+	+	0.0002 μM (ID70)	Raina & Gurtoo (1985)
G	SA9	Retinoic acid (0.0002–2 μM)	Aflatoxin B_1 (0.2 μg/plate)	TA98	+	+	0.0002 μM (ID55)	Raina & Gurtoo (1985)
G	SA0	Retinoic acid (0.0002–2 μM)	Aflatoxin B_1 (0.2 μg/plate)	TA100	+	–	NA	Raina & Gurtoo (1985)
G	SA9	Retinol (2.5–40 μg/plate)	Aflatoxin B_1 (0.5 μg/plate)	TA98	+	+	10 μg/plate (ID50)	Qin & Huang (1985)
G	SA9	Retinoic acid (2.5–40 μg/plate)	Aflatoxin B_1 (0.5 μg/plate)	TA98	+	+	10 μg/plate (ID50)	Qin & Huang (1985)
G	SA0	Retinal (0.1–0.5 μmol/plate)	Aflatoxin B_1 (1.28 nmol/plate)	TA100	+	+	0.1 μmol/plate (ID90)	Bhattarcharya *et al.* (1987)
G	SA0	Retinoic acid (0.1–0.5 μmol/plate)	Aflatoxin B_1 (1.28 nmol/plate)	TA100	+	+	0.1 μmol/plate (ID66)	Bhattarcharya *et al.* (1987)
G	SA0	Retinyl acetate (0.1–0.5 μmol/plate)	Aflatoxin B_1 (1.28 nmol/plate)	TA100	+	+	0.1 μmol/plate (ID50)	Bhattarcharya *et al.* (1987)
G	SA0	Retinyl palmitate (0.1–0.5 μmol/plate)	Aflatoxin B_1 (1.28 nmol/plate)	TA100	+	+	0.5 μmol/plate (ID50)	Bhattarcharya *et al.* (1987)

Table 26 (contd)

End-point[a]	Code[a]	Modulator (tested doses)[b]	Mutagen (tested doses)[b]	*S. typhimurium* strain	S9 mix	Result[c]	Inhibitory dose (IDx)[d]	Reference
G	SA9	Retinyl acetate [No direct treatment – S9 from mice maintained on a vitamin A-deficient diet or on a retinyl acetate-supplemented diet (20 µg/g diet) for 10 weeks]	Aflatoxin B_1 (0.1–0.4 µg/plate)	TA98	+	(+)	NA (ID24)	Qin & Huang (1986)
S	SA9	Retinyl palmitate [no direct treatment – S9 from rats maintained on a retinyl palmitate-normal diet (5 IU/g diet) or a retinyl palmitate-supplemented diet (500 IU/g diet) for 8 days]	Aflatoxin B_1 (2.5–100 ng/plate)	TA98	+	+	NA (ID78)	Decoudu *et al.* (1992)
G	SA9	Retinol (27.5-136 µM)	BP (2.75 µM)	TA98	+	+	27.5 µM (ID40)	Calle & Sullivan (1982)
G	SA9	Retinol (2.5–40 µg/plate)	BP (5 µg/plate)	TA98	+	–	NA	Qin & Huang (1985)
G	SA9	Retinoic acid (2.5–40 µg/plate)	BP (5 µg/plate)	TA98	+	–	NA	Qin & Huang (1985)
G	SA9	Retinyl acetate (2.5–40 µg/plate)	BP (5 µg/plate)	TA98	+	–	NA	Qin & Huang (1985)
G	SA9	Retinyl acetate [No direct treatment – S9 from mice maintained on a vitamin A-deficient diet or on a retinyl acetate-supplemented diet (20 µg/g diet) for 10 weeks]	BP (25–100 µg/plate)	TA98	+	–	NA	Qin & Huang (1986)
G	SA9	Retinyl acetate (80–800 µg/plate)	BP (10 µg/plate)	TA98	+	(+)	800 µg/plate (ID43)	Balansky *et al.* (1994)
S	SA9	Retinyl palmitate (40–4000 µg/plate)	BP (1–1000 µg/plate)	TA98	+	+	400 µg/plate (ID64 with 1 µg BP)	Alzieu *et al.* (1987)

Table 26 (contd)

End-point [a]	Code [a]	Modulator (tested doses) [b]	Mutagen (tested doses) [b]	*S. typhimurium* strain	S9 mix	Result [c]	Inhibitory dose (IDx) [d]	Reference
S	SA9	Retinyl palmitate [No direct treatment – S9 from rats maintained on a retinyl acetate-deficient diet or on a retinyl palmitate diet (20 IU/g diet) for 8 weeks]	BP (50 µg/plate)	TA98	+	(+)	NA (ID37)	Colin *et al.* (1991)
S	SA9	Retinyl palmitate [No direct treatment – S9 from rats maintained on a retinyl acetate-deficient diet or S9 from rats receiving an i.p. injection of retinyl palmitate (750 mg/kg bw) 48 h before sacrifice]	BP (50 µg/plate)	TA98	+	(+)	NA (ID22)	Colin *et al.* (1991)
G	SA9	Retinol (2.8–140 nmol/plate)	6-Methylbenzo[*a*]pyrene (2.8 nmol/plate)	TA98	+	(+)	140 nmol/plate (ID50)	Bayless *et al.* (1986)
G	SA9	Retinol (1.3–65 nmol/plate)	6-Hydroxymethylbenzo-[*a*]pyrene (1.3 nmol/plate)	TA98	+	(+)	26 nmol/plate (ID50)	Bayless *et al.* (1986)
G	SA9	Retinol (0.6–30 nmol/plate)	6–Acetoxymethylbenzo-[*a*]pyrene (0.6 nmol/plate)	TA98	–	–	NA	Bayless *et al.* (1986)
G	SA0	Retinol (2.5–40 µg/plate)	Benz[*a*]anthracene (5 µg/plate)	TA100	+	–	NA	Qin & Huang (1985)
G	SA0	Retinol (2.5–40 µg/plate)	DMBA (20 µg/plate)	TA100	+	–	NA	Qin & Huang (1985)
G	SA0	Retinol (2.5–40 µg/plate)	MCA (5 µg/plate)	TA100	+	+	20 µg/plate (ID50)	Qin & Huang (1985)
G	SA9	Retinol (5–100 µg/plate)	2-Aminofluorene (0.25–1 µg/plate)	TA98	+	+	10 µg/plate (ID100)	Baird & Birnbaum (1979)

Table 26 (contd)

End-point [a]	Code [a]	Modulator (tested doses) [b]	Mutagen (tested doses) [b]	*S. typhimurium* strain	S9 mix	Result [c]	Inhibitory dose (IDx) [d]	Reference
G	SA9	Retinol (2–100 µg/plate)	2-Aminofluorene (0.3–0.6 µg/plate)	TA98	+	§	NA	Busk & Ahlborg (1982a)
G	SA9	Retinol (2–100 µg/plate)	2-Acetylaminofluorene (2 µg/plate)	TA98	+	§	NA	Busk & Ahlborg (1982a)
G	SA9	Retinol (5–500 µg/plate)	2-Aminofluorene (2.5–10 µg/plate)	TA98	+	§	NA	Balbinder *et al.* (1983)
G	SA9	Retinol (2.5–150 µg/plate)	*N*-Hydroxy-2-acetyl-aminofluorene (50 µg/plate)	TA98	+	#	NA	Rondahl *et al.* (1985)
G	SA9	Retinol (2.5–150 µg/plate)	*N*-Hydroxy-2-acetyl-aminofluorene (50 µg/plate)	TA98	-	-	NA	Rondahl *et al.* (1985)
G	SA0	Retinol (0.017–0.525 µmol/plate)	*o*-Aminoazotoluene (5 µg/plate)	TA100	+	+	0.07 µmol/plate (ID50)	Busk & Ahlborg (1982b)
G	SA0	Retinyl acetate (0.017–0.525 µmol/plate)	*o*-Aminoazotoluene (5 µg/plate)	TA100	+	+	0.07 µmol/plate (ID50)	Busk & Ahlborg (1982b)
G	SA0	Retinyl palmitate (0.017–0.175 µmol/plate)	*o*-Aminoazotoluene (5 µg/plate)	TA100	+	(+)	0.175 µmol/plate (ID30)	Busk & Ahlborg (1982b)
G	SA0	Retinol (2–150 µg/plate)	*o*-Aminoazotoluene (7 µg/plate)	TA100	+ (Gerbil)	+	10 µg/plate (ID50)	Victorin *et al.* (1987)
G	SA0	Retinol (2–150 µg/plate)	*o*-Aminoazotoluene (15 µg/plate)	TA100	+ (Mouse)	+	50 µg/plate (ID50)	Victorin *et al.* (1987)
G	SA0	Retinol (2–150 µg/plate)	*o*-Aminoazotoluene (10 µg/plate)	TA100	+ (Hamster)	+	50 µg/plate (ID50)	Victorin *et al.* (1987)
G	SA0	Retinol (2–150 µg/plate)	*o*-Aminoazotoluene (8 µg/plate)	TA100	+ (Rat)	+	150 µg/plate (ID50)	Victorin *et al.* (1987)
G	SA5	Retinol (0.004–0.21 µmol/plate)	Cyclophosphamide (400 µg/plate)	TA1535	+	+	0.105 µmol/plate (ID56)	Busk *et al.* (1984)
G	SA5	Retinyl acetate (0.004–0.21 µmol/plate)	Cyclophosphamide (400 µg/plate)	TA1535	+	+	0.105 µmol/plate (ID70)	Busk *et al.* (1984)

Table 26 (contd)

End-point [a]	Code [a]	Modulator (tested doses) [b]	Mutagen (tested doses) [b]	*S. typhimurium* strain	S9 mix	Result [c]	Inhibitory dose (IDx) [d]	Reference
G	SA5	Retinyl palmitate (0.004–0.21 µmol/plate)	Cyclophosphamide (400 µg/plate)	TA1535	+	(+)	0.21 µmol/plate (ID40)	Busk *et al.* (1984)
G	SA5	Retinol (2.5–40 µg/plate)	Cyclophosphamide (200 µg/plate)	TA1535	+	+	10 µg/plate (ID50)	Qin & Huang (1985)
G	SA9	Retinol (2–150 µg/plate)	Glu–P–1 (0.0075–0.015 µg/plate)	TA98	+	+	25 µg/plate (ID50)	Busk *et al.* (1982)
G	SA9	Retinol (2–150 µg/plate)	Glu–P–2 (0.5–1 µg/plate)	TA98	+	+	20 µg/plate (ID50)	Busk *et al.* (1982)
G	SA9	Retinol (2–150 µg/plate)	Trp-P-1 (0.04–0.08 µg/plate)	TA98	+	+	20 µg/plate (ID50)	Busk *et al.* (1982)
G	SA9	Retinol (2–150 µg/plate)	Trp-P-2 (0.005–0.01 µg/plate)	TA98	+	+	5 µg/plate (ID50)	Busk *et al.* (1982)
G	SA9	Retinol (25–100 µg/plate)	IQ (0.025–0.1 µg/plate)	TA98	+	+	50 µg/plate (ID50)	Ioannides *et al.* (1990)
G	SA9	Retinal (25–100 µg/plate)	IQ (0.1 µg/plate)	TA98	+	(+)	100 µg/plate (ID50)	Ioannides *et al.* (1990)
G	SA9	Retinol (25–100 µg/plate)	MeIQ (0.1 µg/plate)	TA98	+	(+)	100 µg/plate (ID28)	Ioannides *et al.* (1990)
G	SA9	Retinal (25–100 µg/plate)	MeIQ (0.1 µg/plate)	TA98	+	(+)	75 µg/plate (ID50)	Ioannides *et al.* (1990)
G	SA9	Retinol (25–100 µg/plate)	MeIQx (0.1 µg/plate)	TA98	+	+	50 µg/plate (ID50)	Ioannides *et al.* (1990)

Table 26 (contd)

End-point [a]	Code [a]	Modulator (tested doses) [b]	Mutagen (tested doses) [b]	*S. typhimurium* strain	S9 mix	Result [c]	Inhibitory dose (IDx) [d]	Reference
G	SA9	Retinal (25–100 µg/plate)	MeIQx (0.1 µg/plate)	TA98	+	(+)	100 µg/plate (ID50)	Ioannides *et al.* (1990)
G	SA0	Retinol (5–40 µg/plate)	*N*-Nitrosodimethylamine (100 µg/plate)	TA100	+	+	40 µg/plate (ID90)	Huang (1987)
G	SA0	Retinol (5–40 µg/plate)	*N*-Nitrosodiethylamine (100 µg/plate)	TA100	+	+	40 µg/plate (ID60)	Huang (1987)
G	SA9	Retinol acetate (80–800 µg/plate)	Cigarette smoke (43 mL/Lair for 1–5 min)	TA98	+	+	400 µg/plate (ID60)	Balansky *et al.* (1994)
G	SA9	Retinyl palmitate (1–10 µmol/plate)	Cigarette smoke (18 mL/L air for 6 min)	TA98	+	–	NA	Camoirano *et al.* (1994)
G	SA9	Retinoic acid (1–10 µmol/plate)	Cigarette smoke (18 mL/L air for 6 min)	TA98	+	–	NA	Camoirano *et al.* (1994)
G	SA9	Retinol (0.025–0.5 µmol/plate)	Cigarette smoke condensate (100–400 µg/plate)	TA98	+	–	NA	Wilmer & Spit (1986)
G	SA9	Retinoic acid (0.025–0.5 µmol/plate)	Cigarette smoke condensate (100–400 µg/plate)	TA98	+	–	NA	Wilmer & Spit (1986)
G	SA9	Retinyl acetate (0.025–0.5 µmol/plate)	Cigarette smoke condensate (100–400 µg/plate)	TA98	+	–	NA	Wilmer & Spit (1986)
G	SA9	Retinol (50–800 µg/plate)	Cigarette smoke condensate (400 µg/plate)	TA98	+	+	400 µg/plate (ID50)	Romert *et al.* (1994)
G	SA0	Retinol (50–800 µg/plate)	Cigarette smoke condensate (400 µg/plate)	TA100	+	+	100 µg/plate (ID50)	Romert *et al.* (1994)

[a] End-points investigated are: D, DNA damage; G, gene mutation; test codes are given in Appendix 2

[b] Doses of compounds are as reported by the authors

[c] +, inhibition of genotoxicity (> ID50); (+), weak inhibition of genotoxicity (< ID50); –, no inhibition of genotoxicity; #, increase of genotoxicity; §, variable effect, depending on the dose of retinol and on the amount of S9 fraction per plate

[d] Inhibitory dose (IDx), dose inhibiting the genotoxicity by x%, as indicated by the authors or inferred from their data; NA, not applicable.

Abbreviations: BP, benzo[*a*]pyrene; DMBA, 7,12-dimethylbenz[*a*]anthracene; MNU, *N*-methyl-*N*-nitrosourea; MCA, 3-methylcholanthrene; IQ, 2-amino-3-methyl-imidazo[4,5-*f*]quinoline; MeIQ, 2-amino-3,4-dimethylimidazo[4,5-*f*]quinoline; MeIQx, 2-amino-3,8-dimethylimidazo[4,5-*f*]quinoxaline; Glu-P-1, 2-amino-6-methylpyrido[1,2-*a*:3',2'-*d*]imidazole; Glu-P-2, 2-aminodipyrido[1,2-*a*:3',2'-*d*]imidazole; Trp-P-1, 3-amino-3,4-dimethyl-5*H*-pyrido[4,3-*b*]indole; Trp-P-2, 3-amino-1-methyl-5*H*-pyrido[4,3-*b*]indole; MNNG, *N*-methyl-*N*'nitro-*N*-nitrosoguanidine; NNK, 4-(*N*-nitrosomethylamino)-1-(3-pyridyl)-1-butanone

A-deficient diet or a retinyl acetate-supplemented diet were used (Qin & Huang, 1986). On the other hand, higher doses of retinol (Calle & Sullivan, 1982), retinyl acetate (Balansky *et al.*, 1994) and retinyl palmitate (Alzieu *et al.*, 1987) inhibited the mutagenicity of BP in TA98. Moreover, the mutagenic potency of BP, in the presence of liver S9 fractions from Sprague–Dawley rats maintained on a diet lacking retinyl acetate, was higher than in the presence of S9 either from rats maintained for eight weeks on a retinyl acetate-sufficient diet or from rats receiving an intraperitoneal injection of retinyl acetate 48 h before sacrifice (Colin *et al.*, 1991). Retinol was weakly antimutagenic towards two S9-requiring derivatives of BP (6-methylbenzo[*a*]pyrene and 6-hydroxymethylbenzo[*a*]pyrene), whereas it did not affect the mutagenicity of 6-acetoxymethylbenzo[*a*]pyrene (Bayless *et al.*, 1986).

Retinol and retinyl acetate inhibited the mutagenicity of 2-aminofluorene in TA98 following metabolic activation by either rat liver microsomes or S9 fractions (Baird & Birnbaum, 1979). Other studies showed variable effects of retinol on the mutagenicity of 2-aminofluorene and 2-acetylaminofluorene in TA98. In fact, low doses of retinol even increased the mutagenicity of both aromatic amines, whereas high doses did not affect the mutagenicity of 2-acetylaminofluorene and decreased the mutagenicity of 2-aminofluorene (Busk & Ahlborg, 1982a). A similar diphasic effect was observed in testing retinol towards 2-aminofluorene in another laboratory (Balbinder *et al.*, 1983). Retinol also enhanced the mutagenicity of *N*-hydroxy-2-acetylaminofluorene (Rondahl *et al.*, 1985).

Retinol and retinyl acetate and, less effectively, retinyl palmitate decreased the mutagenicity of *o*-aminoazotoluene in TA100 (Busk & Ahlborg, 1982b) and of cyclophosphamide in TA1535 (Busk *et al.*, 1984; Qin & Huang, 1985). In a further study by the same group (Victorin *et al.*, 1987), inhibition of of the activity of *o*-aminoazotoluene by retinol was confirmed when this azo-dye was activated with liver S9 fractions from four rodent species (gerbil, mouse, hamster and rat).

Two studies have demonstrated that retinol and retinal decrease the mutagenicity in TA98 of heterocyclic amines isolated from food pyrolysates. In particular, retinol decreased the mutagenicity of 2-amino-6-methyldipyrido[1,2-*a*:3′,2′-*d*]imidazole (Glu-P-1), 2-aminodipyrido[1,2-*a*:3′,2′-*d*]imidazole (Glu-P-2) and 3-amino-1,4-dimethyl-5*H*-pyrido[4,3-*b*]indole (Trp-P-1) and, with higher efficiency, the mutagenicity of 3-amino-1-methyl-5*H*-pyrido[4,3-*b*]indole (Trp-P-2) (Busk *et al.*, 1982). Both retinol and retinal, when incorporated into the rat liver S9 activation system, caused a dose-related decrease of the mutagenicity of the aminoimidazoazaarenes 2-amino-3-methylimidazo[4,5-*f*]quinoline (IQ), 2-amino-3,4-dimethylimidazo[4,5-*f*]quinoline (MeIQ) and 2-amino-3,8-dimethylimidazo[4,5-*f*]quinoxaline (MeIQx). Several parallel findings led to the conclusion that retinol lowers IQ mutagenicity through inhibition of its cytochrome P450-dependent metabolic activation (Ioannides *et al.*, 1990).

Retinol weakly inhibits the S9-mediated mutagenicity of both *N*-nitrosodimethylamine and *N*-nitrosodiethylamine in TA100 in the presence of mouse liver S9 fractions (Huang, 1987).

Assays of the S9-mediated mutagenicity of cigarette smoke and condensates from it have given conflicting results. In one study, retinol, retinoic acid and retinyl acetate did not affect the mutagenicity of a cigarette smoke condensate in TA98 (Wilmer & Spit, 1986). In contrast, in another laboratory, retinol exerted protective effects in both TA98 and TA100, although the authors noted that occurrence of toxic effects could not be excluded (Romert *et al.*, 1994). The mutagenicity of mainstream cigarette smoke in TA98 was inhibited by retinyl acetate (Balansky *et al.*, 1994) but was unaffected by either retinyl palmitate or retinoic acid (Camoirano *et al.*, 1994).

In the 1–10 μg/mL range, retinol attenuated the differential toxicity of *N*-nitrosodimethylamine and *N*-nitrosopyrrolidine in the *Escherichia coli* strains K-12 343/765 (*uvr*$^+$/*rec*$^+$) and K-12 343/753 (*uvrB*$^-$/*recA*$^-$). In a host-mediated assay in Swiss albino mice, administration of retinol by gavage (250 mg/kg bw) inhibited the differential toxicity in these two *E. coli* strains. Bacteria were injected intravenously and recovered from blood, lungs, liver, spleen, kidneys and testes of mice treated by gavage with *N*-nitrosodimethylamine (80 mg/kg bw) or from liver and spleen of mice treated by gavage with *N*-nitrosopyrrolidine (Knasmüller *et al.*, 1992).

As summarized in Table 27, retinol, retinal, retinoic acid and retinyl esters have been investigated for their ability to influence a variety of genetic and related end-points in mammalian cultured cells. Retinol inhibited the induction of DNA single-strand breaks induced by the nicotine-derived nitrosamine NNK in primary rat hepatocytes (Alaoui-Jamali *et al.*, 1991a). Retinol and retinoic acid did not affect the unscheduled DNA synthesis (UDS) induced by either ethyl methanesulfonate or 254-nm ultraviolet light in primary rat hepatocytes, but were effective in attenuating the UDS induced by DMBA, which requires activation to genotoxic metabolites (Budroe *et al.*, 1987). Retinol increased BP-induced UDS in hamster tracheal epithelium in organ culture. In the same system, retinol did not significantly affect the levels of BP diol epoxide–DNA adducts, as measured by ^{32}P-postlabelling, but reduced the formation of DNA adducts as detected by immunocytochemistry. The authors suggested that, like β-carotene, retinol may protect the respiratory epithelium by enhancing DNA repair activity and removing DNA adducts (Wolterbeek *et al.*, 1995). Retinol decreased the formation of DNA adducts in cultured woodchuck hepatocytes treated with [^{3}H]aflatoxin B_1 (Yu *et al.*, 1994).

Retinol and retinoic acid inhibited the induction of mutations at the HGPRT locus in Chinese hamster ovary cells when DMBA was used as a mutagenic agent, in the presence of an exogenous metabolic activation system (rat liver S9), but not when the direct-acting mutagen ethyl methanesulfonate was used (Budroe *et al.*, 1988).

The protective effects of vitamin A have been extensively investigated in terms of the frequency of sister chromatid exchanges (SCE) in Chinese hamster cells. In V79 cells, no effect was produced on the SCE induced by direct-acting mutagens, including mitomycin C, in the presence of retinol, retinal, retinoic acid and retinyl acetate (Sirianni *et al.*, 1981), or by MNNG and ethyl methanesulfonate in the presence of retinol (Qin *et al.*, 1985). However, retinol significantly inhibited the metabolic deactivation of MNNG in the presence of S9 (Qin *et al.*, 1985). With the exception of the polycyclic aromatic hydrocarbons benz[*a*]anthracene, BP, DMBA and MCA, whose SCE-inducing activity was not affected by retinol (Qin *et al.*, 1985), retinol was protective towards other genotoxic agents requiring metabolic activation. These included cyclophosphamide and aflatoxin B_1 (Sirianni *et al.*, 1981; Qin *et al.*, 1985), *N*-nitrosodimethylamine and *N*-nitrosodiethylamine (Huang, 1987), in the presence of S9 mix, and NNK in primary rat hepatocytes (Alaoui-Jamali *et al.*, 1991a). A delay in the cell cycle was also observed (Huang, 1987). In Chinese hamster epithelial liver cells, which retain the intrinsic capacity to metabolize carcinogens, retinol and retinoic acid weakly inhibited the SCE-inducing activity of cyclophosphamide and DMBA (Cozzi *et al.*, 1990).

Chromosomal aberrations in Chinese hamster V79 cells, in the presence of S9 mix, were significantly inhibited when aflatoxin B_1 and cyclophosphamide were used as clastogenic agents. In contrast, they were significantly enhanced when BP and DMBA were used (Qin *et al.*, 1985).

The morphological transformation of C3H 10T1/2 mouse fibroblasts, pre-treated with MCA seven days earlier, was inhibited by retinol, retinal and retinyl acetate with similar potency. This effect was reversed when cell cultures were further maintained in a retinoid-free medium (Merriman & Bertram, 1979).

In human cultured cells (Table 28), preincubation with retinoic acid for two days did not affect the formation of DNA adducts in endometrioid IGROV$_1$ cells, but enhanced their formation in ovarian carcinoma NIHOVCAR cells at various times (0, 24 or 48 h) after treatment with cisplatin. This effect was accompanied by potentiation of cisplatin toxicity (Caliaro *et al.*, 1997). The mutagenic activity of polycyclic aromatic hydrocarbons, as evaluated by selection against diphtheria toxin, was decreased by vitamin A in human heteroploid epithelial-like (EUE) cells. In particular, retinyl palmitate protected these cells against the mutagenicity of

Table 27. Assay of retinol, retinal, retinoic acid and retinyl esters for ability to inhibit genetic and related effects in cultured animal cells

End-point[a]	Code[a]	Modulator (tested doses)[b]	Genotoxic agent (tested doses)[b]	Cells	Investigated effect	Result[c]	Inhibitory dose (IDx)[d]	Reference
D	DIA	Retinol (69.8 μM)	NNK (1–10 mM)	Primary rat hepatocytes	DNA single-strand breaks	(+)	69.8 μM (ID13)	Alaoui-Jamali *et al.* (1991a)
D	URP	Retinol (1–50 μM)	Ethyl methanesulfonate (200 μg/mL) [1.6 mM]	Primary rat hepatocytes	Unscheduled DNA synthesis	–	NA	Budroe *et al.* (1987)
D	URP	Retinoic acid (1–50 μM)	Ethyl methanesulfonate (200 μg/mL) [1.6 mM]	Primary rat hepatocytes	Unscheduled DNA synthesis	–	NA	Budroe *et al.* (1987)
D	URP	Retinol (1–50 μM)	254 nm UV light (32 J/m^3)	Primary rat hepatocytes	Unscheduled DNA synthesis	–	NA	Budroe *et al.* (1987)
D	URP	Retinoic acid (1–50 μM)	254 nm UV light (32 J/m^3)	Primary rat hepatocytes	Unscheduled DNA synthesis	–	NA	Budroe *et al.* (1987)
D	URP	Retinol (1–50 μM)	DMBA (5 μg/mL) [20 μM]	Primary rat hepatocytes	Unscheduled DNA synthesis	+	1 μM (ID55)	Budroe *et al.* (1987)
D	URP	Retinoic acid (1–50 μM)	DMBA (5 μg/mL) [20 μM]	Primary rat hepatocytes	Unscheduled DNA synthesis	+	1 μM (ID65)	Budroe *et al.* (1987)
D	UIA	Retinol (10 μM)	BP (10 μM)	Hamster tracheal epithelium in organ culture	Unscheduled DNA synthesis	#	NA	Wolterbeek *et al.* (1995)
D	BID	Retinol (10 μM)	BP (10 μM)	Hamster tracheal epithelium in organ culture	BPDE–DNA adducts	(+)	10 μM (ID20)	Wolterbeek *et al.* (1995)
D	BID	Retinol (34–122 μM)	Aflatoxin B_1 (0.08–10 μM)	Woodchuck hepatocytes	DNA adducts	+	34 μM (ID50)	Yu *et al.*, (1994)
G	GCO	Retinol (1–25 μM)	Ethyl methanesulfonate (100 μg/mL) [810 μM]	Chinese hamster ovary (CHO) cells	Mutation at the HGPRT locus	–	NA	Budroe *et al.* (1988)
G	GCO	Retinoic acid (1–25 μM)	Ethyl methanesulfonate (100 μg/mL) [810 μM]	Chinese hamster ovary (CHO) cells	Mutation at the HGPRT locus	–	NA	Budroe *et al.* (1988)

Table 27 (contd)

End-point[a]	Code[a]	Modulator (tested doses)[b]	Genotoxic agent (tested doses)[b]	Cells	Investigated effect	Result[c]	Inhibitory dose (IDx)[d]	Reference
G	GCO	Retinol (1–25 μM)	DMBA (5 μg/mL) [20 μM]	Chinese hamster ovary (CHO) cells + S9	Mutation at the HGPRT locus	+	5 μM (ID63)	Budroe *et al.* (1988)
G	GCO	Retinoic acid (1–25 μM)	DMBA (5 μg/mL) [20 μM]	Chinese hamster ovary (CHO) cells + S9	Mutation at the HGPRT locus	+	5 μM (ID60)	Budroe *et al.* (1988)
G	G9H	Retinyl acetate (100 μg/mL)	Ethyl methanesulfonate (100–1000 μg/mL)	Chinese hamster V79 cells	6-TG-resistance mutation	+	100 μg/mL (ID65)	Kuroda (1990)
S	SIC	Retinol (1–4 μg/mL)	Mitomycin C (0.03 μg/mL)	Chinese hamster V79 cells	Sister chromatid exchanges	–	NA	Sirianni *et al.* (1981)
S	SIC	Retinal (0.25–1 μg/mL)	Mitomycin C (0.03 μg/mL)	Chinese hamster V79 cells	Sister chromatid exchanges	–	NA	Sirianni *et al.* (1981)
S	SIC	Retinoic acid (1–4 μg/mL)	Mitomycin C (0.03 μg/mL)	Chinese hamster V79 cells	Sister chromatid exchanges	–	NA	Sirianni *et al.* (1981)
S	SIC	Retinyl acetate (1–4 μg/mL)	Mitomycin C (0.03 μg/mL)	Chinese hamster V79 cells	Sister chromatid exchanges	–	NA	Sirianni *et al.* (1981)
S	SIC	Retinol (1–8 μg/mL)	Cyclophosphamide (5 μg/mL)	Chinese hamster V79 cells + S9	Sister chromatid exchanges	+	8 μg/mL (ID65)	Huang *et al.* (1982)
S	SIC	Retinol (1–64 μg/mL)	Aflatoxin B_1 (0.2–0.5 μg/mL)	Chinese hamster V79 cells + S9	Sister chromatid exchanges	(+)	32 μg/mL (ID40)	Huang *et al.* (1982)
S	SIC	Retinol (4–32 μg/mL)	*N*-Nitrosodimethylamine (0.5 mg/mL)	Chinese hamster V79 cells + S9	Sister chromatid exchanges	+	32 μg/mL (ID55)	Huang (1987)
S	SIC	Retinol (17.4–139.6 μM)	NNK (20 mM)	Chinese hamster V79 cells + primary rat hepatocytes	Sister chromatid exchanges	+	139.6 μM (ID55)	Alaoui-Jamali *et al.* (1991a)
S	SIC	Retinol (4–32 μg/mL)	*N*-Nitrosodiethylamine (10 mg/mL)	Chinese hamster V79 cells + S9	Sister chromatid exchanges	(+)	32 μg/mL (ID44)	Huang (1987)

Table 27 (contd)

End-point[a]	Code[a]	Modulator (tested doses)[b]	Genotoxic agent (tested doses)[b]	Cells	Investigated effect	Result[c]	Inhibitory dose (IDx)[d]	Reference
S	SIC	Retinol (2–16 μg/mL)	MNNG (0.015 μg/mL)	Chinese hamster V79 cells	Sister chromatid exchanges	–	NA	Qin *et al.* (1985)
S	SIC	Retinol (2–16 μg/mL)	Ethyl methanesulfonate (250 μg/mL)	Chinese hamster V79 cells	Sister chromatid exchanges	–	NA	Qin *et al.* (1985)
S	SIC	Retinol (2–16 μg/mL)	Ethyl methanesulfonate (250 μg/mL)	Chinese hamster V79 cells + S9	Sister chromatid exchanges	–	NA	Qin *et al.* (1985)
S	SIC	Retinol (0.5–2 μg/mL)	Aflatoxin B_1 (0.2 μg/mL)	Chinese hamster V79 cells + S9	Sister chromatid exchanges	+	0.5 μg/mL (ID56)	Qin *et al.* (1985)
S	SIC	Retinol (0.5–2 μg/mL)	Cyclophosphamide (5 μg/mL)	Chinese hamster V79 cells + S9	Sister chromatid exchanges	+	0.5 μg/mL (ID56)	Qin *et al.* (1985)
S	SIC	Retinol (2–16 μg/mL)	Benz[*a*]anthracene (5 μg/mL)	Chinese hamster V79 cells + S9	Sister chromatid exchanges	–	NA	Qin *et al.* (1985)
S	SIC	Retinol (2–16 μg/mL)	Benzo[*a*]pyrene (2 μg/mL)	Chinese hamster V79 cells + S9	Sister chromatid exchanges	–	NA	Qin *et al.* (1985)
S	SIC	Retinol (2–16 μg/mL)	DMBA (2 μg/mL)	Chinese hamster V79 cells + S9	Sister chromatid exchanges	–	NA	Qin *et al.* (1985)
S	SIC	Retinol (2–16 μg/mL)	3-Methylcholanthrene (5 μg/mL)	Chinese hamster V79 cells + S9	Sister chromatid exchanges	–	NA	Qin *et al.* (1985)
S	SIC	Retinol (25 μM)	Cyclophosphamide (1 mM)	Chinese hamster epithelial liver (CHEL) cells	Sister chromatid exchanges	+	25 μM (ID50)	Cozzi *et al.* (1990)
S	SIC	Retinol (25 μM)	DMBA (0.078 μM)	Chinese hamster epithelial liver (CHEL) cells	Sister chromatid exchanges	+	25 μM (ID50)	Cozzi *et al.* (1990)
S	SIC	Retinoic acid (25–50 μM)	Cyclophosphamide (1 mM)	Chinese hamster epithelial liver (CHEL) cells	Sister chromatid exchanges	+	50 μM (ID50)	Cozzi *et al.* (1990)

Table 27 (contd)

End-point[a]	Code[a]	Modulator (tested doses)[b]	Genotoxic agent (tested doses)[b]	Cells	Investigated effect	Result[c]	Inhibitory dose (IDx)[d]	Reference
S	SIC	Retinoic acid (25–50 μM)	DMBA (0.078 μM)	Chinese hamster epithelial liver (CHEL) cells	Sister chromatid exchanges	+	37 μM (ID50)	Cozzi *et al.* (1990)
C	CIC	Retinol (4–32 μg/mL)	Aflatoxin B_1 (2 μg/mL)	Chinese hamster V79 cells + S9	Chromosomal aberrations	+	32 μg/mL (ID56)	Qin *et al.* (1985)
C	CIC	Retinol (4–32 μg/mL)	Cyclophosphamide (150 μg/mL)	Chinese hamster V79 cells + S9	Chromosomal aberrations	+	16 μg/mL (ID77)	Qin *et al.* (1985)
C	CIC	Retinol (4–32 μg/mL)	BP (100 μg/mL)	Chinese hamster V79 cells + S9	Chromosomal aberrations	#	NA	Qin *et al.* (1985)
C	CIC	Retinol (4–32 μg/mL)	DMBA (100 μg/mL)	Chinese hamster V79 cells + S9	Chromosomal aberrations	#	NA	Qin *et al.* (1985)
T	TCM	Retinol (0.05–0.5 μg/mL)	Pre-treatment with 3-methylcholanthrene (2.5 μg/mL)	C3H 10T1/2 mouse fibroblasts	Cell transformation	+	0.05 μg/mL (ID66)	Merriman & Bertram (1979)
T	TCM	Retinal (0.05–0.5 μg/mL)	Pre-treatment with 3-methylcholanthrene (2.5 μg/mL)	C3H 10T1/2 mouse fibroblasts	Cell transformation	+	0.05 μg/mL (ID75)	Merriman & Bertram (1979)
T	TCM	Retinyl acetate (0.005–0.5 μg/mL)	Pre-treatment with 3-methylcholanthrene (2.5 μg/mL)	C3H 10T1/2 mouse fibroblasts	Cell transformation	+	0.05 μg/mL (ID67)	Merriman & Bertram (1979)
T	TCM	Retinol (0.01–1 μM)	Areca nut extracts (2.5–5 mg/mL)	PdPBV-1-transfected C3H 10T1/2 mouse fibroblasts	Cell transformation	+	0.3 μM (ID100)	Stich & Tsang (1989)

[a] End-points investigated are: D, DNA damage; G, gene mutation; S, sister chromatid exchange; C, chromosomal aberration; T, cell transformation; test codes are given in Appendix 2

[b] Doses of compounds are as reported by the authors

[c] +, inhibition of the investigated effect ≥*ID50); (+), weak inhibition of the effect (≤ID50); –, no inhibition of the effect; #, enhancement of the effect; ?, unclear effect*

[d] Inhibitory dose (IDx), dose inhibiting x% of the investigated effect; NA, not applicable.

Abbreviations: BP, benzo[*a*]pyrene; DMBA, 7,12-dimethylbenz[*a*]anthracene; MNNG, *N*-methyl-*N*'nitro-*N*-nitrosoguanidine; NNK, 4-(N-nitrosomethylamino)-1-(3-pyridyl)-1-butanone

Table 28. Assay of retinol, retinal, retinoic acid and retinyl esters for ability to inhibit genetic and related effects in cultured human cells

End-point[a]	Code[a]	Modulator (tested doses)[b]	Genotoxic agent (tested doses)[b]	Cells	Investigated Effect	Result[c]	Inhibitory dose (IDx)[d]	Reference
D	BID	Retinoic acid (1 μM)	Cisplatin (10 μg/mL)	Human ovarian carcinoma NIHOVCAR cells	Pt–DNA adducts	#	NA	Caliaro *et al.* (1997)
D	BID	Retinoic acid (1 μM)	Cisplatin (10 μg/mL)	Human endometrioid $IGROV_1$ cells	Pt–DNA adducts	–	NA	Caliaro *et al.* (1997)
G	GIH	Retinyl palmitate (10 μM)	Benzo[*a*]pyrene (1 μM)	Human heteroploid epithelial-like (EUE) cells	Selection against diphtheria toxin	+	1 μM (ID87)	Rocchi *et al.* (1983)
G	GIH	Retinyl palmitate (10 μM)	3-Methylcholanthrene (1 μM)	Human heteroploid epithelial-like (EUE) cells	Selection against diphtheria toxin	+	1 μM (ID100)	Rocchi *et al.* (1983)
G	GIH	Retinyl palmitate (10 μM)	7,12-Dimethylbenz[*a*]anthracene (1 μM)	Human heteroploid epithelial-like (EUE) cells	Selection against diphtheria toxin	+	1 μM (ID63)	Rocchi *et al.* (1983)
G	GIH	Retinyl acetate (1 μM)	7,12-Dimethylbenz[*a*]anthracene (1 μM)	Human heteroploid epithelial-like (EUE) cells	Selection against diphtheria toxin	+	1 μM (ID72)	Ferreri *et al.* (1986)
G	GIH	Retinyl palmitate (10 μM)	7,12-Dimethylbenz[*a*]anthracene (1 μM)	Human heteroploid epithelial-like (EUE) cells	Selection against diphtheria toxin	+	1 μM (ID56)	Ferreri *et al.* (1986)
S	SHL	Retinol (4 μg/mL)	Melphalan (0.15 μg/mL)	Human lymphocytes	Sister chromatid exchanges	#	NA	Dozi-Vassiliades *et al.* (1985)
S	SHL	Retinol (4 μg/mL)	Caffeine (180 μg/mL)	Human lymphocytes	Sister chromatid exchanges	#	NA	Dozi-Vassiliades *et al.* (1985)

[a] End-points investigated are: D, DNA damage; G, gene mutation; S, sister chromatid exchange; test codes are given in Appendix 2

[b] Doses of compounds are as reported by the authors

[c] +, inhibition of the investigated effect (≥*ID50); (+), weak inhibition of the effect (<ID50); –, no inhibition of the effect; #, enhancement of the effect; ?, unclear effect*

[d] Inhibitory dose (IDx), dose inhibiting x% of the investigated effect; NA, not applicable.

BP, MCA and DMBA (Rocchi *et al.*, 1983). Mutagenicity of the last compound was inhibited to the same extent by retinyl acetate and retinyl palmitate (Ferreri *et al.*, 1986). Retinol even enhanced the ability of melphalan and caffeine to induce SCE in cultured human lymphocytes (Dozi-Vassiliades *et al.*, 1985).

4.3 Mechanism of chemoprevention

Mechanisms by which vitamin A might prevent or delay chemical carcinogenesis remain unclear. Various studies suggest that retinoids inhibit the promotion step of the multistage carcinogenesis process. However, there are some indications for effects on initiation as well.

4.3.1 Inhibition of events associated with carcinogenesis

Several reports described in Section 4.2.3.2 support the hypothesis that retinol and its esters inhibit the action of certain direct-acting mutagens as well as the metabolic activation of some chemical carcinogens to forms that can interact with and damage DNA. In some studies, retinol also induced the activity of detoxifying enzymes (Wang & Higuchi, 1995). These effects may be responsible, at least in part, for anticarcinogenic activity of retinol in inhibiting tumour initiation.

Evidence that retinol has protective effects against the promotion stage of carcinogenesis has come from several studies, which have demonstrated its ability to reverse premalignant lesions, inhibit cell transformation, suppress cell proliferation and DNA synthesis, and alter intercellular communication.

4.3.1.1 Effects on premalignant lesions

Administration of retinyl acetate at the time of removal of the first mammary tumour that developed after female rats had received a single injection of MNU decreased the rate of development of new tumours. Because in this carcinogenesis model the rats develop multiple asynchronous tumours, it is plausible to assume that at the time the first tumour was palpable, many preneoplastic lesions were present in the mammary gland. Therefore, these results suggest that retinyl acetate suppressed the conversion of these putative premalignant lesions to carcinomas (McCormick *et al.*, 1983). In this model, ovariectomy was also effective and the combination of retinyl acetate and ovariectomy was more effective than either agent alone. Thus, there may be a hormone-related effect of retinyl acetate. Further support for this idea comes from a study that showed that retinyl acetate inhibited estrogen-induced mammary carcinogenesis in female ACI rats, without evidence of gross toxicity (Holtzman, 1988). In this study, female rats that received a diet containing retinyl acetate (412 000 IU per kg diet) and then a subcutaneously implanted pellet containing 17α-ethinylestradiol and were maintained on retinyl acetate-containing diet for 24 further weeks developed half as many mammary cancers as rats on a control diet.

In a skin carcinogenesis model using female CD-1 mice with initiation by DMBA and promotion by twice weekly applications of TPA, retinyl palmitate provided in the diet caused a dose-dependent inhibition of the number and weight of papillomas at 21 weeks, reaching 65% in the group given 350 000 IU per kg of diet (Gensler *et al.*, 1987). In male rats given 0.05% BBN as carcinogen followed by 5% sodium saccharin as promoter, a diet containing 0.05% retinyl acetate suppressed saccharin-induced colony growth of bladder cells in soft agar, suggesting that vitamin A has anti-tumour-promoting effects on rat bladder carcinogenesis (Kanamaru *et al.*, 1988).

In a two-stage rat hepatocarcinogenesis model with DEN as the initiator and either 3,3′,4,4′-tetrachlorobiphenyl or 2,2′,4,4′,5,5′-hexachlorobiphenyl as promoter, a diet containing 100 000 IU of retinyl palmitate decreased the number and volume of hepatic foci compared with animals on a diet with little or no retinyl palmitate. Thus, retinyl palmitate protected against preneoplastic changes enhanced by the tumour promoters (Berberian *et al.*, 1995).

One biomarker of genotoxic damage due to carcinogens is the formation of micronuclei in epithelial cells. A reduced frequency of micro-nucleated mucosal cells and remission of leukoplakias was seen following twice weekly administration of vitamin A (100 000 or 200 000 IU per week) for 3–6 months to chewers of tobacco-containing betel quids. The development of new leukoplakias was also inhibited. After vitamin A administration was terminated, micro-nucleated cells and leukoplakia recurred in the oral cavity of chewers who continued to use tobacco throughout the trial period. Vitamin A given at a level of 50 000 IU per week maintained the frequency of micronucleated mucosal cells at low levels for at least 12 months after the trial (Stich *et al.,* 1991a,b).

The mechanism of suppression of tumour promotion is not clear, but may involve inhibition of the transformation of normal cells, or inhibition of proliferation of initiated or premalignant cells such that the premalignant lesion is not converted to a malignant one or the promotion step is prolonged.

Decreased levels of retinol or retinyl esters have been detected in premalignant lesions or tumours. For example, the vitamin A concentration in UV-induced tumours in mouse skin was significantly lower than in perilesional epidermis in mice consuming diets with or without vitamin A supplementation (20 000 IU/kg). The largest difference between the levels in tumour and epidermis was observed in the vitamin A-supplemented group. The low vitamin A content of the tumours was due to a marked reduction in the retinyl ester fraction, whereas the retinol content of the tumours actually increased two-fold. It was suggested that interconversion of retinol to retinyl esters may be disturbed in murine photo-carcinogenesis (Berne *et al.*, 1989). Serum levels of vitamin A were significantly decreased in 50 cases of oral leukoplakia compared with 50 normal controls (Ramaswamy *et al.,* 1996), but intralesional vitamin A levels were not measured in this study. In 34 patients with HPV infection of the cervix and in 40 patients with CIN (cervical intra-epithelial neoplasia) III, retinyl palmitate concentration was extremely low in CIN III tissue compared with normal cervical epithelium and HPV-infected tissue. In this study there was no significant difference in serum vitamin A levels between the two groups. It was concluded that the reduction of retinyl palmitate in CIN III is a local process and that a local supplementation of vitamin A might contribute to prevention of cervical neoplasia (Volz *et al.*, 1995).

4.3.1.2 Inhibition of transformation

As described in Section 4.2.3.1, retinol inhibits the transformation of cultured cells exposed to carcinogens and tumour promoters. Treatment of postconfluent cultures of mouse C3H 10T1/2 fibroblasts with certain carcinogens causes transformation to focus-forming cells, and retinyl acetate inhibits this transformation (Mordan, 1989). Areca nut (used in betel quids) has been linked to the high incidence of precancerous oral lesions and oral cancers in India. The formation of bovine papillomavirus (BPV) DNA-induced transformed foci was enhanced approximately tenfold in cultured mouse C3H 10T1/2 cells transfected with the plasmid pdPBV-1 harbouring BPV DNA and exposed to areca nut extracts. This transformation was completely suppressed when 1 µmol/L retinol was added to the areca nut extract. This was proposed as a mechanism of chemoprevention by vitamin A in betel quid chewers (Stich & Tsang, 1989).

4.3.1.3 Inhibition of DNA synthesis and cell proliferation

The transformation of density-arrested, initiated C3H 10T1/2 cells by certain carcinogens was correlated with the mitogenic response of the preneoplastic cells to platelet-derived or epidermal growth factor. Stimulation by serum of DNA synthesis in carcinogen-treated C3H 10T1/2 cells was inhibited by retinyl acetate, presumably by blockage of the G_0 to G_1 transition in the mitotic response of initiated cells to platelet growth factors (Mordan, 1989).

Retinol inhibited DNA synthesis and growth of MCA-induced squamous cell carcinomas in Swiss male albino mice and basal cell carcinomas in inbred Sprague–Dawley rats (Lupulescu, 1986). In another study, female Sprague–Dawley rats were treated with either solvent, DMBA or MNU at 50 days of age and were placed on a retinyl acetate-containing diet at 57 days of age. [^{3}H]Thymidine incorporation into purified DNA from mammary parenchymal cells was determined. Retinyl acetate effectively inhibited mammary cell DNA synthesis in both MNU- and DMBA-treated animals compared with those on control diet (Mehta & Moon, 1980).

4.3.1.4 Inhibition of ornithine decarboxylase induction

Cell proliferation and transformation require accelerated polyamine biosynthesis and elevated levels of ornithine decarboxylase (ODC), the rate-limiting enzyme in this reaction chain. Tumour promoters enhance ODC activity and retinoids suppress this induction. In an animal model for oral carcinogenesis, DMBA stimulated ODC activity and vitamin A inhibited late-phase ODC induction *in vivo* and prevented carcinogenesis (Calhoun *et al.*, 1989). That retinol also inhibited ODC induction in mouse skin was indicated by the finding that citral (3,7-dimethyl-2,6-octadienal) inhibits the oxidation of retinol to retinoic acid in mouse epidermis on local application. Citral treatment decreased the ability of retinol to inhibit the induction of epidermal ODC activity by TPA (Connor, 1988). In rats, a single intraperitoneal injection of TPA resulted in a transient increase in liver ODC activity. This increase was inhibited when retinyl acetate was injected one hour before TPA (Bisschop *et al.*, 1981). The inhibition by retinoids of the tumour promoter-induced increase in ODC activity was correlated with suppression of carcinogenesis (Verma *et al.*, 1979).

4.3.1.5 Restoration of normal differentiation

Carcinogenesis is characterized by aberrant differentiation, which is manifested by either blockage of cells at an early stage of differentiation or by redirection of differentiation towards an abnormal pathway. Retinol and retinyl esters have been reported to maintain proper differentiation in many epithelial tissues and to reverse abnormal differentiation in premalignant and malignant cells. Vitamin A deficiency is associated with loss of mucociliary differentiation and metaplastic changes to keratinizing squamous epithelium *in vivo* and in long-term rat tracheal organ cultures (Clark *et al.*, 1980). In the presence of retinyl acetate, normal mucociliary epithelium can be maintained for several months in organ culture of tracheal explants. Squamous metaplastic epithelium, which develops in vitamin A-deficient organ cultures, reverts to mucus-secreting tissue (Clark & Marchok, 1979; Clark *et al.*, 1980). The reversal of metaplasia *in vivo* was associated with prevention of lung carcinogenesis (Saffiotti *et al.*, 1967).

4.3.1.6 Restoration of gap junctional communication

An early event in cellular transformation is loss of intercellular communication via gap junctions. Retinol and retinyl esters enhance gap-junctional communication in carcinogen-initiated C3H 10T1/2 cells and suppress neoplastic transformation of these cells. A good correlation between these two events was shown by their overlapping responses to different retinoid doses. These findings led to the proposal that enhanced junctional communication may be an important mechanism for the chemopreventive action of retinol (Hossain *et al.*, 1989). In tracheal epithelial cells cultured in the absence of vitamin A, cigarette-smoke condensate inhibited intercellular communication. However, when retinol was added to tracheal epithelial cells before or simultaneously with exposure to cigarette-smoke condensate, it counteracted the inhibitory effect of the condensate on intercellular communication (Rutten *et al.*, 1988b).

4.3.1.7 Inhibition of prostaglandin production

Excessive production of prostaglandins has been correlated with tumour promotion. Expression of the enzyme cyclooxygenase-2 (Cox-2), which catalyses the synthesis of prostaglandins, can be induced by growth factors and tumour promoters and is up-regulated in transformed cells and tumours. Therefore, Cox-2 inhibition has potential relevance as a mechanism of chemoprevention. A few studies have demonstrated that retinol can suppress prostaglandin biosynthesis and this effect might mediate suppression of the growth of premalignant and malignant cells, thereby inhibiting carcinogenesis. The production of prostaglandin in normal tissues has been found to be regulated by retinol. Production of prostaglandin E_2 from arachidonic acid in bovine seminal vesicles and kidney was considerably inhibited by retinol, whereas the production of hydroxyeicosatetraenoic acid was inhibited to a smaller extent. Thus, it appears that retinol influences both the cyclooxygenase and lipoxygenase pathways (Halevy & Sklan, 1987). Similarly, both retinol and retinoic acid inhibited the oxidation of arachidonic acid to prostaglandin E_2 in squamous carcinoma cells of the tongue (SCC-25) (ElAttar & Lin, 1991). Treatment of oral epithelial cells with TPA enhanced transcription of Cox-2 and increased production of prostaglandin E_2. These effects were inhibited by retinyl acetate and retinoic acid (Mestre *et al.*, 1997).

4.3.1.8 Modulation of cell adhesion and migration

Cell migration and invasion through the basement membrane are important for the conversion of advanced dysplastic lesions to malignant neoplasms. Inhibition of invasion may therefore suppress this conversion. In this context, it is noteworthy that a two-day pretreatment with retinyl acetate (0.09 and 3 μg/mL) inhibited the migration and invasion of A549 human lung carcinoma cells *in vitro* through human amnion basement membrane and the degradation of basement membrane components. This effect was accompanied by a significant decrease in type IV collagenase activity. It has been reported that retinoic acid can inhibit the expression of various basement membrane degradative enzymes (e.g., collagenase, stromelysin) at the level of transcription (Nakajima *et al.*, 1989; Nicholson *et al.*, 1990). These findings suggest that retinol may suppress the expression of invasive phenotype in carcinoma *in situ* and thereby prevent the development of a malignant lesion from a premalignant one (Fazely *et al.*, 1988).

4.3.2 Inhibition of angiogenesis

The progressive growth of solid tumours depends on the development of new blood vessels, a process known as neovascularization or angiogenesis. Tumour cells secrete factors that induce the directed migration and proliferation of endothelial cells from capillaries in the normal tissue, which eventually differentiate and form vessels around and within tumours. In rabbits, intramuscularly injected vitamin A inhibited angiogenesis induced in the eyes by intracorneal implants of carcinoma, and also resulted in inhibition of tumour growth at the implantation site (Arensman & Stolar, 1979). More recent studies with retinyl acetate and retinoic acid have demonstrated anti-angiogenic effects of retinoids in an assay using 4.5-day chorioallantoic membranes of chick embryo (Oikawa *et al.*, 1989). Retinoic acid causes large- and small-vessel endothelial cells to become refractory to stimulation of migration by either tumour-conditioned media or purified angiogenic factors (α-fibroblast growth factor (αFGF), bFGF, vascular endothelial growth factor, PDGF, TGFβ-1 and interleukin-8) without affecting cell proliferation. Retinoic acid (1 mg/kg/day) inhibited a neovascular response to tumour in the cornea of rats (Lingen *et al.*, 1996). These results indicated that the acid can affect directly both tumour cells and endothelial cells and thereby suppress the formation of new blood vessels *in vivo*. Although the latter study was not performed with retinol or retinyl acetate, the data overall suggest that vitamin A may exert its inhibitory effect on carcinogenesis and tumour growth *in vivo* by modifying the normal vascular response to neoplastic tissue.

4.3.3 Modulation of immune responses

Epidemiological studies suggest that vitamin A plays an important role in immune responses in adults and children. Vitamin A deficiency leads to impaired antibody responses to protein antigens, changes in lymphocyte subpopulations and altered T- and B-cell proliferation and function (Semba, 1994; Tomita, 1983). The immune defect caused by vitamin A deficiency may be due to alterations in lymphocyte cell membrane glycoproteins, an adverse effect on helper T-cell function, or some other mechanisms (Rumore, 1993). Vitamin A and its metabolites are immune enhancers that potentiate antibody responses to T-cell-dependent antigens and increase lymphocyte proliferation responses to antigens and mitogens (Semba, 1994). Vitamin A may boost immune responses in the elderly, in persons with high exposure to ultraviolet light, in patients who have undergone surgery, and in persons with parasitic infection (Rumore, 1993). A mechanism to help explain the anticancer action of vitamin A might be immunosuppression during deficiency or immuno-enhancement with high dietary intake. *In vitro*, retinol suppressed

T-lymphocyte functions, whereas high dietary levels of vitamin A enhanced macrophage functions. Enhancement of immune functions by high intake of vitamin A provides a mechanism to explain in part the decreased carcinogenesis (Watson, 1986).

Antitumour effects of vitamin A in mice have been related to immune enhancement in a number of systems. In CBA mice, a diet enriched in retinyl acetate (up to 0.8 g/kg diet) increased the ability of the immune system to respond effectively to tumour antigens and to suppress tumour growth in immunized mice. These effects could be explained partially by an increase in T-cell-mediated cytotoxicity but not by changes in natural killer (NK) cell activity (Malkovsky *et al.*, 1983). Antitumour activity could be increased even without immunization in mice placed on a retinyl acetate-enriched diet for at least three weeks (Malkovsky *et al.*, 1984). Diets with high levels of retinyl palmitate (4000–650 000 IU/kg diet) administered to CD-1 mice for 7 to 10 weeks increased mitogenic response in splenocytes, and enhanced phagocytic ability and tumoricidal activity of peritoneal macrophages, but did not enhance NK activity (Moriguchi *et al.*, 1985).

The administration of retinyl palmitate in the drinking water of BALB/c mice at 200, 500 or 1000 IU per mouse per day increased proliferative response to concanavalin A, *Escherichia coli* lipopolysaccharide and interleukin-2, and the production of lymphokines after 60–90 days. The growth of three distinct transplantable tumours was impaired when the tumour cells were transplanted on day 75 (Forni *et al.*, 1986). Similar results were reported in another syngenic murine tumour system *in vivo* in which intraperitoneal administration of vitamin A suppressed the growth of tumour cells inoculated subcutaneously (Tomita, 1983). [The Working Group was unclear about the nature and stability of the retinyl palmitate preparation that was apparently 'dissolved' into the drinking water.]

More relevant to chemoprevention than the above studies is the report that dietary retinyl palmitate administered at 350 IU/g of diet for 22–30 weeks to CD-1 mice, which had been given an initiating treatment with DMBA followed by TPA promotion, enhanced immune response and prevented skin tumour development. Mice on this diet exhibited an increase in the number of peritoneal macrophages and in their cytotoxic capacity. This enhanced immune response may have contributed to skin tumour prevention (Watson *et al.*, 1987).

Immunomodulatory effects of various retinoids have been demonstrated, both *in vivo* and *in vitro*, in murine and human thymocytes, human lung fibroblasts, Langerhans' cells, tumour cells and NK cells, and peripheral blood mononuclear cells. For example, retinol or retinoic acid (0.1 μmol/L; 48 h) acted as co-stimulators for human peripheral blood mononuclear cells in serum-free medium. Retinol increased the proliferation of such cells from 32 healthy individuals, which had been stimulated with anti-CD3 antibodies 48 h earlier. The increased proliferative response was mediated via the clonotypic T-cell receptor-CD3 complex and correlated with the up-regulation of T-lymphocyte surface adhesion/activation markers (CD18, CD45RO and CD25) and cytokines (interleukin-2 and interferon-gamma) at both the mRNA and protein levels. The authors suggested that retinoids may be used as therapeutic agents in immune system deficiencies that do not affect the clonotypic T-cell receptor (Allende *et al.*, 1997). Lipopolysaccharide-induced release of tumour necrosis factor (TNF) by human peripheral blood monocytes was suppressed in vitamin A-free medium and addition of retinol (1 μmol/L) resulted in the release of TNF-like activity into the culture supernatant after three days of culture (Turpin *et al.*, 1990).

Immune stimulation in humans *in vivo* has been demonstrated in a few studies. Retinyl palmitate was given for up to seven treatment courses during a period of 60 weeks to nine male patients with metastatic unresectable squamous cell carcinoma of the lung. An immune potentiating effect of the vitamin A therapy was indicated by an increase of lymphocyte blastogenesis response to phytohaemagglutinin and increased delayed cutaneous hypersensitivity reactions compared with the pretreatment values (Micksche *et al.*, 1977). Additional aspects of immune enhancement were observed after treatment of patients suffering from chronic lymphocytic leukaemia with vitamin A (100 000 IU daily for two weeks). This resulted in enhancement of antibody-dependent cell-mediated cytotoxicity, NK cell activity and blastogenic response to plant mitogens (Gergely *et al.*, 1988).

These findings suggest that vitamin A may contribute to the prevention of cancer by augmenting an immunological response against tumour cells in the early stages of carcinogenesis. However, it should be noted that a recent report indicated a suppressive effect of supplemental vitamin A (800 μg retinyl palmitate per day) on cell-mediated immune response in an older population (Fortes *et al.*, 1998).

4.3.4 Other mechanisms

Apoptosis may be induced by vitamin A, although current information is limited (Maziere *et al.*, 1997). Vitamin A might also affect any of the processes discussed above by serving as an antioxidant, although many more effective antioxidants, such as vitamin E and ascorbic acid, exist in biological systems.

5. Other Beneficial Effects

5.1 Conditions related to vitamin A deficiency

5.1.1 Night-blindness and xerophthalmia

Moderate deficiency in vitamin A leads to dryness of the conjunctiva of the eyes and decreased night vision, which in severe cases may proceed to irreversible blindness (Tee, 1992). It is implied by the status of retinol as a vitamin that all but the most severe forms of these conditions may be improved by administration of retinol or retinyl esters either as drugs or by dietary means (Olson, 1987; Gerster, 1997). The impact of vitamin A on other conditions of the eye, including macular degeneration and cataract, has been the subject of several studies but no significant effect related to retinol has been observed (Seddon *et al.*, 1994; Sanders *et al.*, 1993; Sperduto *et al.*, 1993; West *et al.*, 1994). In a study of 12 cases treated with vitamin A eyedrops for superior limbic keratoconjunctivitis, ten cases showed improvement, to varying extents (Ohashi *et al.*, 1988). [No systematic studies of this condition were available to the Working Group.]

5.1.2 Growth

Observations of the effect of vitamin A on early child growth are inconsistent. In a field study of 3377 Nepalese children, 12–60 months of age and without signs of xerophthalmia, the participants were given 60 000 μg retinol equivalents (RE) once every four months, or placebo (300 RE). No difference in weight gain or linear growth was observed, except for minor changes in arm circumference and muscle mass (West *et al.*, 1997). However, when xerophthalmic children given 120 000 RE or more at baseline were compared with the non-xerophthalmic children, the former had a significant increase in growth after adjustment for sex, age and measurement status. Although confirmatory studies are needed, the available data indicate that retinol influences growth only in individuals with vitamin A deficiency.

5.1.3 Cystic fibrosis

Retinol levels in plasma are decreased in some patients with cystic fibrosis (Rasmussen *et al.*, 1986). This may lead to overt signs of vitamin A deficiency such as xerophthalmia, decreased night vision or skin abnormalities, which are reversed upon treatment with retinol (Brooks *et al.*, 1990; Rayner *et al.*, 1989). In cystic fibrosis, up to 40% of the dietary retinol may pass unabsorbed and be lost with the stool and thus the patients need supplementation (Ahmed *et al.*, 1990). It has been debated whether dryness of the eye is a sign of vitamin A deficiency in these patients or a manifestation of the disease itself (Morkeberg *et al.*, 1995).

5.1.4 Psoriasis and other skin conditions

Vitamin A has been used to treat a large number of skin disorders, including severe acne (Heller & Schiffman, 1985), psoriasis and pityriasis (Winkelmann *et al.*, 1983). Due to the toxicity of retinol, a number of synthetic retinoids as well as retinal and retinoic acid have replaced retinol and its esters for the treatment of most of these conditions. Corrocher *et al.* (1989) observed a normal plasma level of retinol in psoriatic patients and Rollman and Vahlquist (1985) observed similar retinol levels in skin biopsies from 33 plaque psoriasis patients and 37 healthy control subjects.

Dihydroretinol was, however, significantly increased in samples of both affected and unaffected skin of psoriasis patients. In an open study, 30 psoriasis patients were treated with liarozole, an inhibitor of cytochrome P450-mediated retinol oxidation, for up to 12 months. There was a consistent decrease in symptoms as determined by the Psoriasis Area and Severity Index (PASI) scores with duration of treatment, reaching 87% by 12 months (Dockx *et al.*, 1995). This could indicate a higher demand for vitamin A by these patients. However, skin or serum retinol levels were not determined and thus this possibility has not been confirmed. [No placebo-controlled studies relating retinol with a decrease in PASI scores were available to the Working Group.]

5.1.5 Anaemia

Retinol may influence the uptake or use of iron in anaemic individuals who are vitamin A-deficient. In a randomized, double-blind, placebo-controlled trial, 251 pregnant women from West Java, aged 17–35 years, who had haemoglobin levels of 80–109 g/L, were randomized into four groups, given daily iron (60 mg), retinol (2.4 mg), both or placebo. The supplemented groups all improved significantly with respect to haemoglobin, packed cell volume and transferrin saturation compared with controls. Both iron-supplemented groups improved significantly with respect to serum ferritin, iron, and total iron-binding capacity, whereas retinol-supplemented groups had significantly increased serum retinol. The percentages of women who improved to a level of haemoglobin above the limit of anaemia (110 g/L) were 68%, 35%, 97% and 16%, respectively in the groups supplemented with iron, retinol, both or placebo. The authors concluded that improvement in vitamin A status may contribute to controlling anaemia in pregnant women (Suharno *et al.*, 1993).

5.1.6 Eclampsia and abruptio placentae

Two studies have reported an association between symptoms of eclampsia during pregnancy and low serum levels of vitamin A. Jendryczko and Drozdz (1989) followed 20 pregnant women from 28 weeks of gestation until four weeks after delivery. Blood samples were drawn initially and at delivery. In nine women who developed pre-eclampsia, retinol (263±38 µg/L) and vitamin E levels were significantly lower than in the remaining eleven normo-tensive subjects (396±23 µg/L, $p < 0.02$). In another study of pregnant women aged 14–25 years, retinol levels were significantly lower in seven cases with eclampsia (8.3 mg/dL) and in nine cases with symptoms of pre-eclampsia (15.3 mg/dL) than in their normotensive counterparts (24.2 mg/dL). A similar trend was observed for β-carotene and vitamin E (Ziari *et al.*, 1996). [No information was available to the Working Group on use of vitamin A intervention to prevent eclampsia.]

Retinol levels in venous blood samples from 71 pregnant women with *abruptio placentae* were significantly lower than in 86 pregnant women matched for gestational week. A weaker but overall significant trend was also observed for vitamin E and β-carotene (Sharma *et al.*, 1986). The authors noted that other vitamin deficiencies have been observed in previous studies and suggested that the condition may be caused by multivitamin deficiencies.

5.2 Infectious disease and mortality

Vitamin A is generally believed to be important for resistance to infections (Tee, 1992), but the available literature is more clear with regard to the negative relationship between vitamin A status and mortality in undernourished populations. Up to 1995, seven well documented double-blind placebo-controlled intervention studies had been reported: six showed a beneficial effect of retinol supplementation on child mortality (five were statistically significant) (Bates, 1995). It is important to note that all child mortality studies carried out so far have been conducted in populations in which vitamin A deficiency is prevalent. Moreover, while vitamin A has been shown to lower mortality, subsequent studies have demonstrated a less marked effect of vitamin A on morbidity (Glasziou & Mackerras, 1993).

In two large double-blind placebo-controlled trials in northern Ghana, the influence of vitamin A on mortality and morbidity was specifically addressed (Ghana VAST Study Team,

1993). In the mortality study, 21 906 children aged 6–90 months were randomized in 185 geographical clusters to receive either 200 000 IU retinol equivalents (100 000 IU under 12 months) or placebo, every four months. Mortality was significantly lower in the vitamin A-supplemented clusters than in the placebo clusters (ratio of mean mortality rates, 0.8; 95% CI, 0.7–1.0; $p = 0.03$). Among specific causes of death, only mortality due to acute gastroenteritis was significantly lower in supplemented clusters. There were no sex or age differences in mortality. Also the total numbers of attendances at clinics and of hospital admissions were both significantly lower in supplemented clusters. In the morbidity study, 1455 children aged 6–59 months were assigned on an individual basis to supplementation or placebo as outlined above. There were no differences in the mean daily prevalence of diarrhoea or acute respiratory infections. Of the 18 conditions monitored, only vomiting and refusing food/breast milk were significantly less common in supplemented children.

It is important to distinguish between the influence of infectious diseases on vitamin A status (Olson, 1987) and the possibility that vitamin A prevents infection. In the latter case, it is then necessary to establish the levels of vitamin A which are sufficient for our natural defence systems and to investigate whether high-dose vitamin A has additional effects on specific infections. In the Ghana study, a significant correlation between α1-acid glycoprotein or serum amyloid A, both indicators of infections, and low retinol status was observed, whereas no association was found between serum retinol levels and symptoms of infection (Filteau *et al.*, 1993). The authors' interpretation was that subclinical, underlying infections influence serum retinol levels; they further reported that malaria parasite density was significantly and inversely correlated with plasma retinol, indicating a specific effect of this infection on vitamin A status. Thurnham and Singkamani (1991) also reported a significant negative association between plasma retinol and malaria in a case–control study in Thailand. These authors suggested that increased plasma retinol binding to retinol-binding protein and transthyretin causes increased availability of the vitamin to the tissues, thereby decreasing plasma retinol, while body stores might still be adequate. Thus, plasma retinol may be a doubtful measure of retinol status during malarial infections. In a later cross-sectional study in India, this was supported by the observation that levels of retinol-binding protein, which are influenced by the acute phase response, explain 95% of the variation in plasma retinol in malaria patients (Das *et al.*, 1996). At least seven other cross-sectional or case–control studies have consistently found that plasma levels of retinol were decreased in malaria cases compared with matched healthy controls. In the randomized placebo-controlled study of the effect of retinol on mortality in 21 906 children from Ghana (see above), there was no difference in the malaria mortality rate or fever incidence rate and no correlation between plasma retinol at baseline and subsequent malaria parasitaemia in the placebo group (Binka *et al.*, 1995).

A range of cross-sectional studies and case–control studies have also found an association between infection with various intestinal helminths and low plasma retinol levels. The observation that ascariasis does not influence vitamin A absorption (Ahmed *et al.*, 1993) while treatment with mebendazole may increase plasma retinol levels (Curtale *et al.*, 1994) indicates that helminth infestation *per se* may change retinol distribution without affecting body stores of the vitamin.

An inverse association between infection with human immunodeficiency virus (HIV) and plasma retinol level has been found in several studies. However, a prospective study in a highly endemic area for heterosexual HIV transmission in Rwanda gave no indication of a correlation between baseline retinol levels and the subsequent risk for seroconversion in a group of 119 sexually active women followed over a 24-month period (Moore *et al.*, 1993). In a prospective study of 21 HIV-infected children and 21 controls from France, plasma retinol levels decreased with severity of the disease (Periquet *et al.*, 1995). It has been postulated that HIV infection decreases plasma retinol levels by decreasing the formation and release of retinol-binding protein from the liver, so that body stores of retinol might be adequate while the plasma level remains low (Rosales & Ross, 1996).

In a study of 338 HIV-positive mothers in Malawi, serum retinol concentrations were inversely correlated with risk of HIV transmission to children who survived for more than 12 months ($p < 0.0001$) (Semba *et al.*, 1994). Since serum retinol may reflect severity of disease in the mothers, the result may be a consequence of this association rather than an effect of retinol *per se*. [The Working Group noted that at least four randomized trials are in progress to test vitamin A supplementation in HIV-positive pregnant women in order to resolve this issue.]

The impact of retinol on respiratory infections has been addressed in several studies, with inconsistent outcomes. In a placebo-controlled study of infant morbidity, the impact of 209 μmol vitamin A given immediately after delivery to a group of 50 low-income mothers from Bangladesh was investigated (Roy *et al.*, 1997). A significant decrease was observed in the duration of respiratory tract infections (3.1 days); 95% CI, 2.7–3.5 versus 3.7; 95% CI, 3.3–4.2; $p < 0.03$) and of the mean incidence of febrile illness (0.1; 95% CI, 0.1–0.1 versus 0.3; 95% CI, 0.3–0.3; $p < 0.002$) in breast-fed infants of vitamin A-supplemented mothers. In a randomized controlled trial of 147 pre-school children with frequent respiratory tract infections, supplementation with 450 μg/day of retinol decreased significantly the number of episodes of respiratory symptoms over a period of 11 months (Pinnock *et al.*, 1986). The effect of retinol on established respiratory infection has also been addressed in a few studies. In two multicentre randomized, placebo-controlled studies of 239 and 180 children, respectively, with respiratory syncytial virus infection, there was no evidence of a beneficial effect of vitamin A therapy (Bresee *et al.*, 1996; Dowell *et al.*, 1996). In a randomized study of 24 hospitalized patients with pneumonia in São Paulo, Brazil, who were all immediately treated with penicillin, intervention on day 1 with 200 000 IU of vitamin A did not affect plasma vitamin A on day seven, when all patients were improving. The authors state that these results support the hypothesis that low plasma levels of vitamin A during the acute phase of infection can be independent of vitamin A status (Velasquez Melendez *et al.*, 1995).

Coutsoudis *et al.* (1991) found a significant difference in plasma vitamin A levels in children with measles depending on supplementation with retinol. Such supplementation appears to carry clinical benefit in certain populations. In a randomized placebo-controlled trial of vitamin A treatment on morbidity in children hospitalized with measles in South Africa, Hussey and Klein (1990) observed a significant beneficial action of vitamin A. Similar results were reported previously in a study in Tanzania (Barclay *et al.*, 1987).

5.3 Effects on vascular or heart disease

In a prospective study of antioxidant vitamin intake and coronary heart disease (CHD) among 87 245 nurses (all females) in the United States, the risk of CHD was 0.70 (95% CI, 0.5–0.9) in the highest versus the lowest intake groups for total vitamin A (Manson *et al.*, 1991). [The Working Group noted that these results have been published only in an abstract.] In another prospective study of 34486 postmenopausal women in Iowa, United States, followed for eight years, there was no apparent association between risk for CHD and vitamin A intake from diet or self-administered supplements (Kushi *et al.*, 1996).

The Beta-Carotene and Retinol Efficacy Trial (CARET) was a double-blind, randomized, placebo-controlled primary prevention trial (see Section 4.1.2.1(*b*)), in which retinol (25 000 IU/day) and β-carotene (30 mg/day) or placebo was administered for an average of four years to a group of 18 314 current or former smokers, or asbestos workers, aged 45–69 years. The study was designed primarily as a cancer prevention study, but several end-points were monitored, including various forms of cardiovascular disease and total deaths. There was no improvement in any of these conditions in the intervention group as compared to the placebo group (Omenn *et al.*, 1996b). The intervention group experienced a 17% higher mortality rate (95% CI, 1.0–1.3; $p < 0.05$) and a

26% higher rate of cardiovascular disease deaths (95% CI, 1.0–1.6). The authors concluded that the combination of β-carotene with retinol had no benefit on health within the four-year follow-up period and may have had an adverse effect on cardiovascular disease and overall mortality.

In an intervention trial in Linxian county, China, described fully in Section 4.1.2.1(*a*), subjects receiving retinyl acetate (10 000 IU) with β-carotene showed a significant reduction in deaths from cerebrovascular disease among males (RR, 0.45), but not among females (RR, 0.90).

Administration of retinol (60 000 IU/day) in combination with 300 mg nicotinic acid and 140 mg tocopherol daily decreased LDL cholesterol and marginally increased HDL cholesterol in twelve patients suffering from hypercholesterolaemia (Odetti *et al.*, 1984). A positive correlation between plasma HDL cholesterol and intake of antioxidant vitamins, including intake of vitamin A, has also been observed in subgroups of white women and non-smoking black men in the CARDIA (Coronary Artery Risk Development in Young Adults) study cohort, which comprises 2193 men and 2654 women, 49% blacks and 51% whites, aged 18–30 years, living in the United States (Slattery *et al.*, 1995). Moreover, a single oral supplementation with 20 000 IU of vitamin A increased the *in vitro* oxidation resistance of LDL isolated before and eight hours after supplementation (Livrea *et al.*, 1995).

In a cross-sectional study of 10 359 randomly selected Scottish men and women aged 40–59 years, the risk for subsequent CHD among men was lower in the highest quintiles of intake of total vitamin A, fibre, β-carotene and vitamins C and E, whereas no such relationship was observed for retinol. No significant relationship between total vitamin A or retinol intake and CHD was observed in women (Bolton Smith *et al.*, 1992). In a cross-sectional study of the relationship between coronary artery disease and plasma levels of several vitamins in 72 elderly subjects, vitamin A and E levels were independently and inversely related to the risk of the disease after adjustment for confounders (Singh *et al.*, 1995).

5.4 Other preventive actions

5.4.1 Degenerative conditions of ageing

Some recent reviews have considered the evidence for beneficial antioxidant effects of retinoids in preventive geriatrics (Ward, 1994, 1996). Although there is some theoretical and laboratory evidence that retinol might be protective against degenerative changes in the skin, eye and immune system due to antioxidant action, relevant clinical and epidemiological evidence is scarce.

5.4.2 Arthritis

In a prospective case–control study, Comstock *et al.* (1997) investigated the association between serum levels of antioxidant vitamins and the risk for rheumatoid arthritis and lupus erythematosus. Retinol levels were lower in the serum from patients who subsequently developed either of these conditions. Low plasma levels of vitamin A have also been found in patients with rheumatoid arthritis (Honkanen *et al.*, 1989) and in patients with juvenile rheumatoid arthritis (Bacon *et al.*, 1990) as compared with unmatched controls. Serum levels of retinol were not decreased in cases with spondylitis or ankylosing hyperostosis (Mezes *et al.*, 1986). Finally, it has been reported that in patients with Sjögren's syndrome, supplementation with 100 000 IU of vitamin A daily for 14 days improved immunological performance (Szöcsik *et al.*, 1988).

5.4.3 Other protective antioxidant effects

A mixture of antioxidant vitamins (α-tocopherol, ascorbic acid, vitamin B complex and retinol) given intravenously before operation prevented oedema and lipoperoxidation due to reperfusion damage after revascularization operations of the leg in 24 patients as compared to 27 control patients (Rabl *et al.*, 1995). There was no indication however, that this effect was specifically related to retinol.

5.4.4 Lung function

In a study of 816 current and former asbestos-exposed workers who formed part of the pilot group in the CARET study (see above), lung function determined at baseline was compared with serum retinol levels. There was a significant increase of 70 mL in forced expiratory volume (FEV_1) between the 25th to the 75th percentiles for serum retinol level.

6. Carcinogenicity

6.1 Human studies

The most direct test of carcinogenicity in human populations has been provided by trials of dietary supplementation with vitamin A that are described in detail in Section 4.1.2.

The Beta-Carotene and Retinol Efficacy Trial (CARET; see Section 4.1.2.1(*b*)) included 18 314 American adults, aged 45–74 years, at relatively high risk of lung cancer because of tobacco use or occupational exposure to asbestos. The trial was randomized, double-blinded and placebo-controlled, and the active treatment comprised a combination of 30 mg of β-carotene and 25 000 IU of retinol, taken once a day in a single tablet. The study was halted early, after an average of four years of follow-up, due to an increased occurrence of lung cancer in the active treatment group (RR, 1.3; 95% CI, 1.0–1.6) (Omenn *et al.*, 1996a). The only other cancer that showed increased incidence in the treatment group was leukaemia (26 cases observed; RR, 2.2; 95% CI, 1.0–5.0).

It is not clear how these results should be explained. The randomization process produced study groups that were well matched for the known major risk factors. Compliance with the trial regime was high, as measured both by capsule consumption and by serum vitamin levels (compared with the placebo group, β-carotene levels were more than 10 times higher and retinol levels were raised by about 10% in the active treatment group). The excess lung cancer risk was observed among both asbestos-exposed workers and smokers (although there was a statistically non-significant decrease of 20% among treated former smokers), and applied to all histological types of tumour (with the exception of small cell carcinomas) (Omenn *et al.*, 1996b). If there was indeed an adverse effect of the treatment, it is not possible to distinguish the influences of β-carotene and retinol. However, similar results have been reported from the Finnish ATBC study of chemoprevention among heavy smokers, in which the active treatment included β-carotene (and/or α-tocopherol), without a retinol component. This study included 29 133 males who were current smokers and were followed for a median period of 6.1 years. There was an increase of 16% in the incidence of lung cancer in the group receiving β-carotene (no effect was observed with vitamin E) (ATBC Cancer Prevention Study Group, 1994).

The Working Group was not aware of any other epidemiological study that reported data on vitamin A and incidence of leukaemia.

No intervention study including vitamin A supplementation other than the CARET study has reported an increase in cancer rates. In a study in Linxian County, China (see Section 4.1.2.1(*a*)), 29 584 adults aged 40–69 years were randomly allocated to one of eight study groups to test the effects of four different combinations of vitamins and minerals (Blot *et al.*, 1993). One of these combinations included retinol (5000 IU per day) and zinc (22.5 mg zinc oxide per day). At the end of the study, plasma retinol levels were higher in subjects who received this treatment (mean 54.0 µg/dL compared with 43.0 µg/dL in controls). After five years of follow-up, there was no observed effect on cancer mortality of supplementation with retinol and zinc (RR, 1.0, 95% CI 0.9–1.1). Due to small numbers, lung cancers were not reported separately.

A separate trial in Linxian compared the effects on cancer incidence and mortality of supplementation with a combination of vitamins and minerals (including vitamin A) in 3318 subjects with oesophageal dysplasia (Li, 1993). After six years of follow-up, total cancer mortality was 4% lower in the intervention group (RR, 1.0; 95% CI, 0.7–1.3).

An intervention study with former asbestos workers in Western Australia included two randomly assigned treatment groups (and no placebo) (de Klerk *et al.*, 1998; Musk *et al.*, 1998). 512 participants received β-carotene (30 mg/day) and an equal number received retinol (25 000 IU/day as retinyl palmitate). Median follow-up time was 232 weeks. 54 participants who developed side-effects or abnormal liver function tests suggestive of toxicity were transferred from the retinol group to β-carotene. There were fewer cases of mesothelioma in the retinol-treated group (RR, 0.24; 95% CI, 0.07–0.86), and also fewer lung cancers (RR, 0.7, 95% CI 0.2–2.3). Deaths from other cancers were evenly spread between the treatment groups (RR, 1.0, 95% CI 0.2–3.9).

In a study in the United States, 525 adults with a history of multiple basal cell or squamous cell carcinoma of the skin were randomly assigned to receive oral retinol (25 000 IU/day) or placebo or isotretinoin for three years. New skin cancers occurred more commonly in the retinol-treated group than among those receiving placebo, but the difference was not statistically significant (Levine *et al.*, 1997).

On the basis of a small number of observational studies, there is no evidence that vitamin A in the diet leads to an increase in the overall incidence of cancer, although increased risks have been reported for some sites. For example, several case–control investigations observed higher levels of vitamin A intake among participants with prostate cancer than controls (Kolonel *et al.*, 1987; Graham *et al.*, 1983; Heshmat *et al.*, 1985). However, the retinol and carotenoid components were not always distinguished, the pattern of effect by age varied between these studies, and the findings in one study may have been largely influenced by differential consumption of a single carotenoid-rich food item (papaya) (Le Marchand *et al.*, 1991). Other case–control studies have reported no increase in risk (for example, West *et al.*, 1991), even among men in the sub-category with highest consumption (Rohan *et al.*, 1995). Two cohort studies, both in the United States, have reported on the relationship between vitamin A intake and occurrence of prostate cancer. One found that high intake levels were associated with increased risk among men aged under 75 years, but were protective for older men (Hsing *et al.*, 1990a). The second study found an association between retinol intake from food sources (but not supplements) and prostate cancer, but this applied only to men over the age of 70 years—no association was observed between any measure of vitamin A intake and cancer among younger men (Giovannucci *et al.*, 1995). The CARET study, it should be noted, reported similar incidence of prostate cancer in the active-treatment and placebo groups (RR, 1.0; 95% CI, 0.8–1.3) (Omenn *et al.*, 1996b).

Liver, dairy products and meat are by far the chief sources of retinol. Direct associations between these food groups have been reported with cancer at several sites (e.g., oral cavity, pharynx, oesophagus, colon, rectum, prostate, etc.). However, it should not be assumed that retinol is necessarily responsible for the cancer-enhancing effects of dairy products and meat, since these are also important sources of saturated fat and caloric excess in western populations and it is difficult to control fully for these variables in epidemiological analyses. For example, the observational epidemiological studies of dietary preformed vitamin A suggest that there may be an increased risk of cancers of the upper aerodigestive tract (see Section 4.1.1). This pattern appears to be particularly pronounced in populations with high intake of alcohol (McLaughlin *et al.*, 1988; Gridley *et al.*, 1990). Several observational studies have reported on the effect of supplements: there was a tendency to find a protective effect of vitamin A which, however, in the largest study (Gridley *et al.*, 1992), appeared to be accounted for by vitamin E supplementation (see Section 4.1.1). It is not possible to discount totally the possibility that preformed vitamin A in food sources may increase rates of head and neck cancers, especially in the presence of a carcinogen, but residual confounding by saturated fat or other dietary factors, tobacco or alcohol almost certainly applies in these studies.

Ecological studies shed little light on the carcinogenic potential of vitamin A. There are some populations which may have been exposed, historically, to high levels of vitamin A in the diet (for example, native Alaskans and the Indians and Inuit of northern Canada). However, there are no reliable historical cancer data available, and comparisons based on present cancer rates are likely to be confounded by many other dietary and social factors (Bell *et al.*, 1997); furthermore, historical patterns are not a reliable guide to modern dietary practices (Godel *et al.*, 1996).

In summary, there is not convincing evidence that retinol is carcinogenic.

6.2 Experimental models

Three groups of 50 male and 50 female F344/DuCrj rats were given drinking water containing retinyl acetate in the form of gelatinized beadlets suspended in distilled water at doses of 0.25 or 0.125%. The control group was given 0.25% of placebo beadlets. All surviving animals were killed at 108 weeks. Body weight gain was significantly lower in females of the high-dose group. Malignant phaeochromocytomas developed in 3 (6.1%), 4 (8.0%) and 11 (22.9%) of the male control, low-dose and high-dose groups, respectively. The incidence in the high-dose group was significantly higher ($p < 0.05$) than in controls. One female rat of the low-dose group developed a malignant phaeochromocytoma. Benign phaeochromocytomas developed in 15 (30.6%), 23 (46.0%) and 28 (58.3%) males and in 3 (6.0%), 10 (20.4%) and 20 (41.7%) females of the control, low-dose and high-dose groups, respectively. The incidence in the high-dose groups was significantly different from controls ($p < 0.001$ and $p < 0.01$ for males and females, respectively). No significant difference in tumour incidence in other organs and tissues was observed (Kurokawa *et al.*, 1985).

Four groups of 200 female Sprague-Dawley rats, six weeks of age, were administered vitamin A (retinyl acetate/palmitate 50 : 50) at dose levels of (1) 3.9, (2) 16.9, (3) 75 and (4) 150 IU/g of diet for life (168 weeks). At death, all animals were necropsied and major organs and tissues examined histopathologically. A higher incidence of mammary adenocarcinomas was observed: (1) 11/200 (5.5%); (2) 27/200 (13.5%); (3) 26/200 (13.0%) and (4) 30/200 (15.0%). The numbers of mammary adenocarcinomas per 100 animals were as follows: (1) 7.5, (2) 16.0, (3) 16.0 and (4) 18.5. There was no dose–response relationship in the three supplemented groups. [The Working Group noted that the incidence of tumours in other tissues and organs was not reported] (Soffritti *et al.*, 1996).

Certain retinoic acid metabolites that have been approved as drugs, e.g., Accutane®, are known to cause haemangiosarcoma in mice (see *Physicians' Desk Reference*, 1997). No published reports of studies using retinol were identified.

7. Other Toxic Effects

7.1 Adverse effects

7.1.1 Human studies

Toxic effects due to hypervitaminosis A occur in the skin, the circulation (e.g., plasma proteins), internal organs (e.g., liver), the nervous system and the musculo-skeletal system. The manifestations of acute and chronic toxicity vary with dose and body mass, age (paediatric, adult, and elderly), sex and reproductive status (pregnant, lactating), disease conditions (e.g., liver or renal impairment; nutritional status) and concurrent drug administration or environmental chemical exposures. Toxicities associated with acute and chronic excess of vitamin A intake have been extensively reviewed (National Research Council, 1989; US Food and Drug Administration, 1976; Underwood, 1986; Olson, 1987; Hathcock *et al.,* 1990).

Approximately 10–15 cases of toxic reactions to vitamin A are reported per year in the United States, usually due to doses of over 100 000 IU retinol per day (Meyers *et al.*, 1996). Reported cases of overt signs of hypervitaminosis A resulting from food intake and/or supplements have been summarized graphically by Bendich and Langseth (1989) in time blocks from 1850 through 1987. Except for the periods 1952–55 and 1970–72, when infant supplements and treatments for dermatological disorders were introduced, the numbers of cases per year appear consistent with that reported by Meyers *et al.* (1996). In clinical trials, particularly those in which adults are enrolled for cancer preventive studies, eligibility criteria and frequent clinical evaluations tend to limit the occurrence of the more severe side-effects of hypervitaminosis A and the less severe effects are rapidly reversible.

Acute toxicity from large doses, relative to body mass, is more common in young children than in adults and is frequently associated with erroneous or over-zealous administration of supplements. In controlled settings, the frequency of acute toxicity has been evaluated in infants and young children to whom vitamin A (≥25 000 IU) was being administered in an effort to reduce childhood morbidity and mortality associated with vitamin A deficiency

(Florentino *et al.*, 1990; Stansfield *et al.*, 1993; Rahman *et al.*, 1995). Retinol distributes to maternal milk and doses of vitamin A given to lactating women with an inadequate vitamin A status improve that of nursing infants. However, 2000 IU of vitamin A has been safely and effectively administered, with plasma monitoring, to premature infants at risk for bronchopulmonary dysplasia (Robbins & Fletcher, 1993). Acute toxicity, in the context of organogenesis (teratogenesis), is well established through animal studies and case reports of fetal malformations (central nervous system, cardiovascular, palate and ear) following ingestion of ≥25 000 IU/day (≥0.4 μmol/kg bw/day) during pregnancy in humans (Schardein, 1993) (see also Section 7.2.2). Although a teratogenic threshold for vitamin A supplements of 10 000 IU/day has been suggested (Rothman *et al.*, 1996), this is not consistent with other data on teratogenicity (Mills *et al.*, 1997) and the study has been criticized on several scientific grounds (see Section 7.2.1) (Brent *et al.*, 1996; Khoury *et al.*, 1996; Watkins *et al.*, 1996; Werler *et al.*, 1996).

Information concerning the common toxicities associated with chronic administration of low doses of vitamin A to healthy adults is available from the Beta-Carotene and Retinol Efficacy Trial (CARET), a primary cancer prevention study (see Section 4.1.2.1(*b*)). No effect on liver function was observed after more than three years' administration of 25 000 IU retinol per day (*c.* 0.4 μmol/kg bw/day) with or without β-carotene (30 mg) in the pilot studies preceding CARET (Goodman *et al.*, 1993; Omenn *et al.*, 1993a). Only a negligible increase in serum triglyceride levels was observed in the CARET vanguard cohort of 1845 heavy smokers and asbestos-exposed workers, representing 10 184 person-years of intervention (Omenn *et al.*, 1994a). No other common toxicities were cited.

In the context of secondary cancer prevention, daily doses of 300 000 to 600 000 IU vitamin A as retinol for several months have usually been required to produce signs of hypervitaminosis A, although intake as low as 50 000 IU/day has been reported to be toxic after >18 months (Gossel & Bricker, 1994). Interestingly, 300 000 IU retinyl palmitate in an emulsion formulation (A-mulsin®, Mucos Pharma, Munich, Germany) given daily for twelve months to patients with resected stage I non-small-cell lung cancer did not produce major hepatic toxicity in the completed Italian adjuvant trial (Pastorino *et al.*, 1993). Serum levels of γ-glutamyltranspeptidase (GGT) rose during treatment, but were significantly higher only after two years (149 versus 57 IU/L). Serum triglyceride levels increased 63% over the first year of treatment and were significantly higher than those of controls at 8 and 12 months (Pastorino *et al.*, 1991; Infante *et al.*, 1991). The majority of adverse events were dermatological (dryness, desquamation, itching).

7.1.1.1 Mucocutaneous toxicity

Vitamin A is important in the differentiation of the skin, hair and mucous membranes and has been used in dermatology for many years (Peck & Di Giovanna, 1994). Side-effects of systemic vitamin A administration are common, as observed in the adjuvant trial above, but are reversible: dry and scaly skin (desquamation), mouth or lip fissures or chapping (cheilitis), dryness of mucous membranes (including conjunctivitis), brittle nails, skin rashes and erythema, and hair loss (alopecia) (Bendich & Langseth, 1989; Hathcock *et al.*, 1990). Emollients can reduce the discomfort of some of these symptoms.

Topical application causes similar focal reactions but typically not systemic reactions. Both retinyl acetate and retinoic acid have been evaluated as topical treatments for chemoprevention and they produce similar toxicities. After treatment of skin with retinoic acid (0.001–0.1% [unknown volume]) for up to 22 months, the most common adverse events were peeling, erythema and a burning sensation (Thorne, 1992; Mitchell *et al.*, 1995). Both retinoids have been further investigated as intravaginal treatments for cervical intraepithelial neoplasia (CIN) (Mitchell *et al.*, 1995). In a phase I/II trial, CIN I/II patients applied 3, 6, 9 or 18 mg retinyl acetate or placebo intravaginally for seven days beginning on day 5 of three sequential menstrual cycles (Romney *et al.*, 1985). Frequent severe adverse events at the highest dose were vulvar irritation and itching and 14% of all treated patients had vaginal burning during the trial. The most common general complaints were fatigue and irritability. Phase I/II trials evaluated the safety of retinoic acid applied to a sponge and inserted in a cervical cap or diaphragm. Doses of 0.05–0.2% (5 mL/day) for four days commonly produced vaginal irritation, ulceration and discharge, but no evidence of systemic toxicity (Surwit *et al.*, 1982). In a second study, the same group evaluated a range of doses from 0.05% (1 mL, or approx. 0.002 μmol/day) for four days; the maximum tolerated dose was 0.372% (1 mL/day) (Meyskens *et al.*, 1983). A subsequent phase II study using this dose for induction and maintenance (2 days during months 3, 6, and 9) found mild local effects (cervical inflammation, vaginal discharge and itching) more frequent during induction (Graham *et al.*, 1986). Mild systemic effects (dry skin, chapped lips, mood change, headache and fever) were also noted, although a previous pharmacokinetic study failed to detect retinoic acid in serum up to 24 h after a one-day insertion at the same dose (Peng *et al.*, 1986).

7.1.1.2 Circulatory toxicity

Vitamin A affects lipid metabolism. Hypervitaminosis A may cause hypertriglyceridaemia, possibly due to increases in VLDL. Patients given 300 000 IU retinyl palmitate for 12 months had a mean serum triglyceride level of 283 mg/dL (n = 138) versus 179 mg/dL in 145 control patients (Pastorino *et al.*, 1991) Increases in cholesterol and apoprotein B and decreases in HDL cholesterol are also common (Marsden, 1989). Although the effects are reversible, they have implications for acute pancreatitis and atherosclerotic cardiovascular disease (Armstrong *et al.*, 1994). In the CARET vanguard cohort of 1845 participants, retinyl palmitate (25 000 IU) produced only negligible increases in serum triglyceride levels during five years (Omenn *et al.*, 1994b).

Due to effects on other organs, there may also be other changes in measures of physiological chemistry and haematology. Increase in serum alkaline phosphatase and hypercalcaemia may reflect alterations in bone cell biology. Approximately three-fold increases in GGT have also been reported (Infante *et al.*, 1991). Petechia and haemorrhage, such as bleeding nose or gums, have been reported as symptoms (Bendich & Langseth, 1989). Hypothrombinaemia related to vitamin K deficiency may be due to competitive intestinal absorption (McCarthy *et al.*, 1989).

7.1.1.3 Internal organ toxicity

(a) Liver

About 90% of the total vitamin A is stored in the liver, the majority (= 75%) as retinyl esters in lipid droplets of stellate cells (see Section 3.2) (Blaner & Olson, 1994; Hathcock *et al.*, 1990). Excess storage of vitamin A may result in fatty liver. Hepatomegaly and palpable or tender liver were mentioned in 16% of case reports of hypervitaminosis A (Bendich & Langseth, 1989). Viral hepatitis may precipitate symptoms of hypervitaminosis A, possibly due to low levels of retinol-binding protein. Protein malnutrition, particularly in children and the elderly, may predispose to hypervitaminosis A, also due to low levels of retinol-binding protein. In a study of 41 patients with vitamin A hepatoxicity (Geubel *et al.*, 1991), there were 17 cases of cirrhosis, 10 of mild chronic hepatitis, five of noncirrhotic portal hypertension and nine of increased storage. The authors concluded that vitamin A consumption in the low therapeutic range might be an appreciable cause of liver disease. Pre-existing liver disease may predispose individuals to vitamin A toxicity. Additional case reports indicate that in countries where vitamin A is available as a supplement, hypervitaminosis A should be investigated in cases of liver dysfunction, such as portal hypertension of unknown origin (Dubois *et al.*, 1991; Kowalski *et al.*, 1994).

(b) Gastrointestinal tract

Nausea and vomiting were the most commonly reported symptoms of hypervitaminosis A, occurring in 34% of cases (Bendich & Langseth, 1989). Anorexia, diarrhoea and weight loss may also occur. Adverse events of these types are rapidly reversible upon cessation of vitamin A administration. Symptoms of fatigue, malaise, lethargy, somnolence, weakness and irritability were also commonly reported (Bendich & Langseth, 1989).

7.1.1.4 Neurological toxicity

Headache is a common symptom associated with hypervitaminosis A and may occur transiently with supplement doses. More severe reactions include elevated pressure of the cerebrospinal fluid, cranial hypertension, altered vision, and papilloedema (Bendich & Langseth, 1989; Hathcock *et al.*, 1990). Vitamin A toxicity should also be considered with the diagnosis of pseudotumor cerebri (Benrabah *et al.*, 1995; Moskowitz *et al.*, 1993; Sharieff & Hanten, 1996; Hathcock *et al.*, 1990). There are case reports of drug interactions: headache, visual disturbance, optic disc oedema, and intracranial hypertension in patients combining vitamin A with minocyclin (a synthetic tetracycline) (Benrabah *et al.*, 1995; Moskowitz *et al.*, 1993; Sharieff & Hanten, 1996; Hathcock *et al.*, 1990). In prophylactic treatment of vitamin A deficiency, among 100 infants who received 25 000 IU vitamin A and 98 who received placebo concurrently with three sequential doses of diphtheria/pertussis/tetanus (DTP)/oral polio vaccination, there were eight versus one transient episodes of bulging fontanelles without associated symptoms and without significant increases in serum retinol levels (Rahman *et al.*, 1995). Among 2471 Haitian children, 1–6 years old, randomized to receive placebo or 100 000 IU (30 mg) or 200 000 IU (60 mg) of vitamin A, symptoms of headache, nausea and/or vomiting were dose-related and occurred in 12–24 h (Florentino *et al.*, 1990).

7.1.1.5 Musculo-skeletal toxicity

Hypervitaminosis A is known to cause demineralization of bone, periosteal calcification and hypercalcaemia in all age groups (Peck & Di Giovanna, 1994; Frame, 1974). Retinoid metabolites used in dermatology have caused altered bone remodelling, demineralization and closure of epiphyses. Disseminated idiopathic skeletal hyperostosis, including calcification of tendons and ligaments in the spine and elsewhere, can also occur (Peck & Di Giovanna, 1994). Vitamin A may interact with vitamin D and parathyroid hormone to stimulate osteoclastic activity.

Bone and joint pain and myalgia are listed as commonly associated symptoms of hypervitaminosis A (Bendich & Langseth, 1989; Hathcock *et al.*, 1990). However, only two case reports in the recent literature have described these symptoms, in a 59-year old woman and in an eight-year old boy with renal failure (Doireau *et al.*, 1996; Romero *et al.*, 1996). Mechanistic research is being conducted in animal models (see below).

7.1.2 Experimental studies

The single-dose acute toxicity of vitamin A and its analogues in laboratory rodents is summarized in Table 29 (Kamm *et al.*, 1984; Kelloff *et al.*, 1996). In young monkeys, the LD_{50} for retinyl acetate was 168 mg (0.56 x 10^6 IU) retinol/kg bw. No animals receiving the equivalent of 100 mg (0.33 x 10^6 IU) retinol/kg bw died (Hathcock *et al.*, 1990).

As in humans, vitamin A can be toxic to laboratory animals due to bioaccumulation when it is administered chronically at low daily doses. In rats, symptoms of hypervitaminosis A have been produced by retinol doses as low as 3 mg/day (10 000 IU/day) after a few days to several weeks (Hathcock *et al.*, 1990). The toxicities generally reflected those seen in humans and occurred in the skin, circulation (e.g., plasma proteins), internal organs (e.g., liver) and musculo-skeletal system. No studies in animals have modelled the human neurological toxicity. Efficacy and toxicity at low doses are mediated by metabolism of vitamin A to retinoic acid metabolites that bind to the RAR and RXR hormone receptor classes (see Section 3.1) and activate gene expression. Receptor-selective agonists/antagonists are being developed in an attempt to separate efficacy and toxicity. Homozygous RAR-γ mutant mice have increased resistance to toxicity (Look *et al.*, 1995). Toxicity at high doses may also be due to overloading of the capacity of transport molecules, with the result that free vitamin A

Table 29. Oral LD_{50} values for retinol and retinyl esters in mice and rats

Retinoid	Species	LD_{50} (mg/kg bw)
Retinol	Mouse	2570
Retinyl acetate	Mouse	4100
Retinyl palmitate	Mouse	6060
	Rat	7910

exerts a cytotoxic, detergent-like effect on membranes.

The LD_{50} rank-order of the vitamin A esters and metabolites is reflected in their long-term toxicity. Retinyl palmitate, at 250 times the human recommended dietary allowance (RDA), produced no adverse effects in rats given up to 27.5 mg/kg bw/day (50 000 IU/kg bw/day) or dogs given up to 13.8 mg/kg bw/day (25 100 IU/kg bw/day) for 10 months. However, retinoic acid administered to rats and dogs at doses of 5 and 50 mg/kg bw/day for 13 weeks showed toxicity (Kamm *et al.*, 1984). Rats in the low-dose group displayed hair loss, dermal and mucosal alterations, inhibition of spermatogenesis and weight loss. At the high dose, serum transaminase and alkaline phosphatase activities were elevated, total protein declined and 20% of the animals died. Similar signs were seen in the dogs; however, mortality at the high dose was 50%. In mice, doses of 150–250 mg/kg bw/day caused alopecia, weight loss and skin and membrane changes after five days.

7.1.2.1 Mucocutaneous toxicity

The commonly observed effects of retinoids on the skin of laboratory animals include erythema, epidermal thickening, scaling, loosening of the stratum corneum, increases in transepidermal water loss and conjunctivitis (Armstrong *et al.*, 1994). The effect is more pronounced on smooth and bare skin. Alopecia is also seen. Ophthalmological changes are more common with the retinoid metabolites. Cellular proliferation is increased, resulting in hyperplasia, particularly in the stratum spinosum (acanthosis), and hypergranulosis occurs. Vitamin A causes a broad spectrum of biological effects in the epidermis, including decreased numbers of tono-filaments and desmosomal attachments, increased gap junction proliferation, suppressed expression of epidermal transglutaminase and cornification, altered pattern of keratin expression towards fetal K19 and K13 forms and decreased total keratin content, and altered cell surface proteins and receptors (Peck & Di Giovanna, 1994). The effects are dose- and substance-specific, so that the histology of epidermal hyperplasia on the dorsal skin of hairless mice can be used to rank-order natural and synthetic retinoids by potency (Connor *et al.*, 1986). Retinol and retinyl palmitate have been extensively evaluated for toxicity in mice and rats, as well as clinically, and are considered to be safe as cosmetic ingredients in products containing 0.1–1.0% (Cosmetic Ingredient Review Expert Panel of the American College of Toxicology, 1987).

7.1.2.2 Circulatory toxicity

Elevations of serum levels of triglycerides, cholesterol and alkaline phosphatase and decreases in blood erythrocyte count and haemoglobin concentration have been reported, but vary with the form of vitamin A (Armstrong *et al.*, 1994). Hypertriglyceridaemia was induced in rats by doses of 33 mg retinol per day (110 000 IU/day) and by 550–1100 mg retinyl palmitate per day (1–2 x 10^6 IU/day), but in another study was not produced by a dose of 185 mg (336 000 IU) retinyl palmitate/100 g body weight/day (Hathcock *et al.*, 1990). The increase in cholesterol is less consistent and varies with the form of vitamin A. Alkaline phosphatase increases are also variable and may represent activity from bone osteoblasts and/or from the liver. Other reported serum enzyme changes (e.g., alanine aminotransferase (ALAT), aspartate aminotransferase, GGT) are associated with liver function. With respect to haematological changes, retinyl acetate at a dose of 0.5% in the diet reduced prothrombin to 65% and kaolin-activated partial thromboplastin times to 28% of control values; this dose was considered to have relatively weak haemorrhagic effects in the rat (Takahashi, 1995). The haemorrhagic action of retinyl acetate and other vitamin A compounds was prevented by dietary vitamin K supplementation (McCarthy *et al.*, 1989).

7.1.2.3 Internal organ toxicity

(a) Liver

In rats, after six months of dietary supplementation with 328 mg retinyl palmitate/kg, hepatic levels of the ester were increased ten-fold compared with vehicle-control animals (Grubbs *et al.*, 1990). Hypervitaminosis A causes fatty infiltration of rodent liver. Tissues such as adipose, kidney, testes, lung and bone marrow may also take up significant amounts of lipid and undergo histological changes.

In Kupffer cells isolated from male rats treated for 3–7 days with 75 mg/kg bw/day of retinol by oral gavage once daily, respiratory and phagocytic activity and the release of reactive oxygen species, tumour necrosis factor alpha and prostaglandin E_2 were elevated (Hoglen *et al.*, 1997). Also in rats, excessive intake of vitamin A for seven days caused activation of Kupffer cells and induced accumulation of lipid drop-lets in fat-storing cells, as well as proliferation of these cells (Lettinga *et al.*, 1996). Increased alkaline phosphatase pointed to activation of retinyl ester transport across bile canalicular membranes, while changes in metabolic enzyme markers suggested decreases in purine breakdown, antioxidant capacity, phagocytotic capacity and ammonia regulation. However, no cell damage was apparent.

With regard to drug interactions, the effect of vitamin A on ethanol-induced liver toxicity has been investigated in efforts to develop a model of human alcoholic liver disease. However, the role of vitamin A as a major risk factor in the pathogenesis of alcoholic liver fibrosis has not been established. Liver fibrosis, characterized by perivenular fibrosis and central vein thickening, was elicited in Sprague-Dawley rats when ethanol and retinyl acetate (up to 29 000 IU per litre of liquid diet) were incorporated into the diet for nine months (Leo & Lieber, 1983). Other investigators, using a similar experimental design, failed to produce fibrosis, as measured histologically or as increased collagen, after 16 months of treatment. They tested two different strains of rats (BN/BiRij and WAG/Rij), which develop fibrosis after carbon tetrachloride treatment (Bosma *et al.*, 1991; Seifert *et al.*, 1991). There was evidence of steatosis (fatty degeneration), round cell inflammatory infiltration and elevations in liver enzymes and serum lipids. However, neither group observed the characteristic histological picture of human alcoholic hepatitis in connection with hypervitaminosis A.

Pretreatment of rats with a single high dose of vitamin A (250 000 IU) led to increased hepatoxicity of vinylidene chloride (Wijeweera *et al.*, 1996). Vitamin A treatment activated Kupffer cells and induced CYP2E1 which, in turn, potentiated vinylidene chloride metabolism and induced an increase in plasma ALAT *in vivo*, an increase in potassium ion leakage from liver slices *in vitro* and histological evidence of centrilobular necrosis. Similarly, vitamin A pretreatment for seven days potentiated the hepatotoxicity of carbon tetrachloride (ElSisi *et al.*, 1993a,b,c). Other investigators found that when vitamin A (12 500 IU retinyl palmitate twice a week for four weeks) was given during carbon tetrachloride treatment of rats, parenchymal cell damage and fibrosis were enhanced, whereas vitamin A post-treatment after carbon tetrachloride strongly reduced fibrosis (Knook *et al.*, 1995). Conversely, in mice, retinol pretreatment at 75 mg/kg bw/day for seven days protected against increases in ALAT and histopathological necrosis induced by carbon tetrachloride and phalloidin, but potentiated the toxicity of allyl alcohol, acetaminophen and D-galactosamine (Rosengren *et al.*, 1995). The results of drug interaction studies in rats and mice indicate that there are species differences in the effect of vitamin A on the liver and that the timing of vitamin A administration may also affect the hepatotoxicity of the drug or chemical.

(b) Gastrointestinal tract

In rat intestine, vitamin A doses up to ten times the RDA for rats (4 μmol/kg) for seven days did not cause disturbance in absorptive cell processes (Suzuki *et al.*, 1995). However, at higher doses (100 times the RDA), the unesterified retinol/cellular retinol binding protein ratio (type II) was > 3, while at 1000 times the RDA the ratio was > 19 and lecithin:retinol acyltransferase activity was significantly elevated. In hamster, retinyl acetate, administered as 250 IU/g of diet, produced gallstones and elevations of serum ALAT (Cardenas *et al.*, 1991). Systemic effects of hypervitamosis A on the upper gastrointestinal epithelium have also been described. When rats were given daily intraperitoneal injections of 150 IU vitamin A per gram body weight for 10 days, there was histological evidence of hyperplasia and hypertrophy of the oesophageal epithelium, with increased mitoses and numbers of immature cells (Oliveira *et al.*, 1990). The alterations were more evident in the lower third of the oesophagus.

(c) Other organs

Extensive foci of degenerative myocardial fibres, associated with electrocardiogram changes, were reported in rats treated with vitamin A equivalent to 3 or 6 mg (10 000 or 20 000 IU) retinol/kg bw/day for three months (Hathcock *et al.*, 1990). Fatty changes and haemosiderosis in the spleen, glomerulonephritis and necrotizing nephrosis in the kidney, and testicular atrophy in adults and degenerative testicular changes in weanlings have been described (Kamm *et al.*, 1984).

7.1.2.4 Musculo-skeletal toxicity

Demineralization, thinning of the long bones, cortical hyperostosis, periostosis and premature closure of the epiphyses have been described in animals treated with high doses of vitamin A. In adult cats, confluent exostoses in the cervical spine were observed (Peck & Di Giovanna, 1994). Retinyl acetate fed to rats at doses of 8.5–13.6 mg retinol/day (28 300–45 300 IU) caused a limping gait and fractures. Bone mineralization, determined as bone-ash, was normal, so the toxicity was associated with alterations in the bone matrix (Hathcock *et al.*, 1990). Mice fed retinyl acetate (75–300 μg daily) in the diet for 3–16 months developed radiographic and histological evidence of arthritis and periarticular bone formation similar to diffuse idiopathic skeletal hyperostosis (Boden *et al.*, 1989). Retinyl palmitate fed at 60, 200 or 350 IU/g diet for 23 weeks caused dose-related increases in bone fractures, osteoporotic lesions, metaphyseal flares and bone deformities in mice treated with DMBA and TPA (Forsyth *et al.*, 1989). The bone toxicity of hypervitaminosis A has also been demonstrated in dogs, cats, calves and hogs (Kamm *et al.*, 1984).

7.2 Reproductive and developmental effects

7.2.1 Human studies

There are case reports of malformations following very high intakes of vitamin A early in pregnancy (Rosa *et al.*, 1986). The estimated doses vary from 25 000 IU to 500 000 IU, and the adverse outcomes include a range of abnormalities of the central nervous system, kidneys and urinary system and adrenal gland, some of which are similar to abnormalities seen in offspring of animals dosed with vitamin A (Monga, 1997). On their own, these case reports do not provide strong evidence of cause and effect, as the doses, patterns of ingestion and constellation of abnormalities vary considerably. However, suspicion that there is an effect is raised by laboratory studies showing teratogenic effects of vitamin A in all species tested, although the doses required vary considerably between species. Moreover, it is well known that synthetic chemicals with vitamin A activity are powerful human teratogens. For example, isotretinoin, a derivative of retinoic acid, introduced in the early 1980s for oral treatment of acne, was associated with an almost ten-fold increase in the occurrence of major malformations when mothers took the drug in the first month of pregnancy (Lammer *et al.*, 1985).

Three case–control studies have investigated the role of vitamin A as a human teratogen. A Spanish study compared 11 293 cases of congenital malformation (excluding chromosomal abnormalities) with 11 193 controls, matched for sex, hospital and day of birth (Martínez-Frías & Salvador, 1990). Maternal intake of vitamin A from diet and supplements during the pregnancy was assessed by questionnaire. Few women (16 with birth defects, 14 controls) had intakes above 10 000 IU per day, and no increased risk was observed in this group (RR, 1.1; $p = 0.4$). The risk was increased in the highest-dose group (above 40 000 IU; 11 cases, 4 controls); this finding bordered on significance (RR, 2.7; $p = 0.06$) and was stronger for women exposed in the first two months of pregnancy (RR, 4.0; $p = 0.19$; 4 cases, 1 control) than for those exposed in the last five months of gestation (RR, 2.0; $p = 0.35$; 4 cases, 2 controls).

A study in the United States included 2658 infants with malformations of structures derived from cranial neural crest cells (Werler *et al.*, 1990), as animal experiments have indicated that this tissue is particularly sensitive to effects of retinoids *in utero*. The control group included a similar number of infants with other malformations. Vitamin A supplementation was defined as daily use, for at least seven days, of retinol with or without vitamin D, or of fish oils. Relative risk estimates were 2.5 (95% CI, 1.0–6.2) for use in the first month of pregnancy, 2.3 (95% CI, 0.9–5.8) in month 2, and 1.6 (95% CI, 0.6–4.5) in month 3. There was a slight and statistically non-significant increase in risk associated with use of multivitamins containing vitamin A. No information was obtained on dose provided by these supplements nor on vitamin A intake from diet.

In a study of all pregnancies in California and in Illinois, United States, between 1985 and 1987, infants with neural tube defects (n = 548) were compared with infants with other major malformations (n = 387) and normal controls (n = 573) (Mills *et al.*, 1997). There was no evidence of an increased risk of neural tube defects or other major malformations associated with high doses of vitamin A (greater than 10 000 IU) (RR for major malformations, 0.7; 95% CI, 0.3–2.0). Similar results were obtained when the cases were restricted to cranial neural crest defects. The odds ratios were slightly greater when intake from supplements only was considered rather than supplements plus dietary sources, but the differences were small, all risk estimates being close to unity, and were statistically non-significant. High intakes were uncommon: fewer than 1% of participants had vitamin A exposures estimated to be greater than 15 000 IU per day.

Data from a population-based case–control study of major birth defects in the 1980s were subsequently re-analysed to search for an association between vitamin A intake and occurrence of cranial neural crest defects (Khoury *et al.*, 1996). Exposure was defined as use of vitamin A, alone or as a component of multivitamin supplements, for three days per week or more frequently, in the period from one month before conception to the end of the first trimester of pregnancy. There was no evidence of an increased risk associated with use of vitamin A supplements (RR, 0.5; 95% CI, 0.2–1.3). It was estimated that the women taking these supplements seldom received doses above 10 000 IU per day. The relative risk in women who took only vitamin A was 0.6 (95% CI, 0.2–1.4).

The findings of Rothman *et al.* (1995) prompted a review of data from the Californian Birth Defects Monitoring Program, to compare use of vitamin A supplements by mothers of children with specific defects (orofacial clefts and conotruncal heart defects) with that of control women (Shaw *et al.*, 1996). The data were collected from a number of case–control studies conducted in the late 1980s, at which time it is thought that vitamin A supplements contained 10 000–15 000 IU retinol. There was no evidence of increased exposure among the cases compared with the controls in this analysis (for orofacial clefts, RR, 0.6, 95% CI 0.2–1.6; for conotruncal heart defects, none of the 207 case mothers took supplements).

In a cohort study, 22 748 women in the United States were recruited in the second trimester of pregnancy and information was obtained by telephone interview on diet and use of vitamin supplements (Rothman *et al.*, 1995). Information on the outcome of pregnancy was obtained from questionnaires mailed to obstetricians, or if the obstetricians did not reply, from the women themselves. It was estimated that about 2% (n = 455) of the women had total daily intake of vitamin A above 10 000 IU. The prevalence of all birth defects was twice as great in women taking 15 000 IU or more per day compared with those in the lowest-intake category (< 5000 IU per day) (prevalence ratio 2.2, 95% CI, 1.3–3.8). There was a more marked effect for neural crest defects (excluding neural tube anomalies), particularly among women whose excess vitamin A intake came from supplements: for intakes above 10 000 IU compared with less than 5000 IU, the prevalence ratio was 4.8 (95% CI, 2.2–10.5). This is consistent with data from studies of human volunteers, showing that exposure to retinoic acid was markedly lower after consumption of liver than after taking supplements of the same retinol equivalent dose (Buss *et al.*, 1994), presumably reflecting differences in the extent of oxidation of retinol to retinoic acid depending on the form in which the retinol is presented. The increased prevalence of abnormalities was apparent only among women with relatively high vitamin A intake around the time of conception or in the first six weeks of pregnancy; no effect was associated with high intake confined to later stages of pregnancy.

It has been pointed out that the study by Rothman *et al.* relied on birth defect data reported by physicians and mothers, that the category of 'neural crest defects' was very broad and that the prevalence of major defects in the cohort was less than would be expected (Brent *et al.*, 1996). Unless there was differential misclassification with respect to vitamin A intake, these sources of error would not cause an apparent effect to be reported when one did not exist. However, the findings in the cohort study were based on relatively small numbers (for example, a total of 10 defects among women taking > 10 000 IU/day) and have not been replicated.

The study by Rothman *et al.* (1995), despite its limitations, provides the strongest evidence available that retinol may act as a teratogen in human populations. If it does, the critical question is then: at what level of intake does the effect occur? It has been argued on the basis of the non-human primate data and the case–control findings in human populations that teratogenic effects are unlikely to occur below about 30 000 IU per day (Miller *et al.*, 1998). However, Rothman *et al.* (1996) have stated that further analysis of the cohort data provides evidence for an effect in the range of 10 000–20 000 IU per day, with an approximately four-fold increase in prevalence of defects compared with the lowest-dose category. It should be noted also that a number of the case–control studies used as controls infants with malformations other than neural crest-derived lesions. Therefore, if there is a relationship between vitamin A and a wide range of malformations, as suggested by the cohort study, these case–control investigations may have underestimated the effect of vitamin A.

Evidence of safety of intakes below 10 000 IU, at least when given in conjunction with folic acid, is provided by a randomized controlled trial in Hungary of vitamin supplementation in early pregnancy (Czeizel & Dudás, 1992). In this study, the active agent contained vitamin A (4000 or 6000 IU) and folic acid; the observed rates of both neural tube defects and of other major malformations were lower in the vitamin user group than in subjects taking a control capsule. [The Working Group noted that since folic acid deficiency may be an important cause of certain malformations, the safety of vitamin A alone is difficult to ascertain on the basis of this study.]

7.2.2 Experimental studies

7.2.2.1 Effects on embryonic development

(a) Vitamin A deficiency

The importance of vitamin A for embryonic development was first demonstrated in the 1930s, when pregnant pigs fed a diet deficient in vitamin A were found to give birth to offspring that were blind and had severe malformations, such as cleft palate and cleft lip (Hale, 1933; Kalter & Warkany, 1959). In rats, vitamin A deficiency before and during gestation leads to increased embryolethality and a wide variety of abnormalities in the live offspring, including malformations of the eyes, urogenital system, respiratory tract, heart and great vessels. Administration of retinol to vitamin A-deficient rats during midgestation is essential for prevention of late fetal death as well as for delivery and neonatal survival, and retinoic acid cannot replace retinol in these functions (Wilson *et al.*, 1953). These results suggest that retinol itself or one of its metabolites, other than all-*trans*-retinoic acid, may be responsible for late developmental events in gestation (Thompson *et al.*, 1964; Takahashi *et al.*, 1975; Wellik & DeLuca, 1995; Wellik *et al.*, 1997).

(b) Retinoid excess

The first report on the teratogenicity of excess vitamin A appeared in the early 1950s. Oral doses of about 60 mg retinol/kg bw administered to pregnant rats daily during gestational days 2 to 16 resulted in high rates of embryolethality and severe fetal malformations, such as exencephaly, cleft lip and palate and eye defects (Cohlan, 1953). Subsequent studies in many animal species have consistently shown embryotoxic effects of excess of vitamin A or retinoic acid at doses that do not cause overt signs of maternal toxicity (Geelen, 1979; Agnish & Kochhar, 1993). Furthermore, the embryotoxic effects of retinoids are not restricted to mammals, but can also be induced in other vertebrate classes, such as birds (Tickle *et al.*, 1982), amphibians (Durston *et al.*, 1989) and fishes (Holder & Hill, 1991).

The teratogenic effects of retinoids cover a wide spectrum and show marked stage-specificity. For example, exposure of the early postimplantation embryo can result in craniofacial, central nervous system, cardiovascular and thymus defects, whereas exposure at later stages of development is associated with defects of the limbs, palate and genitourinary tract (Kalter & Warkany, 1961; Shenefelt, 1972; Kistler, 1981; Sulik *et al.*, 1995).

Studies with synthetic retinoids in rodents have revealed interesting structure–activity relationships. For example, the presence of an acidic terminus group and a polyene side-chain of more than five carbon atoms or an aromatic system are important structural requirements for the teratogenic activity of retinoids. Modifications of the β-ionone ring of retinoids, such as hydroxylation or oxygenation at C-4, affect the teratogenic activity of retinoic acid to only a small extent. Finally, the *cis–trans* configuration of the side-chain can be of great significance; thus 13-*cis*-retinoic acid is only marginally active, although all-*trans*-retinoic acid is highly active in rodent species (Kraft *et al.*, 1987; Wilhite *et al.*, 1989).

(c) Molecular basis for the role of retinoids in embryonic development

Significant progress has been made in the last decade towards elucidating the role of retinoids in normal and abnormal embryonic development. The many investigations in this field can be roughly divided into the following categories (presented in part in Tzimas, 1996).

(i) Endogenous retinoids: The retinoids that occur naturally in the developing embryo (Table 30) have been analysed by methods such as HPLC or either HPLC alone or gas chromatography combined with mass spectrometry. Endogenous retinoic acid and retinol have been identified in the embryo of all species examined to date, including birds (Thaller & Eichele, 1987; Scott *et al.*, 1994; Dong & Zile, 1995), rodents (Collins *et al.*, 1994; Tzimas *et al.*, 1995; Satre & Kochhar, 1989), rabbits (Tzimas *et al.*, 1996a), primates, including humans (Hummler *et al.*, 1994; Kraft *et al.*, 1993), *Xenopus* (Durston *et al.*, 1989) and zebrafish (Costaridis *et al.*, 1996). Notably, there is a concentration gradient of retinoic acid across the anterior–posterior axis of the developing chick limb bud, with highest concentrations posteriorly (Thaller & Eichele, 1987; Scott *et al.*, 1994). A similar gradient from the forebrain (lowest) to the spinal cord (highest) of the early mouse embryo has also been reported (Horton & Maden, 1995). Using an alternative approach, Hogan *et al.* (1992) examined the capacity of embryonic tissues to convert radiolabelled retinol to retinoic acid *in vitro* and found that the Hensen's node and the primitive streak of the early mouse embryo are more important sites of all-*trans*-retinoic acid synthesis than more anterior tissues (Costaridis *et al.*, 1996).

In addition, 3,4-didehydroretinol and 3,4-didehydroretinoic acid are endogenously found in avian (Scott *et al.*, 1994) and rabbit embryos (Tzimas *et al.*, 1996a), and 3,4-didehydroretinol is also present in the embryo of monkeys (Tzimas, 1996) and humans (Sass, 1994). Surprisingly, none of these retinoids occurs physiologically in the embryos of mice or rats (Collins *et al.*, 1994; Tzimas *et al.*, 1995).

Table 30. Endogenous concentrations of plasma retinoids in several species[a]

Retinoid	Rat[b]	Cynomolgus monkey[c]	Rabbit[d]	Human[e]
All-*trans*-retinoic acid	0.4 ± 0.03	0.5 ± 0.3	1.4 ± 0.3	1.3 ± 0.6
13-*cis*-retinoic acid	n.d.	n.d.	1.7 ± 1.1	0.9 ± 0.2
Retinol	100 ± 42.4	219 ± 12.6	826 ± 140	477 ± 71.0
Retinyl palmitate	102 ± 19.5	104 ± 46.4	35.6 ± 13.3	10.5 ± 7.1

[a] Concentrations are expressed in ng/mL (means ± SD); measured by HPLC
[b] Pregnant Wistar rats on gestational day 12. Data from Collins *et al.* (1994)
[c] Pregnant cynomolgus monkeys on gestational day 31. Data from Tzimas (1996)
[d] Pregnant Swiss hare rabbits on gestational day 12. Data from Tzimas *et al.* (1996a)
[e] Nonpregnant female volunteers. Data from Peiker *et al.* (1991)
n.d., not determined

Other endogenous embryonic retinoids include all-*trans*-4-oxoretinoic acid and all-*trans*-4-oxoretinal in *Xenopus* embryos (Pijnappel *et al.*, 1993; Blumberg *et al.*, 1996) and all-*trans*-retinal in *Xenopus* (Durston *et al.*, 1989) and zebrafish (Satre & Kochhar, 1989) embryos. 9-*cis*-Retinoic acid has been tentatively identified in *Xenopus* embryos (Kraft *et al.*, 1994), but this finding has been questioned (Blumberg *et al.*, 1996). None of these retinoids was detected in the embryo of mammalian or avian species, suggesting that either they do not play a significant physiological role, at least at the developmental stages examined, or they elicit biological effects at concentrations which are lower than the detection limits of the analytical methods used.

To allow retinoid determination in small tissue segments of early embryos, the more sensitive reporter gene assays have been employed; these assays make use of transgenic mice carrying a reporter gene which is under the transcriptional control of a retinoic acid response element (RARE) (Rossant *et al.*, 1991; Mendelsohn *et al.*, 1991; Balkan *et al.*, 1992) or cell lines transfected with a retinoic acid-driven reporter gene (Wagner *et al.*, 1992; Chen *et al.*, 1992a, 1994). The response of the reporter systems is assumed to reflect the presence of all-*trans*-retinoic acid or other retinoids that induce the expression of the reporter gene, but cannot be considered conclusive with respect to the chemical identity of the retinoids. Despite this caveat, studies using such methods have clearly demonstrated the existence of some 'hot spots' of embryonic retinoid concentrations, such as the Hensen's node of the chicken embryo (Chen *et al.*, 1992b); furthermore, anterior–posterior gradients of retinoid concentrations were found in early neurula *Xenopus* embryos (Chen *et al.*, 1994) and the central nervous system tissue of rat embryos (Wagner *et al.*, 1992), with highest levels posteriorly rather than anteriorly. It will be important to complement these reporter gene studies with direct chemical identification and quantitation of endogenous retinoids.

(ii) Cellular retinoid-binding proteins and retinoid receptors: The cellular retinoid-binding proteins and the retinoid receptors (see Section 3.1) display characteristic spatial and temporal patterns of expression during mouse and chicken embryogenesis (Giguere, 1994; Mendelsohn *et al.*, 1992). CRABP-I is abundantly expressed in the mesenchyme of the hindbrain, the cranial neural crest cells and the limb buds, reflecting the structures of the embryo that are susceptible to retinoic acid-induced teratogenicity, whereas CRBP is found in the epithelium of the same regions. In contrast, the expression of CRABP-II is more widespread and not restricted to the retinoid-sensitive embryonic regions (Ruberte *et al.*, 1992; Gustafson *et al.*, 1993; Lyn & Giguere, 1994; Vaessen *et al.*, 1990; Maden, 1994). RAR-α and RXR-β are widely distributed, whereas the other receptors are temporally and spatially restricted (Giguere, 1994; Mangelsdorf *et al.*, 1994).

The role of CRABP-I and -II during embryonic development has been subject of controversy. One hypothesis is that CRABP-I (and perhaps CRABP-II as well) regulates the cytoplasmic levels of retinoic acid by binding the majority of this acid or enhancing the rate of its catabolism, thus allowing only small amounts of free ligand to enter the nucleus and activate the retinoid receptors (Napoli, 1994; Ruberte *et al.*, 1992). This would be consistent with data from studies with cell lines, which showed that overexpression of CRABP-I reduced the ability of retinoic acid to stimulate RAR-mediated gene transcription (Boylan & Gudas, 1991). Alternatively, CRABP-I may shuttle its ligand to the nucleus (Takase *et al.*, 1986); this hypothesis has recently been supported by the demonstration of nuclear localization of CRABP-I in mouse embryonic cells (Gustafson *et al.*, 1996). However, other studies have shown that mutant mice deficient in either CRABP-I or CRABP-II, or both, are essentially normal, both during development and in adult life, and are as susceptible to the teratogenic effects of retinoic acid as their wild-type littermates (Gorry *et al.*, 1994; de Bruijn *et al.*, 1994; Fawcett *et al.*, 1995; Lampron *et al.*, 1995). However, the double-knockout mice exhibit increased mortality by six weeks of age compared with wild-type controls. It remains to be determined whether the absence of CRABPs affects susceptibility to vitamin A deficiency (Li & Norris, 1996).

The physiological role of RARs in embryonic development has been studied by targeted modification of certain members of the RAR family (Lohnes *et al.*, 1995). Notably, most congenital defects of the fetal vitamin A deficiency syndrome were observed after combined disruption of various genes within the RAR family, but not in RAR single mutants, suggesting functional redundancy between the members of the RAR family. Other studies have shown the significance of RXR-α for heart and eye morphogenesis (Kastner *et al.*, 1994; Sucov *et al.*, 1994) and of RXR-β for normal spermatogenesis (Kastner *et al.*, 1996). In addition, combined disruption of RXR-α and RAR isoforms resulted in even more severe phenotypes, indicating that RAR/RXR-α heterodimers mediate retinoid signalling *in vivo* (Kastner *et al.*, 1994, 1997).

(iii) Regulation of morphogenesis and gene expression by retinoids: The fundamental role of retinoids in vertebrate embryonic development has been further emphasized by studies that examined the effects of retinoids on pattern formation of structures of the embryonic body such as the central nervous system, the vertebral column, and limbs (Hofmann & Eichele, 1994). For example, retinoic acid released from a bead implanted at the anterior margin of a chick limb bud can alter the normal digit pattern and even cause pattern duplications (Tickle *et al.*, 1982). Thus, retinoic acid mimics the zone of polarizing activity, which is a group of cells located at the posterior region of the limb bud that is well known to evoke the development of additional digits when grafted at the anterior edge of another limb bud (Tickle *et al.*, 1975). The polarizing activity of retinoic acid in this system and the demonstration of its physiological occurrence in limb tissue (Thaller & Eichele, 1987) have led to the speculation that retinoic acid is the endogenous morphogen of limb development. Morphogens are thought to be distributed in gradients and determine the fate of cells in a concentration-dependent manner.

The results of more recent studies have, however, challenged the proposed existence of a concentration gradient for morphogenetically active retinoids. First, the endogenous concentrations of 3,4-didehydroretinoic acid do not form a gradient across the anterior–posterior axis of the chicken limb bud (Scott *et al.*, 1994), although this retinoid is as potent as all-*trans*-retinoic acid in inducing pattern duplications after local application to the anterior margin of the limb bud (Thaller & Eichele, 1990). Second, in contrast to the situation in the chick limb bud, retinoic acid does not display an anterior–posterior concentration gradient in the mouse limb bud (Scott *et al.*, 1994; Ang *et al.*, 1996). Third, immunohistochemical analysis of a monoclonal antibody raised against retinoic acid revealed that this acid is distributed in the peripheral rather than the core mesenchyme of the developing chick limb bud (Tamura *et al.*, 1990). Thus, the small posterior tissue segment (one-fourth of the limb) assayed by Thaller and Eichele (1987) and Scott *et al.* (1994) would contain less core mesenchyme with a low retinoic acid concentration than the larger anterior segment, and the anterior–posterior gradient of retinoic acid (Thaller & Eichele, 1987; Scott *et al.*, 1994) may therefore be an artefact.

Other studies have also challenged the validity of retinoic acid being the proximate morphogen of the zone of polarizing activity, based on differential effects of retinoic acid and the zone of the polarizing activity at the molecular level (Noji *et al.*, 1991), as well as the discovery of several signalling molecules, such as the sonic hedgehog protein (shh), which act downstream of retinoic acid (Riddle *et al.*, 1993; Ogura *et al.*, 1996). Therefore, retinoic acid seems to be an important but intermediate signal of limb morphogenesis.

Recent investigations have focused on the effects of all-*trans*-retinoic acid on the expression of growth factors within the developing embryo, such as homeotic genes (*hox* genes), the *shh* gene and members of the fibroblast growth factor (FGF) and TGFβ families. The products of these genes are believed to play important roles in determining the developmental fate of many embryonic structures, such as the rhombomeres of the hindbrain and the limb bud (Gudas, 1994; Means & Gudas, 1995). Retinoic acid activates the expression and alters the spatial pattern of expression of many of these genes, as shown in cell culture systems and in developing embryos. This up-regulation may result from transcriptional activation via the RAR/RXR pathway, as the identification of RAREs in several *hox* genes suggests, or, indirectly, as a result of induction by *shh*. Furthermore, null mutations of some *hox* genes in mice induce phenotypes similar to the teratogenic phenotypes induced by retinoids. These findings suggest that alteration of the expression of *hox* genes is part of the mechanism of retinoid teratogenicity (Gudas, 1994; Means & Gudas, 1995).

(d) Interspecies variations in retinoid teratogenesis

The relative teratogenic potencies of retinoids used in human therapy have been investigated in numerous animal species. In general, retinoids induce qualitatively similar patterns of abnormalities in every species tested, depending on the dose and the developmental stage at the time of exposure to the drug. Unlike the spectrum of defects, the doses of retinoids required to induce teratogenic effects often show pronounced interspecies variation. Table 31 lists the lowest reported teratogenic doses of retinol in various species. This information has been obtained mainly from studies in which vitamin A was administered to animals by gavage daily during the period of organogenesis, although in some studies with monkeys, the treatment began before the onset of organogenesis, and the drug was administered twice daily on the last two to four days of the dosing period.

Table 31. Lowest reported teratogenic doses of vitamin A following oral administration

	Retinol dose[a]	
Species	mg/kg	IU/kg
Mouse[b]	25	83 000
Rat[b]	50	167 000
Rabbit[b]	5.5	18 000
Cynomolgus monkey [c]	6	20 000
Human[d]	(0.2–1.5)[e]	700–5000

[a] Doses of retinyl palmitate are expressed as retinol
[b] From experiments with daily dosing throughout organogenesis (Tzimas *et al.*, 1994; Collins *et al.*, 1994; Agnish & Kochhar, 1993; Agnish *et al.*, 1990)
[c] Daily dosing with 13-*cis*-retinoic acid and all-*trans*-retinoic acid began before the onset of organogenesis, followed by dosing twice daily on the last 2–4 days of the dosing period (Hummler et al., 1990; Hendrickx & Hummler, 1992). Retinol was dosed daily from gestational day 16 to 27 (Hendrickx *et al.*, 1997)
[d] The numbers indicated refer to the therapeutic dose of 13-*cis*-retinoic acid (Lammer *et al.*, 1985) or the estimated doses of retinol obtained via supplementation and food
According to case reports (Rosa, 1993)

The lowest teratogenic doses of retinol in mice and rats are at least one order of magnitude higher than in rabbits, cynomolgus monkeys and humans.

Much effort has been expended to determine the reasons for the marked interspecies variations. It is generally accepted that a direct embryotoxic effect of a drug is determined by pharmacodynamic factors, such as the inherent activity of the drug and the intrinsic sensitivity of the embryo, as well as pharmacokinetic factors that determine the extent of embryonic exposure to the drug and its active metabolites (Wilson, 1977; Nau, 1986).

(e) Influence of placenta type on transplacental distribution of retinoids

In rodents, the type of placenta changes with gestational age. In the rat, for instance, the choriovitelline (yolk-sac) placenta is formed after angiogenesis of the chorionic placenta. Another type of placenta, the chorioallantoic placenta, differentiates from gestational day 11.5 and gradually becomes functional from day 12 onward (Beck, 1976; Garbis-Berkvens & Peters, 1987; Jollie, 1990). Most information on the transplacental distribution of retinoids in rodents is derived from studies performed at mid-organogenesis stages, such as gestational day 11 in mice and day 12 in rats, before full development of the chorioallantoic placenta. In contrast, development of the chorioallantoic placenta in the monkey takes place much earlier during gestation and is already complete at the time when measurements of embryonic retinoid concentrations can be performed (Beck, 1976). Therefore, it was previously hypothesized that the relatively extensive placental transfer of 13-*cis*-retinoic acid to the monkey embryo, as compared to rodent embryos at midgestation, was related to the type of placenta (Hummler *et al.*, 1994). A recent study further addressed this question by comparing the placental transfer of 13-*cis*-retinoic acid in mice and rats at gestational ages at which the chorioallantoic placenta is either starting to differentiate (day 11 for mice and day 12 for rats) or well established (day 14 for mice and day 16 for rats) and found more efficient transfer at the later than earlier gestational ages (Tzimas *et al.*, 1995).

(f) Duration of retinoid exposure is a major determinant of teratogenic outcome

Interspecies comparison of the transplacental pharmacokinetics of all-*trans*-retinoic acid and 13-*cis*-retinoic acid has not only helped to explain the marked interspecies variations of the lowest teratogenic doses of 13-*cis*-retinoic acid, but has also shown that embryonic AUC values of the corresponding retinoic acid isomer are similar across species after equipotent dosing regimens. In contrast, this was not the case for the C_{max} values. These results point out the importance of prolonged exposure to retinoids for induction of teratogenicity, rather than short-lived exposure reflected by relatively high C_{max} and rapid elimination. Other investigations have also addressed this issue by various approaches, as described later in this section.

The aforementioned postulate is in harmony with results of other studies, which have shown that the elevation of RAR-β2 expression above physiological levels in retinoid-sensitive regions of the mouse embryo is a specific marker of retinoid-induced teratogenicity (Harnish *et al.*, 1990). Thus, the elevation in RAR-β2 expression in mouse embryos must persist for at least 6 to 9 h after administration of teratogenic doses of all-*trans*- or 13-*cis*-retinoic acid to result in dysmorphogenesis, whereas the proportional extent of the increase in RAR-β2 expression did not correlate with the teratogenic outcome (Soprano *et al.*, 1994). Thus, the hypothesis that prolonged embryonic exposure to active retinoids — even if obtained by relatively low concentrations — is the decisive determinant of the teratogenic potency of retinoids has been confirmed by two different approaches, one based on pharmacokinetics, and one based on the effects of retinoids at the molecular level.

7.2.2.2 Interspecies comparison of the metabolism and bioactivation of vitamin A following teratogenic doses

(a) Mouse

The metabolism of vitamin A in mice following doses of different teratogenic activity has been examined in four studies (Kochhar *et al.*, 1988; Eckhoff *et al.*, 1989; Collins *et al.*, 1992; Tzimas *et al.*, 1996a,b).

Kochhar *et al.* (1988) reported plasma and embryonic pharmacokinetic data for retinoids following a highly teratogenic oral dose of 200 mg retinol/kg bw or a nonteratogenic oral dose of 100 mg/kg to ICR mice on gestational day 11. Notably, substantial concentrations of all-*trans*-retinoic acid, all-*trans*-4-oxoretinoic acid and 13-*cis*-retinoic acid were measured in maternal plasma and embryos after the teratogenic dose, whereas little if any acidic retinoids were detected following the nonteratogenic dose. Furthermore, a marked increase in retinol concentrations in maternal plasma and embryos was observed (up to 36-fold and 8-fold, respectively). Retinyl esters were not determined in this study due to limitations of the analytical method.

Eckhoff *et al.* (1989) reported transplacental pharmacokinetics of retinoids following administration of a highly teratogenic oral dose of 100 mg retinol/kg bw or a nonteratogenic dose of 10 mg/kg to NMRI mice on gestational day 11. High concentrations of all-*trans*-retinoic acid (C_{max} values of 593 ng/mL plasma and 327 ng/g embryo) and all-*trans*-4-oxo-retinoic acid (C_{max} values of 174 ng/mL plasma and 143 ng/g embryo) were determined after the teratogenic dose. However, in contrast to the results of Kochhar *et al.* (1988), the plasma concentrations of 13-*cis*-retinoic acid were much lower (< 10% of those of all-*trans*-retinoic acid) and no 13-*cis*-retinoic acid was found in the embryo, findings which were reproduced in subsequent experiments with this strain of mice (Collins *et al.*, 1992; Tzimas *et al.*, 1996b). The lower concentrations of 13-*cis*-retinoic acid found in this study as compared to that of Kochhar *et al.* (1988) may be due to a strain difference. It should also be noted that after doses of 100 mg/kg, the C_{max} of retinol was 40-fold (plasma) and 13-fold (embryo) higher than physiological concentrations. In addition, levels of retinyl esters in both plasma and embryos were markedly increased after the 100 mg/kg dose. In contrast, the increase in plasma and embryonic concentrations of retinol and retinyl esters was much less after administration of the 10 mg/kg dose. The formation of all-*trans*-retinoic acid and all-*trans*-4-oxoretinoic acid was very limited after the nonteratogenic dose, and the concentrations of these retinoids were much less than 10% of those obtained after the ten-fold higher dose (Eckhoff *et al.*, 1989).

Furthermore, 14-hydroxy-4,14-retro-retinol (14-HRR) was identified by Tzimas *et al.* (1996b) as a major metabolite of vitamin A in plasma, maternal and embryonic tissues of pregnant NMRI mice following administration of a teratogenic dose of retinol on gestational day 11. Concentrations of 14-HRR increased relatively slowly to their maximum and decreased slowly afterwards, in contrast to the rapid increase and subsequent elimination of all-*trans*-retinoic acid and all-*trans*-4-oxo-retinoic acid. Embryonic concentrations of 14-HRR were two- to five-fold higher than those in plasma, but it remains to be elucidated whether this is due to extensive transplacental passage of 14-HRR and/or to synthesis from retinol occurring *in situ* in the embryo.

The major question which arises from the results of these studies is whether retinol itself or some of its metabolites are responsible for the teratogenic effects observed after retinol administration. The discovery of RARs and their participation in the mediation of retinoid action in a wide variety of biological systems make plausible the assumption that RAR-binding of all-*trans*-retinoic acid and all-*trans*-4-oxo-retinoic acid mediates retinol-induced teratogenicity, at least in part.

Two lines of evidence suggest that exposure solely to all-*trans*-retinoic acid or its 4-oxo metabolite cannot explain the teratogenic effects of retinol treatment:

First, when NMRI mice were treated with teratogenic doses of either all-*trans*-retinoic acid (Kraft *et al.*, 1989) or retinol (Eckhoff *et al.*, 1989), embryonic exposure to all-*trans*-retinoic acid was substantially higher following all-*trans*-retinoic acid administration than after treatment with retinol, although the dosing regimen with all-*trans*-retinoic acid was less teratogenic than that with retinol.

Table 32. Area under the curve (AUC) values of retinoids in plasma and embryos of mice and rates of skeletal anomalies following administration of a teratogenic dose of retinol with or without pretreatment with 4-methylpyrazole[a]

Parameter	Retinol[b]	Retinol + 4-methylpyrazole[c]
AUC values in plasma[d]		
Retinol	9.48	8.50
All-*trans*-retinoic acid	3.75	0.156
All-*trans*-4-oxoretinoic acid	1.56	0.112
AUC values in embryos[d]		
Retinol	9.08	7.69
All-*trans*-retinoic acid	3.43	0.547
All-*trans*-4-oxoretinoic acid	1.50	0.310
Teratogenicity[e]		
Forelimb anomalies	55.6%	31.3%[f]
Hindlimb anomalies	43.9%	24.0%[f]
Craniofacial anomalies	56.0%	31.3%[f]

[a] From Collins *et al.* (1992)
[b] Following a single oral administration of 50 mg retinol/kg bw to pregnant mice on gestation day 11
[c] Following a single oral administration of 50 mg retinol/kg bw and pretreatment with an intraperitoneal dose of 100 mg 4-methylpyrazole/kg before retinol administration to pregnant mice on gestation day 11
[d] AUC values are expresssed in mg x h/g and were calculated for the time interval 0–8 h post-treatment.
[e] Percentage of fetuses affected
[f] Significantly lower than in the group receiving retinol alone (χ^2, $p < 0.01$)

Second, in a further study, the oxidative metabolism of retinol was blocked by pretreatment of pregnant NMRI mice with 4-methylpyrazole before retinol administration (Collins *et al.*, 1992). This led to a drastic reduction in the generation of all-*trans*-retinoic acid and all-*trans*-4-oxoretinoic acid and in the total embryonic exposure to these retinoids. Teratogenic effects, however, were reduced only partially (Table 32). However, the total embryonic exposure to retinol and 14-HRR was not affected by 4-methylpyrazole.

These results show that all-*trans*-retinoic acid is only in part responsible for the teratogenic effects induced by retinol treatment in mice, as proposed earlier (Kochhar *et al.*, 1988; Eckhoff *et al.*, 1989) and suggest that retinol may participate in eliciting teratogenicity.

(b) Rat

Retinoid profiles in maternal plasma and embryos of Wistar rats at gestational day 12 were determined after a teratogenic dosing regimen, consisting of six daily oral administrations of 90 mg retinyl palmitate/kg bw on days 7–12 (Collins *et al.*, 1994). In addition, retinoid pharmacokinetics have been examined after a single oral administration of 90 mg/kg on gestational day 12 (Tzimas, 1996); this dose is not expected to be teratogenic when given only once (Piersma *et al.*, 1996). The plasma concentrations of all-*trans*-retinoic acid and 13-*cis*-retinoic acid were in the low ng/mL range and increased over endogenous levels only sporadically following either single or multiple daily dosing with retinyl palmitate. All-*trans*-4-oxoretinoic acid and 13-*cis*-4-oxoretinoic acid were found in rat plasma at higher concentrations than the retinoic acid isomers, but only after multiple dosing. Retinyl β-glucuronide and 14-HRR were also identified in rat plasma, and exposure to these retinoids seemed to increase during long-term administration of retinyl palmitate.

As observed in the maternal plasma, embryonic concentrations of all-*trans*-retinoic acid were not significantly elevated over endogenous levels after either the single-dose or the multiple-dose regimen. Thus, the AUC of all-*trans*-retinoic acid in the embryo in the multiple-dose experiment was only 21% above the 'endogenous' AUC value obtained by extrapolation of the endogenous concentration over a 24-h period. Embryonic exposure to retinyl β-glucuronide, 13-*cis*-retinoic acid and the 4-oxo isomers was also relatively low or negligible, in contrast to the relatively high embryonic exposure to 14-HRR, retinol and retinyl esters.

These results clearly show that embryonic exposure to metabolically generated all-*trans*-retinoic acid is negligible following a single dose or during long-term administration of retinyl palmitate. Thus, the pattern of embryonic retinoids in the rat is very different following administration of the lowest teratogenic doses of either all-*trans*-retinoic acid or retinyl palmitate. Following treatments with retinyl palmitate, rat embryos were highly exposed to retinol and 14-HRR, and to a very small extent to all-*trans*-4-oxoretinoic acid and 13-*cis*-retinoic acid. On the other hand, after all-*trans*-retinoic acid administrations, rat embryos were exposed mainly to all-*trans*-retinoic acid and to a minor degree to all-*trans*-4-oxoretinoic acid and 13-*cis*-retinoic acid. This divergence between two dosing regimens with approximately equal teratogenic potency suggests that retinoids other than all-*trans*-retinoic acid are responsible for the teratogenic potency of retinyl palmitate.

Tembe *et al.* (1996) reached a similar conclusion about the role of the acidic retinoids in retinol-induced teratogenicity, after comparing the profiles of retinoids in maternal plasma of rats at gestational day 10 following different doses of either all-*trans*-retinoic acid or retinol. Doses of 500 mg retinol/kg bw induced gross structural malformations in all fetuses, and plasma concentrations of all-*trans*-retinoic acid and all-*trans*-4-oxo-retinoic acid reached 250 and 50 ng/mL, respectively. However, both the concentrations and the AUC values of the acidic retinoids were < 10% of the corresponding values seen after administration of an equipotent dose of all-*trans*-retinoic acid (50 mg/kg). It should be noted that the doses used were in the upper range of the dose–response curve, in contrast to the lowest teratogenic doses of all-*trans*-retinoic acid and retinyl palmitate used in the study of Collins *et al.* (1994).

(c) Rabbit

A single study has been reported dealing with the transplacental pharmacokinetics of retinoids in pregnant rabbits following administration of vitamin A (Tzimas *et al.*, 1996a). Retinyl palmitate was given orally to pregnant Swiss hare rabbits at a dose level of 10 mg/kg bw once daily on gestational days 7–12, and retinoid profiles in plasma and embryos were determined after the last dosing on day 12. This dosing regimen was within the teratogenic dose range and was clearly embryotoxic, based on the high resorption rate determined on gestational day 12 during sample collection.

Retinol and several of its esters were the predominant retinoids in both plasma and embryos. The major polar metabolite of retinol in plasma was 9,13-di-*cis*-retinoic acid, but its embryonic concentrations were about 6% of those in plasma. Other major plasma retinoids were retinyl β-glucuronide and 13-*cis*-4-oxo-retinoic acid, neither of which was detected in the embryo due to their limited placental transfer. 9-*cis*- and 13-*cis*-retinoic acid and 14-HRR were found in plasma at trace amounts; among those minor metabolites, only 14-HRR was found in measurable amounts in the embryo (C_{max} 37.4 ng/g). Finally, levels of all-*trans*-retinoic acid were very low in maternal plasma, and this was reflected by its AUC, which was only 2.4% of that of 9,13-di-*cis*-retinoic acid. In contrast, embryonic concentrations of all-*trans*-retinoic acid were about two-fold higher than endogenous levels.

The embryonic exposure to retinoids following the teratogenic dosing regimen with retinyl palmitate was compared with that observed after a teratogenic dosing regimen with all-*trans*-retinoic acid (Table 33). The similarity of the potency of the two dosing regimens is consistent with the fact that the AUC values of both all-*trans*-retinoic acid and all-*trans*-4-oxo-retinoic acid in the embryo were virtually identical in the two studies. It has therefore been suggested that the embryonic exposure to all-*trans*-retinoic acid and all-*trans*-4-oxo-retinoic acid is sufficient to explain the embryotoxic effects of dosing with retinyl palmitate in the rabbit (Tzimas *et al.*, 1996a). Rabbit embryos were also considerably exposed to retinol, but in view of the identical levels of exposure to all-*trans*-retinoic acid and all-*trans*-4-oxoretinoic acid after the two dosing regimens, retinol does not seem to play a significant role in the teratogenicity of retinyl palmitate in this species. Finally, the relatively low exposure to 14-HRR after dosing with retinyl palmitate suggests that this retinoid makes little contribution to the mediation of the embryotoxic effects of the applied dosing regimen in the rabbit.

Table 33. Area under the curve (AUC) values of retinoids in embryos of rabbits following roughly equipotent dosing regimens with all-*trans*-retinoic acid or retinyl palmitate[a]

Retinoid	All-*trans*-retinoic acid (6 mg/kg body wt per day)	Retinyl palmitate (10 mg/kg body wt per day)
All-*trans*-retinoic acid	954 (404)[b]	929 (379)[b]
All-*trans*-4-oxo-retinoic acid	276	217
13-*cis*-Retinoic acid	83	–[c]
9,13-Di-*cis*-retinoic acid	–[c]	136
14-Hydroxy-4,14-retro-retinol	–[c]	271
Retinol	6720 (1104)[b]	9051 (3435)[b]

[a] AUC values are expressed in ng x h/g and were calculated for the time interval 0–24 h after the last of six daily oral administrations of 6 mg all-*trans*-retinoic acid/kg bw or 10 mg retinyl palmitate/kg to rats from gestation day 7 to 12 (Tzimas *et al.*, 1994, 1996)

[b] The values in brackets represent only the excess of all-*trans*-retinoic acid or retinol over the endogenous concentrations

[c] Below limit of detection

(d) Monkey

The few data on retinoid metabolism following vitamin A administration to cynomolgus monkeys (Eckhoff *et al.*, 1990, 1991b; Eckhoff, 1991) were published before the determination of the lowest teratogenic dose of vitamin A in this species (Hendrickx *et al.*, 1997).

Eckhoff *et al.* (1990, 1991b) examined the plasma profiles of retinoids in nonpregnant cynomolgus monkeys following increasing oral doses of vitamin A (2, 10 and 50 mg retinol/kg bw), given in either an oil-based vehicle or a detergent-based vehicle. A wide variety of polar retinoids, including all-*trans*- and 13-*cis*-retinoic acid, all-*trans*- and 13-*cis*-4-oxoretinoic acid, all-*trans*-retinoyl-β-glucuronide and retinyl β-glucuronide, were identified as plasma metabolites of retinol. It remains to be elucidated whether and, if so, to what extent, retinol is metabolized to 14-HRR and 9,13-di-*cis*-retinoic acid in cynomolgus monkeys. The relative abundance of some of the retinoid meta-bolites was shown to be dose- and vehicle-dependent. For example, exposure to the acidic retinoids (all-*trans*- and 13-*cis*-retinoic acid, all-*trans*- and 13-*cis*-4-oxoretinoic acid) was increased overproportionally to the dose between 2 and 10 mg/kg (with the detergent-based vitamin A preparation) and between 10 and 50 mg/kg (with the oil-based preparation). Concentrations of retinol, retinyl esters and the polar metabolites tended to be higher after dosing with the detergent-based vehicle (Eckhoff *et al.*, 1991b).

The same investigators further compared plasma retinoid profiles in pregnant and nonpregnant female monkeys after a single oral dose of 5 mg retinol/kg bw dissolved in a detergent-based vehicle (Eckhoff, 1991). Surprisingly, the C_{max} values of most of the polar metabolites of retinol were much lower in pregnant than nonpregnant animals. It was hypothesized that the pregnant monkey has a more limited capacity to metabolize retinol, compared with nonpregnant animals, although the possibility of decreased absorption of retinol during pregnancy cannot be ruled out (Eckhoff, 1991).

Finally, in a further experiment, embryonic levels of retinoids were determined in pregnant monkeys following a single oral dose of 5 mg retinol/kg bw (n = 1) or 25 mg/kg (n = 2) during midgestation (Eckhoff, 1991). The results provide a very limited basis for estimation of embryonic retinoid exposure after dosing with vitamin A, but suggest that substantial embryonic exposure to retinoids may have occurred only after administration of the 25 mg/kg dose, and that, with the exception of the glucuronides, all metabolites which were measured in the plasma were also present in the embryo. In addition, embryonic concentrations of retinol and retinyl esters were highly elevated above endogenous levels (Eckhoff, 1991).

The teratogenic activity of vitamin A in cynomolgus monkeys has only recently been reported (Hendrickx *et al.*, 1997). Oral administration of daily doses of retinol (6 to 24 mg/kg bw) to the dams on gestational days 16–27 resulted in manifestation of embryolethality and retinoid-typical fetal anomalies in the craniofacial region, heart and thymus. The lowest teratogenic dose was 6 mg/kg bw; a dose of 2.25 mg/kg did not induce any observable fetal anomalies. It would therefore be valuable to examine plasma and embryonic retinoid profiles following these dosing regimens, in order to identify the retinoids which may be responsible for the observed teratogenicity.

(e) Human

The metabolism of vitamin A in humans *in vivo* has been examined following vitamin A (retinyl palmitate) supplementation (Eckhoff *et al.*, 1991a; Tang & Russell, 1991; Buss *et al.*, 1994; Peiker *et al.*, 1991; Chen *et al.*, 1996b) as well as consumption of fried liver (Buss *et al.*, 1994; Arnhold *et al.*, 1996) or other meals rich in vitamin A and provitamin A. In these studies, concentration profiles of retinoids were monitored in the plasma of volunteers following a single or long-term administration of vitamin A.

All-*trans*-retinoic acid, 13-*cis*-retinoic acid and 13-*cis*-4-oxoretinoic acid are physiological constituents of human plasma (Eckhoff & Nau, 1990a; Tang & Russell, 1990). Furthermore, these metabolites, together with all-*trans*-4-oxoretinoic acid, have been identified as plasma metabolites of exogenously administered vitamin A (Eckhoff *et al.*, 1991a; Tang & Russell, 1991; Buss *et al.*, 1994). 9-*cis*- and

9,13-di-*cis*-retinoic acid and 14-HRR have been detected in human plasma after liver consumption (Arnhold *et al.*, 1996); these retinoids were not searched for in previous studies (Eckhoff *et al.*, 1991a; Tang & Russell, 1991; Peiker *et al.*, 1991). Neither retinyl β-glucuronide nor any isomer of retinoyl β-glucuronide or 4-oxoretinoyl β-glucuronide was detected in human plasma after vitamin A intake (Eckhoff *et al.*, 1991a; Arnhold *et al.*, 1996), and it is not known whether these glucuronides are excreted in the urine.

With respect to the quantitative pattern of plasma retinoids following vitamin A intake, the results of the human studies can be summarized as follows:

(i) Plasma levels of retinyl esters increase substantially over baseline values following vitamin A supplementation or liver consumption (Eckhoff *et al.*, 1991a; Buss *et al.*, 1994). In contrast, a relatively low increase of retinol concentrations over endogenous values was seen only after vitamin A intake at doses corresponding to 0.8 mg retinol/kg bw or higher (Buss *et al.*, 1994; Arnhold *et al.*, 1996).

(ii) Plasma concentrations of 13-*cis*- and 9,13-di-*cis*-retinoic acid and 13-*cis*-4-oxo-retinoic acid were elevated to a much higher degree than those of all-*trans*- and 9-*cis*-retinoic acid, all-*trans*-4-oxoretinoic acid and 14-HRR after vitamin A intake (Eckhoff *et al.*, 1991a; Tang & Russell, 1991; Buss *et al.*, 1994; Arnhold *et al.*, 1996). Concentrations of retinoic acid isomers reached their peak about 1–3 h earlier than retinyl esters in some studies (Eckhoff *et al.*, 1991a; Buss *et al.*, 1994); this was proposed to result from oxidation of free retinol which escaped esterification in the intestinal mucosa cells after absorption and reached the liver via the portal blood.

(iii) A steady-state plasma concentration of 13-*cis*-4-oxoretinoic acid was reached upon long-term administration of vitamin A (Eckhoff *et al.*, 1991a; Chen *et al.*, 1996b), whereas a steady-state for 13-*cis*-retinoic acid was found only in one study (Chen *et al.*, 1996b). All other retinoids were rapidly eliminated from the blood during the period between daily doses.

(iv) Controversy exists about the extent of the increase of plasma concentrations of all-*trans*-retinoic acid following vitamin A intake. For instance, the ratios of the C_{max} versus the endogenous concentration (C_{end}) of all-*trans*-retinoic acid were 35 and 62 after pharmacological doses of 0.8 and 2.3 mg retinol/kg, respectively, in one study (Buss *et al.*, 1994), but only 3.9 after a dose of 2.25 mg retinol/kg in another (Tang & Russell, 1991). Following vitamin A supplementation with less than 0.8 mg retinol/kg bw as well as after liver consumption, the C_{max} of all-*trans*-retinoic acid was only 1.3- to 3-fold higher than the C_{end} (Eckhoff *et al.*, 1991a; Buss *et al.*, 1994; Arnhold *et al.*, 1996). In contrast, no elevation of all-*trans*-retinoic acid levels over the C_{end} was observed after consumption of meals rich in vitamin A and provitamin A, corresponding to an intake up to 170 000 IU (Chen *et al.*, 1996b). A possible explanation is the inclusion of plant sources of carotenoids in the composition of the menu; however, the conversion of carotenoids to all-*trans*-retinoic acid may be much more limited than the generation of the latter from retinol.

(v) Exposure to all-*trans*-retinoic acid was markedly lower after liver consumption than after supplementation with the same dose (Buss *et al.*, 1994). Thus, the plasma AUC of all-*trans*-retinoic acid after liver consumption (corresponding to a dose of 2.3 mg retinol/kg bw) was about 13% of that after administration of the same dose as a supplement. This phenomenon was not observed, at least to this extent, for the other polar retinoids. The reason for this discrepancy is not clear; differences in the milieu of the intestinal lumen depending on the material ingested (liver versus galenic formulation) may perhaps affect the extent to which retinol becomes available for oxidation to all-*trans*-retinoic acid.

(f) Interspecies comparison of vitamin A metabolism and risk of vitamin A exposure in humans

(i) Interspecies comparison of vitamin A metabolism: The metabolism of exogenously administered retinol and retinyl esters is qualitatively similar across species and comprises esterification of retinol with fatty acyl moieties, oxidation to retinoic acid isomers and their 4-oxo metabolites,

hydroxylation to 14-HRR (not yet shown in monkeys) and β-glucuronidation of retinol and all-*trans*-retinoic acid (not yet shown in mice and humans) (see also Section 3.2).

However, there are pronounced interspecies differences in terms of the relative exposure to individual retinoids. In Table 34, the polar metabolites of retinol in five species are categorized as major and minor ones, depending on the relative contributions of their plasma AUC values to the total AUC of all polar retinoids. This evaluation was based on pharmacokinetic data derived after teratogenic dosing regimens (for mice, rats and rabbits) (Eckhoff *et al.*, 1989; Tzimas *et al.*, 1994, 1996a; Collins *et al.*, 1994) or dosing regimens suspected to be teratogenic (for monkeys and humans) (Eckhoff *et al.*, 1991a,b; Buss *et al.*, 1994; Arnhold *et al.*, 1996). The following conclusions can be drawn:

(1) The conversion of retinol to all-*trans*-retinoic acid and the further oxidation to all-*trans*-4-oxoretinoic acid are much more extensive in mice and monkeys than in rats, rabbits and humans. This conclusion is, however, based on plasma data; the total body burden of the all-*trans*-retinoids may be higher in rats, rabbits and humans, because of possible interspecies differences in the volume of distribution.

(2) 9,13-Di-*cis*-retinoic acid is the predominant polar metabolite of vitamin A in rabbits and a major one in humans, but it is not present in rats, mice, or monkeys.

(3) The formation of 14-HRR is more extensive in mice and rats than in rabbits and humans (no information about this metabolic pathway in monkeys is available).

(4) Two of the three major plasma metabolites of vitamin A in humans are major retinoids also in rabbits (9,13-di-*cis*-retinoic acid and 13-*cis*-4-oxoretinoic acid) and monkeys (13-*cis*-retinoic acid and 13-*cis*-4-oxoretinoic acid), whereas only 13-*cis*-4-oxoretinoic acid is a major plasma retinoid in rats. In contrast, concentrations of 13-*cis*-retinoic acid in mouse plasma were very low, and the other two retinoids were not formed at all. Notably, the sum of the plasma AUC values of 9,13-di-*cis*-retinoic acid and 13-*cis*-4-oxoretinoic acid in

Table 34. Interspecies comparison of vitamin A metabolism based on plasma area under the curve (AUC) values of retinoid metabolites following dosing with vitamin A

Category[a]	Mouse	Rat	Rabbit	Monkey	Human
Major metabolites	All-*trans*-retinoic acid All-*trans*-4-oxo-retinoic acid 14-Hydroxy-retro-retinol	13-*cis*-4-Oxoretinoic acid 14-Hydroxy-retro-retinol Retinol glucuronide All-*trans*-4-oxo-retinoic acid	9,13-Di-*cis*-retinoic acid 13-*cis*-4-Oxoretinoic acid Retinyl glucuronide	All-*trans*-retinoic acid 13-*cis*-Retinoic acid All-*trans*-4-Oxo-retinoic acid 13-*cis*-4-oxoretinoic acid Retinoyl glucuronide Retinoyl glucuronide	13-*cis*-4-Oxoretinoic acid 13-*cis*-Retinoic acid 9,13-Di-*cis*-retinoic acid
Minor metabolites	13-*cis*-Retinoic acid Retinyl glucuronide Retinoyl glucuronide	All-*trans*-retinoic acid 13-*cis*-Retinoic acid 9-*cis*-Retinoic acid	13-*cis*-Retinoic acid All-*trans*-retinoic acid 9-*cis*-Retinoic acid All-*trans*-4-oxoretinoic acid 14-Hydroxy-retro-retinol	9-*cis*-retinoic acid all-*trans*-4-oxo-retinoic acid	All-*trans*-retinoic acid 9-*cis*-Retinoic acid All-*trans*-4-oxo-retinoic acid 14-Hydroxy-retro-retinol

[a] The categorization to major and minor metabolites is based on the ratio of the plasma AUC value of individual retinoids to the sum of the AUC values of all polar retinoids; ratios <0.1 led to characterization of a metabolite as 'minor'. For these calculations, AUC values were corrected for different molecular masses.

rabbits accounted for 83% of the sum of AUC values of all polar metabolites of retinol. This is very close to the relative contribution of 13-*cis*-4-oxoretinoic acid, 13-*cis*-retinoic acid, and 9,13-di-*cis*-retinoic acid in humans (87%), whereas the corresponding percentages were lower for 13-*cis*-retinoic acid and 13-*cis*-4-oxoretinoic acid in monkeys (18–60%, depending on the dose of retinol administered) and for 13-*cis*-4-oxoretinoic acid in rats (33%).

Finally, great interspecies variations exist in the degree of the increase in plasma retinol levels above endogenous levels following teratogenic dosing regimens with vitamin A. Rabbits and monkeys appear to be more similar to humans than are mice or rats with respect to the relative increase of plasma retinol. However, since the monkey data were derived from experiments performed with nonpregnant monkeys, additional studies with pregnant monkeys are required to address the similarity of humans to monkeys.

From all these comparisons, it seems that among the species tested so far, the rabbit shares the most similarities to humans with respect to maternal metabolism of vitamin A.

(ii) The proximate retinoid teratogens of vitamin A dosing are different across species: Data on embryonic exposure to retinoids following teratogenic dosing regimens with vitamin A in various species strongly suggest that the proximate retinoid teratogens of vitamin A differ across species. Thus, retinol and 14-HRR are the most probable candidates in this regard in rats, whereas all-*trans*-retinoic acid (and to a smaller extent all-*trans*-4-oxoretinoic acid) seems to be the ultimate teratogen in rabbits (Table 33). The relative contributions of retinol and its polar metabolites to the teratogenicity of vitamin A could not be dissociated in the mouse and cynomolgus monkey (Table 32).

The different pathways of metabolic activation of retinol in rats compared with rabbits may well explain why the lowest teratogenic dose of retinol is about nine-fold higher in rats than in rabbits (Table 31). This may result from the limited, if any, embryonic exposure of the rat embryo to all-*trans*-retinoic acid (Collins *et al.*, 1994); in contrast, the rabbit embryo is substantially exposed to all-*trans*-retinoic acid (Tzimas *et al.*, 1996a). However, a threshold of embryonic exposure to retinol and 14-HRR, resulting in teratogenic effects, may exist, and this seems to be attained in rats after the teratogenic dose (Collins *et al.*, 1994).

(iii) Risk of vitamin A exposure in humans: Information on the teratogenicity, metabolism and bioactivation of vitamin A in various animal species may be utilized for a rational risk assessment of vitamin A exposure of humans. Due to the wide interspecies differences in the bioactivation of retinol, it is necessary to know which species is most appropriate for comparison of human and animal data. For this purpose, several parameters should be compared between animal species and humans, such as the lowest teratogenic doses of vitamin A, the endogenous pattern of retinoid metabolism, and the metabolism and pharmacokinetics of retinoids following administration of vitamin A.

First, the lowest teratogenic doses of vitamin A in rabbits and cynomolgus monkeys, rather than other species, are quite close to those suspected to be teratogenic in humans, namely 10 mg retinyl palmitate/kg bw (equivalent to 5.5 mg retinol/kg) in rabbits, 6 mg retinol/kg in monkeys, and 0.2–1.5 mg retinol/kg in humans (cf. Table 31). An even lower teratogenic threshold dose (10 000 IU/day) has been suggested in an epidemiological study (Rothman *et al.*, 1995), but the validity of the estimate has been questioned (see Section 7.2.1).

Second, the pattern of endogenous plasma retinoids in rabbits resembles that in humans with respect to the presence of all-*trans*-retinoic acid and 13-*cis*-retinoic acid at concentrations of 1–2.5 ng/mL as well as the high abundance of retinol and much lower concentrations of retinyl esters (Tzimas *et al.*, 1996a; Eckhoff *et al.*, 1991a). In comparison, much lower physiological concentrations of retinoic acid isomers and a higher ratio of esterified versus nonesterified retinol have been measured in the plasma of mice, rats and monkeys (Hummler *et al.*, 1994; Eckhoff *et al.*, 1991b; Collins *et al.*, 1994; Tzimas *et al.*, 1995).

Third, among all species examined, the available data suggest that rabbits share the most similarities to humans with respect to maternal retinoid metabolism following dosing with vitamin A. The close similarity between rabbits and humans comprises the following points:

(i) The fairly low relative increase in plasma retinol concentrations after dosing with vitamin A.

(ii) The predominant plasma retinoic acid isomer is not the all-*trans* form; instead, 9,13-di-*cis*-retinoic acid is the main retinoic acid isomer in rabbit plasma, while both 13-*cis*-retinoic acid and 9,13-di-*cis*-retinoic acid are major retinoids in human plasma, at least following liver consumption (Tzimas *et al.*, 1996a; Eckhoff *et al.*, 1991a; Buss *et al.*, 1994; Arnhold *et al.*, 1996).

(iii) 13-*cis*-4-Oxoretinoic acid is a major plasma retinoid in both rabbits and humans, with similar steady-state concentrations and systemic exposure levels (Tzimas *et al.*, 1996a; Eckhoff *et al.*, 1991a; Buss *et al.*, 1994; Arnhold *et al.*, 1996; Chen *et al.*, 1996b).

(iv) Plasma levels of 14-HRR are low in both species (Tzimas *et al.*, 1996b; Arnhold *et al.*, 1996).

(v) Plasma concentrations of all-*trans*-retinoic acid are marginally elevated in both species after dosing with vitamin A. For example, plasma concentrations of all-*trans*-retinoic acid in rabbits after the last vitamin A administration were in most cases 1.3- to 2.3-fold higher than endogenous levels (Tzimas *et al.*, 1996a). Similarly, the plasma C_{max} of all-*trans*-retinoic acid in humans after liver consumption was 1.6- to 2.9-fold higher than endogenous concentrations (Buss *et al.*, 1994; Arnhold *et al.*, 1996), whereas the relative increase in plasma all-*trans*-retinoic acid after supplementation was similar after doses up to 0.25 mg retinol/kg (Eckhoff *et al.*, 1991a).

Fourth, retinoid pharmacokinetic profiles are similar in both species. In particular, apparent steady-state concentrations were reached for all retinoids in rabbit plasma following repeated daily dosing with vitamin A. Similarly, steady-state concentrations of 13-*cis*-4-oxoretinoic acid and 13-*cis*-retinoic acid were observed in human plasma during long-term administration of vitamin A supplements (Eckhoff *et al.*, 1991a; Chen *et al.*, 1996b).

Overall, therefore, it appears that the rabbit is the most appropriate species for extrapolation of embryonic exposure data for human risk assessment (Tzimas *et al.*, 1996a). Remarkably, despite the very low systemic exposure of rabbits to all-*trans*-retinoic acid, the embryonic exposure to this acid following dosing with vitamin A was substantial and probably sufficient to account for the embryotoxic effects of the dosing regimen used (Table 33). Two sources of all-*trans*-retinoic acid in the rabbit embryo after maternal dosing with vitamin A are possible. First, all-*trans*-retinoic acid can efficiently be transferred from the maternal circulation to the embryo, a process which may be mediated by embryonic CRABP-I or -II. Notably, specific binding of all-*trans*-retinoic acid to human embryonic proteins (probably CRABPs) has been reported (Nau, 1990), in agreement with findings in rodent and avian embryos (Scott *et al.*, 1994; Ruberte *et al.*, 1992; Gustafson *et al.*, 1993; Lyn & Giguere, 1994; Vaessen *et al.*, 1990; Maden, 1994). Second, and perhaps more relevant in the rabbit, all-*trans*-retinoic acid can be produced locally from retinol in the embryo (Tzimas *et al.*, 1996a). Several enzymes have been proposed to catalyse this process, but their expression in rabbit and human embryonic tissues has not been investigated. The available data for the rabbit, together with numerous similarities between rabbits and humans, do not rule out the possibility of substantial exposure of the human embryo to all-*trans*-retinoic acid, in spite of the marginal increases in plasma concentrations of all-*trans*-retinoic acid in vitamin A-exposed pregnant women.

The human risk for embryotoxic effects induced by vitamin A dosing may be further enhanced due to exposure to 13-*cis*-retinoic acid and 13-*cis*-4-oxoretinoic acid. Only limited amounts of these retinoids were found in the rabbit embryo following administration of retinyl palmitate (Tzimas *et al.*, 1996a). However, in humans, higher embryonic exposure might occur, especially if these retinoids are transferred across the human placenta more readily than across the rabbit placenta. This hypothesis is based on the more extensive transfer of the two 13-*cis*-retinoids across the monkey placenta than the rodent placenta and the close similarities of the placentas of humans and monkeys (Tzimas *et al.*, 1996a; Beck, 1976).

7.2.2.3 Role of vitamin A in reproduction, in particular spermatogenesis

Animals maintained on a vitamin A-deficient diet can be rescued by treatment with all-*trans*-retinoic acid and most of the symptoms of vitamin A deficiency are relieved except for those related to vision and reproduction. Retinoic acid cannot be reduced to retinal and therefore the cofactor of rhodopsin cannot be produced, resulting in eye defects. Vitamin A-deficient rats supplemented regularly with retinoic acid fail to reproduce (Thompson *et al.*, 1964); they continue their normal estrous cycles, mate with healthy males, and become pregnant, but invariably resorb their fetuses around gestational day 15. Retinol must be administered before day 10 to rescue the fetuses (Wellik & DeLuca, 1996). Retinoic acid cannot substitute for retinol in spermatogenesis, probably because retinoic acid cannot cross the blood–testis barrier (made up mostly by Sertoli cells), and little uptake of radiolabelled retinoic acid by the rat testes occurs (Blaner & Olson, 1994). The testis appears to be quite an exceptional organ in this regard, since all-*trans*-retinoic acid transfers well into most other organs, in particular the well perfused liver and brain. It is thought that all-*trans*-retinoic acid is the active retinoid metabolite in spermatogenesis, but because of its poor uptake, the testis is dependent on vitamin A as a precursor for retinoic acid. This view is supported by the finding that injection of large doses of retinoic acid into the testes can restore spermatogenesis (van Pelt & de Rooij, 1991).

Although CRABP-I and -II as well as CRBP-I are present in the testis in a very specific distribution, the function of these proteins remains unclear and knock-out of these proteins does not effect development or adult life, including fertility (Gorry *et al.*, 1994; Lampron *et al.*, 1995). This is also true for transthyretin-deficient mice, although they do have very low retinol serum levels. The roles of RBP and CRBP remain speculative, but may reside in transfer, metabolism and storage of retinol.

Male null mutant mice in which either the RAR-α, the RAR-β or the RXR-β gene was deleted are sterile. Deletion of the RAR-α gene resulted in degeneration of seminiferous epithelium (Lufkin *et al.*, 1993), and mutation of the RAR-γ gene in squamous metaplasia of the glandular epithelia of the seminal vesicles (Lohnes *et al.*, 1993). Mutation of the RXR-β gene resulted in failure of spermatid release within the seminiferous epithelia; female mice were fertile (Kastner *et al.*, 1996). Lipid accumulation was found in the Sertoli cells, perhaps due to heterodimerization of the RXR-β with one of the PPARs. Deletions of the RAR-β, RXR-α and RXR-γ genes did not result in infertility or effects on spermatogenesis. It thus appears that RAR-β and RXR-β are the primary signalling receptors in the germ cells and Sertoli cells, respectively. The importance of RXR-β also suggests that 9-*cis*-retinoic acid may be essential in spermatogenesis and this isomer was indeed identified in epididymal fluids. Recently, 9-*cis*-retinol dehydrogenase was found in the human testis (Mertz *et al.*, 1997) and this could possibly play a role in the generation of 9-*cis*-retinoic acid from 9-*cis*-retinol. Further-more, an extracellular binding protein for all-*trans*-retinoic acid was identified in the epididymis. This indicates a very special role for all-*trans*-retinoic acid and possibly its 9-*cis* isomer in sperm maturation, because in all other tissues or fluids only intracellular, but not extracellular binding proteins for retinoic acid were identified.

7.2.2.4 Possible metabolic basis of retinoid-induced teratogenicity

The teratogenicity induced by vitamin A is not associated with embryonic exposure to all-*trans*-retinoic acid in all cases. Teratogenic activity of vitamin A in mice and rats cannot be explained by embryonic exposure to all-*trans*-retinoic acid only; retinol and 14-HRR may be involved in these species. The results implicate 13-*cis*-retinoic acid and 13-*cis*-4-oxoretinoic acid as well as retinol and 14-HRR as possible proximate teratogens.

It is currently believed that retinoid toxicity (including teratogenicity) results from interaction of active retinoids with RARs and RXRs (Armstrong *et al.*, 1994). Contradictory information exists on the binding of retinol to RARs; no appreciable binding was reported in two studies (Crettaz *et al.*, 1990; Keidel *et al.*, 1992), whereas Repa *et al.* (1993) showed that retinol is one order of magnitude less potent than all-*trans*-retinoic acid in binding to RARs, and the binding observed was not the result of metabolism to all-*trans*-retinoic acid during the binding experiment. Finally, 14-HRR does not bind to any of the known retinoid receptors (Ross & Hämmerling, 1994).

The apparent differences in the lowest teratogenic doses of vitamin A in rats and rabbits probably result from interspecies differences in the bioactivation of retinol. Thus, teratogenic dosing regimens with vitamin A led to significant embryonic exposure to all-*trans*-retinoic acid in the rabbit, at levels similar to those obtained after dosing with all-*trans*-retinoic acid. In contrast, rat embryos were appreciably exposed to retinol and 14-HRR, but not to all-*trans*-retinoic acid, following vitamin A administration. Therefore, different retinoids may be responsible for vitamin A-induced teratogenicity in different species. The relative contributions of retinol and its metabolites to the teratogenicity induced by excess vitamin A in mice, monkeys and humans cannot yet be fully evaluated.

Among all the species examined to date, the rabbit appears the most similar to the human with respect to the endogenous retinoid profile and the pattern of plasma retinoids following vitamin A intake. Therefore, the marginal systemic exposure to all-*trans*-retinoic acid observed in humans after vitamin A supplementation or liver consumption does not rule out the possibility of high embryonic exposure to this retinoid, as is the case in rabbits. The potential involvement of 13-*cis*-retinoic acid and 13-*cis*-4-oxoretinoic acid, both of which are major retinoids in human plasma after vitamin A intake, in the induction of teratogenic effects should also be considered. Therefore, a teratogenic risk of high vitamin A intake in humans cannot at present be excluded.

7.3 Genetic and related effects

7.3.1 Human studies

As reported in Section 4.1.3, phase II chemoprevention studies have shown the ability of vitamin A, either alone or in combination with other agents, to decrease the frequency of micronuclei in cells of individuals exposed to genotoxic agents. Moreover, molecular epidemiology studies have provided evidence for an inverse relationship between either the dietary intake or serum/plasma levels of vitamin A and certain intermediate biomarkers, such as levels of aromatic DNA adducts in cells of smokers (see Section 4.1.3).

One study evaluated the detection rate of the major aflatoxin B_1–DNA adduct, i.e., aflatoxin B_1–N^7-guanine, in the urine of healthy males in Taiwan. After adjusting for chronic hepatitis B surface antigen (HBsAg) carrier status and other potential confounders, no association was found between adduct levels and the plasma levels of retinol. In the same study, this biomarker was positively associated with plasma levels of α-carotene and β-carotene and inversely correlated with plasma levels of lycopene (Yu *et al.*, 1997).

7.3.2 Experimental studies

Published data concerning the assessment of genetic and related effects of retinol, retinal, retinoic acid, retinyl acetate and retinyl palmitate *in vitro* and/or *in vivo* are summarized in Table 35 and represented diagrammatically in Appendix 4. Most data were generated in studies evaluating the ability of these compounds to modulate genetic and related effects produced by genotoxic agents (see Sections 4.2.2 and 4.2.3.2).

Retinol failed to revert the *Salmonella typhimurium his*⁻ strains TA1538, in the absence of S9 mix, and, irrespective of the addition of the exogenous metabolic system, TA1535, TA98, TA100 and TA102 (Baird & Birnbaum, 1979; White & Rock, 1981; Qin & Huang, 1985; Wilmer & Spit, 1986). In one study, however, retinol was reported to be mutagenic in strain TA104, in the presence of S9 mix (Han, 1992) [The Working Group noted that this result contrasts with the lack of mutagenicity of retinyl palmitate and retinoic acid in the same strain (see below)]. Retinol induced the mitochondrial mutation to respiratory deficiency (*petite*) mutation in *Saccharomyces cerevisiae* strain 6-81, but was not mutagenic to nuclear genes, as shown by the lack of reversion to methionine prototrophy (Cheng & Wilkie, 1991). Retinol did not affect a variety of endpoints in cultured mammalian cells, including DNA single-strand breaks (Alaoui-Jamali *et al.*,

1991a) and unscheduled DNA synthesis in primary rat hepatocytes (Budroe *et al.*, 1987), hypoxanthine phosphoribosyl transferase (HGPRT) mutation in Chinese hamster ovary (CHO) cells (Budroe *et al.*, 1988), 6-TG^R mutation (Ferrari *et al.*, 1989; Kuroda, 1990), sister chromatid exchanges (Sirianni *et al.*, 1981; Huang *et al.*, 1982; Qin & Huang, 1985; Alaoui-Jamali *et al.*, 1991a) and chromosomal aberrations (Qin & Huang, 1985) in Chinese hamster V79 cells, sister chromatid exchanges in Chinese hamster epithelial liver (CHEL) cells (Cozzi *et al.*, 1990) and morphological differentiation in mouse melanoma B-16 cells (Hazuka *et al.*, 1990). Retinol significantly decreased the 'spontaneous' chromosome instability, measured in terms of frequency of chromatid bridges and fragments at anaphase and telophase, in mouse C127 cells transformed by bovine papillomavirus DNA (Stich *et al.*, 1990). In contrast to these negative results, retinol produced a statistically significant increase in sister chromatid exchanges in cultured human lymphocytes (Dozi-Vassiliades *et al.*, 1985) [The Working Group noted the quite small difference in mean SCE/cells ± SE in controls (9.9 ± 0.3) and retinol-treated cells (11.7 ± 0.3)].

The genotoxicity of retinal was investigated in a single study which showed its lack of influence on the frequency of sister chromatid exchanges in Chinese hamster V79 cells (Sirianni *et al.*, 1981).

Retinoic acid failed to revert *S. typhimurium* strains TA1535, TA98, TA100 and TA102, irrespective of the presence of S9 mix (Qin & Huang, 1985; Wilmer & Spit, 1986) and TA104, in the absence of an exogenous metabolic system (Han, 1992; De Flora *et al.*, 1994). Retinoic acid did not induce unscheduled DNA synthesis in primary rat hepatocytes (Budroe *et al.*, 1987), HGPRT mutation in CHO cells (Budroe *et al.*, 1988), sister chromatid exchanges in Chinese hamster V79 cells (Sirianni *et al.*, 1981) or CHEL cells (Cozzi *et al.*, 1990). Retinoic acid displayed the same potency as retinol in attenuating the intrinsic chromosome instability in mouse C127 cells transformed by bovine papilloma-virus DNA (Stich *et al.*, 1990).

Irrespective of the presence of S9 mix, retinyl acetate did not affect the 'spontaneous' mutation frequency in *S. typhimurium* strains TA1535, TA98, TA100 and TA102 (Qin & Huang, 1985; Wilmer & Spit, 1986). It did not induce mutations in human heteroploid epithelial-like EUE cells (Ferreri *et al.*, 1986) or sister chromatid exchanges in Chinese hamster V79 cells (Sirianni *et al.*, 1981). Administration of retinyl acetate to C57BL/6J mice with the diet (20 mg/kg diet) for 10 weeks did not affect the frequency of sister chromatid exchanges in bone marrow cells (Qin & Huang, 1986).

Retinyl palmitate did not revert *S. typhimurium* strain TA104 (without S9 mix) (De Flora *et al.*, 1994). It was mutagenic, as measured by selection against diphtheria toxin, in human heteroploid epithelial-like EUE cells (Ferreri *et al.*, 1986) and it failed to induce DNA single-strand breaks, as evaluated by alkaline elution assay, when given for eight weeks in the diet (500 IU/g diet) of Sprague–Dawley rats. When given by gavage (32 mg/kg bw) twice a week for seven weeks, it did not affect the frequency of micronuclei in bone marrow cells of NMRI mice (Busk *et al.*, 1984) or in bone marrow cells of Swiss albino mice after a single oral administration (150 IU) of vitamin A [unspecified] (Rao *et al.*, 1986). Studies performed in a single laboratory showed the ability of retinyl palmitate to induce chromosomal aberrations in mouse cells *in vivo*. In particular, after treatment of Swiss albino mice with 132 IU/kg bw/day for 14 days, retinyl palmitate increased total chromosomal aberrations [1.6 times] (not significant) in bone marrow cells and [2.0 times] in spermatocytes (Kumari & Sinha, 1994). Under the same conditions but extending the treatment period to 14 weeks, retinyl palmitate increased the frequency of micronuclei [2.1 times] (not significant) in polychromatic and normochromatic erythrocytes from bone marrow, and total chromosomal aberrations [2.9 times] ($p < 0.002$) in bone marrow cells and [2.6 times] ($p < 0.002$) in spermatocytes (Sinha & Kumari, 1994). As reported in the same studies, the frequency of spermatozoa showing abnormal head morphology was unchanged after 14 days but was significantly enhanced ($p < 0.002$) after 14 weeks of treatment with retinyl palmitate.

Table 35. Genetic and related effects of retinol, retinal, retinoic acid and retinyl esters in *in vitro* and *in vivo* test systems

End-point*	Code*	Test system	Result[a]		Dose[b] (LED or HID)	Reference
			Without exogenous metabolic system	With exogenous metabolic system		
Retinol						
G	SA0	*Salmonella typhimurium* TA100, reverse mutation	–	–	40 µg/plate	Qin & Huang (1985)
G	SA2	*Salmonella typhimurium* TA102, reverse mutation	–	–	40 µg/plate	Qin & Huang (1985)
G	SA5	*Salmonella typhimurium* TA1535, reverse mutation	–	–	40 µg/plate	Qin & Huang (1985)
G	SA8	*Salmonella typhimurium* TA1538, reverse mutation	–	0	100 µM	White & Rock (1981)
G	SA9	*Salmonella typhimurium* TA98, reverse mutation	0	–	200 µg/plate	Baird & Birnbaum (1979)
G	SA9	*Salmonella typhimurium* TA98, reverse mutation	–	–	40 µg/plate	Qin & Huang (1985)
G	SA9	*Salmonella typhimurium* TA98, reverse mutation	0	–	0.5 µmol/plate	Wilmer & Spit (1986)
G	SA4	*Salmonella typhimurium* TA104, reverse mutation	+	0	1 µmol/plate	Han (1992)
G	SCF	*Saccharomyces cerevisiae* 6–81, mitochondrial (petite) mutation	+	0	4 mg/mL	Cheng & Wilkie (1991)
G	SCR	*Saccharomyces cerevisiae* 6–81, reverse mutation	–	0	4 mg/mL	Cheng & Wilkie (1991)
D	DIA	DNA single-strand breaks in primary rat hepatocytes	–	0	139.6 mM	Alaoui-Jamali *et al.* (1991a)
D	URP	Unscheduled DNA synthesis in primary rat heptocytes	–	0	50 µM	Budroe *et al.* (1987)
G	GCO	HGPRT mutation in Chinese hamster ovary (CHO cells)	–	–	50 µM	Budroe *et al.* (1988)
G	G9H	6-TG[R] mutation in Chinese hamster V79 cells	–	–	50 µM	Ferrari *et al.* (1989)
G	G9H	6-TG[R] mutation in Chinese hamster V79 cells	–	0	100 µg/mL	Kuroda (1990)
S	SIC	Sister chromatid exchanges in Chinese hamster V79 cells	–	0	4 µg/mL	Sirianni *et al.* (1981)
S	SIC	Sister chromatid exchanges in Chinese hamster V79 cells	–	–	32 µg/mL	Huang *et al.* (1982)
S	SIC	Sister chromatid exchanges in Chinese hamster V79 cells	–	–	16 µg/mL	Qin *et al.* (1985)
S	SIC	Sister chromatid exchanges in Chinese hamster V79 cells	0	–	139.6 mM	Alaoui-Jamali *et al.* (1991a)
S	SIC	Sister chromatid exchanges in Chinese hamster epithelial liver (CHEL) cells	–	0	25 µM	Cozzi *et al.* (1990)
C	CIC	Chromosomal aberrations in Chinese hamster V79 cells transformed by bovine papillomavirus DNA	–	–	32 µg/mL	Qin *et al.* (1985)
–	–	Chromosome instability in mouse C127 cells	*	0	0.5 µM(ID50)	Stich *et al.* (1990)
–	–	Morphological differentiation, mouse B-16 melanoma cells	–	0	18.6 µM	Hazuka *et al.* (1990)
S	SHL	Sister chromatid exchanges in cultured human lymphocytes	(+)	0	4 µg/mL	Dozi-Vassiliades *et al.* (1985)

Table 35 (Contd)

End-point*	Code*	Test system	Result[a]		Dose[b] (LED or HID)	Reference
			Without exogenous metabolic system	With exogenous metabolic system		
Retinal						
S	SIC	Sister chromatid exchanges in Chinese hamster V79 cells	–	0	1 μg/mL	Sirianni *et al.* (1981)
Retinoic acid						
G	SA0	*Salmonella typhimurium* TA100, reverse mutation	–	–	40 μg/plate	Qin & Huang (1985)
G	SA2	*Salmonella typhimurium* TA102, reverse mutation	–	–	40 μg/plate	Qin & Huang (1985)
G	SA5	*Salmonella typhimurium* TA1535, reverse mutation	–	–	40 μg/plate	Qin & Huang (1985)
G	SA9	*Salmonella typhimurium* TA98, reverse mutation	–	–	40 μg/plate	Qin & Huang (1985)
G	SA9	*Salmonella typhimurium* TA98, reverse mutation	0	–	0.5 μmol/plate	Wilmer & Spit (1986)
G	SAS	*Salmonella typhimurium* TA104, reverse mutation	–	0	10 μmol/plate	Han (1992)
G	SAS	*Salmonella typhimurium* TA104, reverse mutation	–	0	4 μmol/plate	De Flora *et al.* (1994)
D	URP	Unscheduled DNA synthesis in primary rat hepatocytes	–	0	50 μM	Budroe *et al.* (1987)
G	GCO	HGPRT mutation in Chinese hamster ovary (CHO) cells	–	–	50 μM	Budroe *et al.* (1988)
S	SIC	Sister chromatid exchanges in Chinese hamster V79 cells	–	0	4 μg/mL	Sirianni *et al.* (1981)
S	SIC	Sister chromatid exchanges in Chinese hamster epithelial liver (CHEL) cells	–	0	50 μM	Cozzi *et al.* (1990)
–	–	Chromosome instability in mouse C127 cells transformed by bovine papillomavirus DNA	*	0	0.5 μM(ID50)	Stich *et al.* (1990)
Retinyl acetate						
G	SA0	*Salmonella typhimurium* TA100, reverse mutation	–	–	40 μg/plate	Qin & Huang (1985)
G	SA2	*Salmonella typhimurium* TA102, reverse mutation	–	–	40 μg/plate	Qin & Huang (1985)
G	SA5	*Salmonella typhimurium* TA1535, reverse mutation	–	–	40 μg/plate	Qin & Huang (1985)
G	SA9	*Salmonella typhimurium* TA98, reverse mutation	–	–	40 μg/plate	Qin & Huang (1985)
G	SA9	*Salmonella typhimurium* TA98, reverse mutation	0	–	0.5 μmol/plate	Wilmer & Spit (1986)
G	GIH	Diphtheria toxin mutation in human heteroploid epithelial-like (EUE) cells	–	0	1 μM	Ferreri *et al.* (1986)
S	SIC	Sister chromatid exchanges in Chinese hamster V79 cells	–	0	10 μg/mL	Sirianni *et al.* (1981)
S	SVA	Sister chromatid exchanges in mouse bone marrow cells	–	NA	20 mg/kg diet for 10 weeks	Qin & Huang (1986)

Table 35. (Contd)

End-point*	Code*	Test system	Result[a]		Dose[b] (LED or HID)	Reference
			Without exogenous metabolic system	With exogenous metabolic system		
Retinyl palmitate						
G	SAS	*Salmonella typhimurium* TA104, reverse mutation	–	0	4 µmol/plate	De Flora *et al.* (1994)
D	DVA	Single-strand breaks in rat hepatocytes	NA	–	500 IU/g diet for 8 weeks	Decoudu *et al.* (1992)
G	GIH	Diphtheria toxin mutation in human heteroploid epithelial-like (EUE) cells	–	0	10 µM	Ferreri *et al.* (1986)
M	MVM	Micronuclei in mouse peripheral blood erythrocytes	–	NA	132 IU/kg bw/day for 14 weeks	Sinha & Kumar (1994
M	MVM	Micronuclei in mouse bone marrow cells	–	NA	150 IU (single administration)	Rao *et al.* (1986)
M	MVM	Micronuclei in mouse bone marrow cells	–	NA	32 mg/kg bw by gavage twice a week for 7weeks	Busk *et al.* (1984)
C	CBA	Chromosomal aberrations in mouse bone marrow cells	–	NA	132 IU/kg bw/ day for 14 days	Kumari & Sinha (1994)
C	CBA	Chromosomal aberrations in mouse bone marrow cells	+	NA	132 IU/kg bw/ dayfor 14 weeks	Sinha & Kumari (1994)
C	CCC	Chromosomal aberrations in mouse spermatocytes	(+)	NA	132 IU/kg bw/ day for 14 days	Kumari & Sinha (1994)
C	CCC	Chromosomal aberrations in mouse spermatocytes	(+)	NA	132 IU/kg bw/day for 14 weeks	Sinha & Kumari (1994)

[a] Result: +, positive; (+), weak positive; –, negative; 0, not tested; NA, not applicable (in vivo assay); *, inhibition of the investigated end-point
[b] LED, lowest effective dose; HID, highest ineffective dose; ID50, dose inhibiting the 50% of the investigated effect. The units are as reported by the authors.
*See Appendix 2 for codes; – test or end-point is not defined and is not shown in the activity profile.

8. Summary of Data

8.1 Chemistry, occurrence and human exposure

The components of vitamin A—retinol and retinyl esters—are lipophilic compounds that are inherently unstable, being sensitive to light, heat and oxygen. In the presence of light, their all-*trans*-tetraene double-bond systems can isomerize to provide a mixture of *trans* and *cis* isomers. Heat also affects double-bond stability and reactivity, and oxygen causes the formation of oxygenated species. Being hydrophobic, retinol and its esters (such as the acetate and palmitate) are insoluble in water and plasma unless associated with proteins.

Vitamin A is metabolically derived from carotenoids having at least one terminus consisting of a cyclohexenyl ring. β-Carotene, with two such terminal rings, is the most active precursor. Vitamin A activity is reduced by minor structural variations in retinol structure, such as double-bond isomerization or introduction of another ring double bond at the 3-position, but is eliminated by significant changes, such as double-bond saturation. Esterification does not reduce activity unless intestinal absorption is impaired. Retinal has activity similar to that of retinol because it is readily reduced; however, while active in regulating cell differentiation, retinoic acid is inactive in supporting vision and reproduction because it cannot be converted back to retinol or retinal.

Human intake of vitamin A is mainly in the form of the provitamin carotenoids and retinyl esters, which are found most abundantly in foods of plant tissue and animal origin, respectively. These forms are converted to retinol in the body. The average recommended daily intake of vitamin A is approximately 0.6–1.0 mg retinol for men and 0.5–0.8 mg retinol for women. However, in treatment of disorders related to vitamin A deficiency such as xerophthalmia, single doses are much higher. On the worldwide scale, vitamin A deficiency has been identified as a severe public health problem.

Retinyl esters, particularly the palmitate and acetate, are found in vitamin A supplements (as a micronutrient) and fortified foods, as well as in cosmetics used to enhance a youthful appearance, based on the efficacy shown by retinoic acids against adverse dermatological conditions. Carotenoids are also used in nutritional supplements and fortified foods. Supplemental retinyl esters and carotenoids have been investigated in trials for cancer prevention.

Measurement of plasma retinol is most commonly used to assess vitamin A status. However, a relative dose–response test probably gives more accurate information on total concentrations of vitamin A in the body. High-performance liquid chromatography is the method of choice for these and other analyses of vitamin A in biological samples.

8.2 Metabolism and kinetic properties in humans and animals

Retinyl esters are hydrolysed in the intestine to retinol, which appears to be absorbed by binding to a mucosal cell transporter. Many yellow, orange, red and green fruits and vegetables, as well as sea plants and fishes, contain carotenoids, some of which serve as precursors of vitamin A. After being incorporated into lipid micelles and absorbed by intestinal cells, provitamin A carotenoids are primarily cleaved in the centre to form one or two molecules of retinal. Retinal is then largely reduced to retinol. Thereafter, the metabolism of vitamin A derived either from retinyl esters or from provitamin A carotenoids follows the same pathway.

Retinol within intestinal cells is esterified, incorporated into chylomicra and transported via the lymph into the general circulation. A portion of the triglyceride fraction of chylomicra is hydrolysed by lipoprotein lipase, producing much smaller chylomicron remnants that contain retinyl esters, some retinol, and carotenoids. These remnants are removed from the circulation by receptor-mediated uptake, primarily by the liver but also by adipose tissue, bone marrow and other tissues.

Within the liver as well as other organs, stellate cells are the major storage sites for retinyl esters. Retinol is released from the liver primarily as a 1:1 complex with retinol-binding protein (RBP), which further combines with transthyretin. The concentration of holo-RBP in the plasma is homeostatically controlled over a wide range of total body reserves of vitamin A. The uptake of retinol by peripheral tissues may occur by interaction of unbound retinol with membranes and possibly in some tissues by formation of a complex with a cell-surface receptor for holo-RBP.

Within cells, retinol may be oxidized to retinal and then to retinoic acid, esterified with long-chain fatty acids, oxidized at other positions, or conjugated with glucuronic acid. Most of these enzymatic transformations occur when retinoids are complexed with cellular retinoid-binding proteins. All forms of vitamin A and retinoic acid may also undergo double-bond isomerization. Retinol and retinoic acid may also be degraded by stepwise oxidative cleavage of the polyene chain.

Vitamin A is highly conserved in humans and animals by recycling, in which vitamin A released from the liver is taken up by peripheral tissues and then returned to the liver. The kinetics of this rapid and extensive process have been carefully studied in both humans and animals. The irreversible loss of vitamin A from the body is directly related to the total body stores.

Vitamin A functions in vision as 11-*cis*-retinal, in cell differentiation as all-*trans*- and 9-*cis*-retinoic acids; in the immune response, probably primarily as retinoic acid; and in embryonic development both as retinol and as retinoic acid. Retinol and its metabolites serve as ligands for different functional proteins, with opsins in the eye and with the nuclear receptors RAR and RXR in developing and differentiating cells. The interactions of retinoids with these nuclear receptors seem to be most closely associated with their normal functions, as well as with possible events leading to unregulated cellular proliferation.

Most of the biochemical and molecular details regarding vitamin A physiology have been obtained through study of animal models. Much of this information has come from studies in the rat, a model which, with respect to basic transformations in vitamin A physiology, closely resembles man. However, studies of vitamin A transport and metabolism are increasingly being carried out in the mouse model, primarily because of the development of transgenic and knockout technologies and the increasing availability of suitable transgenic mouse strains. Although less frequently reported, vitamin A transport and metabolism have also been studied in many other species, including most commonly rabbits, pigs, ferrets and chickens. Studies of these species have provided information which is directly relevant to the human situation. The validity of data obtained from animal models for describing the human situation must necessarily depend on the physiological or medical context of the study.

In dosing studies on humans, concentrations of metabolic intermediates in plasma and tissues are markedly affected by the vitamin A formulation employed, inasmuch as the nature of the matrix or carrier, rate of release of vitamin A, and the types of solubilizers and stabilizers used vary. In addition, the patterns of metabolites of vitamin A differ markedly between species. Thus, metabolic transformations are qualitatively similar but quantitatively different among species.

8.3 Cancer-preventive effects

8.3.1 Human studies

There is no evidence from human studies that vitamin A has a generalized cancer-preventive effect. Observational studies have generally been based on estimates of preformed vitamin A in the diet, with some information from older studies that reported only total vitamin A; a small number of studies related use of vitamin A supplements to cancer risk. Measurements of serum retinol are relatively uninformative in well nourished populations due to the strong homeostatic controls that modulate plasma levels of retinol. Intervention studies have been conducted with vitamin A doses ranging from approximately 50 to 250% of typical total vitamin A dietary intakes, except for one high-dose study, although the period of supplementation has not extended beyond five years, and duration of follow-up has been limited. Summarized below are the results of studies on vitamin A in relation to specific cancers.

(a) Lung cancer
No association has been found between dietary intake of preformed vitamin A and risk of lung cancer in many observational studies. Data from a large randomized placebo-controlled trial among North American smokers and asbestos-exposed workers suggested, if anything, an adverse effect on lung cancer incidence of a combination of retinol with β-carotene. In a randomized, placebo-controlled trial of a combination of β-carotene and retinol among former asbestos-exposed workers, no significant reduction in sputum atypia was observed. In one trial in treated lung cancer patients, supplementation with high-dose retinol was associated with a reduction in second primary lung cancers.

(b) Mesothelioma
The risk of mesothelioma was reduced in an intervention trial among Australian asbestos miners given retinol, as compared with those given β-carotene. Mesothelioma risk was not affected by retinol in combination with β-carotene in a North American trial.

(c) Upper aerodigestive tract
Case–control studies have suggested either a modest direct association with high dietary intake of retinol or no association. Two Chinese intervention trials did not show a beneficial effect on oesophageal cancer when retinol was given in addition to zinc or a multivitamin preparation. There was a statistically significant effect on head and neck cancers in a trial in which retinol was given in combination with β-carotene to heavy smokers and asbestos-exposed workers. Leukoplakia of the mouth shows a marked positive phenotypic response to preformed vitamin A, but the original cellular phenotype returns in a considerable proportion of cases after cessation of treatment. Whether treatment with preformed vitamin A reduces or delays the progression of these lesions to carcinoma is not known. This work was performed in populations that may have been vitamin A-deficient, the series were small and original lesions could recur after treatment. Its meaning remains unclear.

(d) Gastric cancer
No association has been found between dietary intake of retinol and risk of gastric cancer in many observational studies. No beneficial effect was detected in two intervention studies in China, where retinol was given in addition to either zinc or a multivitamin preparation.

(e) Colorectal cancer
No association between dietary intake of retinol and risk of colorectal cancer has been found in many observational studies, nor in the one available intervention study.

(f) Skin cancer
No association has been found between dietary intake of retinol and risk of skin cancer in a small number of observational studies. An intervention study in the United States showed no beneficial effect of retinol as compared to placebo on the incidence of basal-cell carcinoma. With respect to squamous-cell carcinoma of the skin, a risk reduction was found in relatively moderate-risk individuals, but not in high-risk subjects.

(g) Breast cancer
No association between dietary intake of retinol and risk of breast cancer has been found in many observational studies, mainly of postmenopausal women, nor was a significant association found in one intervention trial. There is a lack of information to indicate presence or absence of effects in premenopausal women.

(h) Prostate cancer
No consistent association has been found between dietary intake of retinol and risk of prostate cancer in many observational studies, nor in the one available intervention study.

(i) Bladder cancer
No association has been found between dietary intake of retinol and risk of bladder cancer in many observational studies and in the one available intervention study.

(j) Cervical cancer
No association has been found between dietary intake of retinol and risk of cervical dysplasia or

invasive cervical cancer in many observational studies.

8.3.2 Experimental studies

(a) Lung

The chemopreventive effects of retinyl esters on lung carcinogenesis have been studied in rats and hamsters. In one study in rats, retinyl acetate caused a dose-dependent inhibition of lung carcinogenesis. Of three studies in Syrian golden hamsters, one was inconclusive and two showed no protective effect.

(b) Mammary gland

The preventive effects of retinyl esters on mammary carcinogenesis were studied in mice and rats. Of two studies conducted in mice, one showed no protective effect, whereas the other study showed enhanced tumour development. Nine studies were performed in rats using different chemical carcinogens. In eight of these, retinyl acetate protected against mammary carcinogenesis, but in one study the result was inconclusive. The protective effect was enhanced when retinyl acetate treatment was combined with other agents such as selenium or butylated hydroxytoluene or with ovariectomy.

(c) Urinary bladder

The preventive efficacy of retinyl esters was assessed in three rat studies. In one, retinyl acetate protected against bladder carcinogenesis, whereas in two, retinyl palmitate was not protective.

(d) Skin

The preventive effects of retinyl esters on mouse skin carcinogenesis were studied in five experiments. Papilloma development induced by chemical carcinogens was inhibited by retinyl palmitate in two studies, while skin carcinoma development was not affected in another study. In two studies on skin tumour induction by ultraviolet irradiation, treatment was ineffective or inconclusive. In a third study, skin carcinoma induction by ultraviolet radiation was enhanced by retinol.

(e) Other organs

In studies of tumour development in the oesophagus, colon and thyroid, retinyl ester treatment either was ineffective or gave equivocal results. In some organs, including forestomach, colon and bladder, vitamin A deficiency led to increased susceptibility to chemical carcinogenesis.

(f) In-vitro models

In vitro, retinol and retinyl acetate were found to inhibit the proliferation and to modulate the differentiation of a large number of untransformed, transformed and malignant rodent and human cells derived from many different histological types of tissue. Growth inhibition was dose- and time-dependent and reversible. Studies with keratinocytes and tracheobronchial epithelial cells indicated that retinyl acetate can modulate cell proliferation, suppress squamous cell differentiation and enhance mucus cell differentiation. Retinol may reduce cell proliferation by arresting the cell cycle. Similarly, the anchorage-independent growth of human fibroblasts induced by growth factors was inhibited by retinol. In contrast, the response of haematopoietic stem cells to certain growth factors was potentiated by retinol or retinyl acetate.

The effects of retinol and/or some of its metabolites on cell proliferation and differentiation are thought to be mediated by interaction with nuclear retinoic acid receptors, which are members of the steroid thyroid hormone receptor superfamily that are *trans*-acting modulators of gene transcription.

(g) Inhibition of genetic and related effects

Vitamin A and its natural derivatives were evaluated in short-term tests *in vitro* and *in vivo* as modulators of genetic and related effects induced by over 50 physical and chemical agents.

In most but not all studies, vitamin A did not affect the genotoxicity of direct-acting compounds. With genotoxic agents that need to be activated metabolically by cells, vitamin A showed consistent protective effects towards mycotoxins, such as aflatoxin B_1, heterocyclic amines isolated from food pyrolysis products, and nitrosamines present in tobacco smoke and polluted air. The results were inconsistent or equivocal when vitamin A was challenged with other classes of procarcinogens, including polycyclic aromatic hydrocarbons, aromatic amines and some complex mixtures.

8.3.3 Mechanisms of cancer-prevention

Vitamin A may prevent or delay carcinogenesis at both the initiation and promotion steps. However, the mechanisms through which these effects may be exerted have not been fully elucidated. Although retinol can activate the nuclear retinoid receptors either directly or through some of its metabolites, information on which retinoid-regulated genes are the proximal mediators of the above effects of retinol is scarce. Plausible mechanisms based on findings in cultured cells and animal models include modulation of cell properties (cell proliferation, differentiation, communication, adhesion, migration and invasion) or host properties (immune response, angiogenesis). Analysis of these mechanisms in the context of a chemoprevention trial is required for validation of their relevance.

8.4 Other beneficial effects

Vitamin A relieves the symptoms of vitamin A deficiency, including night-blindness and mild cases of xerophthalmia, whereas more severe cases are irreversible. In populations in which clinically apparent vitamin A deficiency is common, a number of intervention trials have shown that vitamin A supplementation reduces child mortality and morbidity. In relatively well nourished populations, evidence of benefit with vitamin A supplement use is inconsistent. Conditions such as arthritis and many infectious diseases have not been consistently improved by vitamin A supplements. These conditions may often involve changes in vitamin A distribution rather than overt deficiency. Psoriasis and other skin conditions may improve with vitamin A treatment, but less toxic analogues of retinol have been effectively used for the last 25 years. Based on results from observational studies and a large intervention study (CARET), retinol together with β-carotene does not seem to be protective against heart disease. In conclusion, preformed vitamin A has not been unambiguously shown to be protective against any conditions other than the direct effects of vitamin A deficiency.

8.5 Carcinogenic effects

8.5.1 Human studies

A large number of observational epidemiological studies on the relation between dietary retinol and cancer risk have not shown consistent evidence of increased cancer rates. Two trials of vitamin A and primary skin cancer have shown no sign of increased risks of squamous or basal cell carcinoma. Similarly, two trials in China and one in Australia reported no evidence of increases in overall cancer incidence or mortality. One study (CARET) reported an increased risk of lung cancer among high-risk individuals taking a vitamin A supplement in combination with β-carotene. Findings from another trial (the ATBC study) suggest that this apparent adverse effect may be largely attributable to the β-carotene component of the supplement rather than to retinol.

8.5.2 Experimental animals

Retinyl esters were evaluated for carcinogenicity by long-term oral administration in one study with female rats and in one study with male and female rats.

In the study with female rats, a higher incidence of mammary adenocarcinomas was observed in rats fed diets supplemented with high levels of mixtures of retinyl acetate and retinyl palmitate; no dose–response relationship was observed. In the other study, the incidence of benign phaeochromocytomas increased in both males and females with increasing levels of retinyl acetate. The incidence of malignant phaeochromocytomas was significantly increased in high-dose males.

8.6 Toxic effects

8.6.1 Human studies

Toxicity due to hypervitaminosis A occurs in the skin, the circulation (e.g., plasma proteins), internal organs (e.g., liver), the nervous system, and the musculo-skeletal system. Side-effects of systemic vitamin A administration commonly encountered in the skin include desquamation, cheilitis, brittle nails, skin rashes and alopecia. Circulatory side-effects may include hypertriglyceridaemia, serum enzyme increases and hypothrombinaemia. Hepatomegaly and palpaple or tender liver have been reported. Viral hepatitis, protein energy malnutrition and pre-existing liver disease may predispose individuals to vitamin A toxicity. Nausea and vomiting, anorexia, diarrhoea, weight loss, fatigue, malaise, lethargy, somnolence, weakness and irritability are also commonly reported.

Headache may occur transiently with supplement doses. More severe reactions include elevated cerebrospinal fluid pressure, cranial hypertension, pseudotumor cerebri, altered vision and papilloedema. Drug interactions may occur in patients combining vitamin A with minocyclin (a synthetic tetracycline). Hypervitaminosis A is known to cause demineralization of bone, periosteal calcification and hypercalcaemia, in all age groups. Bone and joint pain and myalgia are commonly associated symptoms.

There have been few studies of the effects in pregnancy of retinol itself, although teratogenic effects of 13-*cis*-retinoic acid and synthetic retinoids are well documented. Case–control studies and a trial of multivitamin supplementation reported no increase in the risk of malformations associated with increased intake of vitamin A during pregnancy, but one cohort study did observe an association with major defects.

8.6.2 Experimental studies

The toxicities elicited by vitamin A in laboratory animals generally reflect those seen in humans and occur in the skin, the circulation, internal organs, and the musculo-skeletal system. No studies in animals have modelled the human neurological toxicities.

The commonly observed effects of retinoids on the skin of laboratory animals include erythema, epidermal thickening, scaling, loosening of the stratum corneum, increases in transepidermal water loss, alopecia and conjunctivitis. Elevations in rodent serum lipid profiles, enzyme activities and coagulation times have been reported. Hypervitaminosis A causes fatty infiltration of the rodent liver and up-regulates Kupffer cell activity. The results of drug interaction studies in rats and mice indicate that there are species differences in the effects of vitamin A on the rodent liver and that the timing of vitamin A administration may also affect the hepatotoxicity of the drug or chemical. Altered intestinal absorptive processes, gallstones, degeneration of myocardial fibres with associated electrocardiographic changes, fatty changes and haemosiderosis in the spleen, glomerulonephritis and necrotizing nephrosis in the kidney, and testicular atrophy in adult and degenerative testicular changes in weanling rodents have also been described. Demineralization, thinning of the long bones, cortical hyperostosis, periostosis, limping gait, fractures, osteoporotic lesions and premature closure of the epiphyses have been described in numerous animal species.

Retinol, retinal, retinoic acid and retinyl esters gave negative results in the large majority of studies evaluating induction of genetic and related effects in bacteria, yeast, mammalian cultured cells and animal models.

Vitamin A (retinol, retinyl esters) was teratogenic in a number of experimental animal studies. The doses needed to elicit a frank teratogenic response were, however, much higher than those expected in human therapy, prophylaxis or nutrition.

Mice and rats not only need extremely high doses to elicit a teratogenic effect, but also exhibit a very different metabolic pattern as compared to humans. Thus, rats and mice are poor models for the human. In the rabbit, much lower doses are sufficient to induce developmental defects. Also, the endogenous retinoid plasma pattern is very similar to that seen in humans after vitamin A administration.

Highly active retinoids have been found in human plasma after vitamin A exposure (supplementation, liver consumption). Their plasma concentrations and AUC values were in some instances in the same range as those found after administration of embryotoxic doses to rabbits, currently the most appropriate experimental animal model. Thus, a teratogenic risk of supplementation and liver consumption in humans can at present not be excluded on the basis of experimental studies. It is not known if a safe threshold dose or exposure exists with regard to developmental defects.

9. Recommendations for future research

The assessment of the literature presented in this handbook led to formulation of the following recommendations for future research:

1. To study the mechanism of action of retinol and its metabolites at the molecular and genetic levels in relation to carcinogenesis;

2. To identify new nontoxic conjugates and formulations of retinol and retinyl esters that may show cancer-preventive properties;

3. To consider the conduct of randomized prevention trials of longer duration among particularly high-risk groups such as asbestos-exposed individuals and former lung cancer patients;

4. To evaluate exposure biomarkers useful in epidemiological studies and clinical trials;

5. To continue the follow-up of the terminated intervention trials to assess the long-term effects of the intervention agents.

It is becoming clear that the effects of retinol metabolites such as the retinoic acids on their nuclear receptors are modulated, either directly or indirectly, by other important nuclear receptors and their ligands (glucocorticoids, estrogen, thyroid hormones, vitamin D and prostaglandins), other transcription factors and intermediary proteins. The retinoid signalling system is even more complex in that there are at least two classes of retinoid receptors and three subtypes of each class that in the presence of their ligands can activate or repress retinoic acid responsive elements on genes. Depending on the dimeric partner and response element, receptors can be affected differently by their natural or synthetic ligands. Thus, much remains to be learned on the molecular mechanisms controlling these processes, the interaction of the different pathophysiological factors involved at cellular and tissue levels, and how such environmental factors as asbestos, tobacco, bidi smoking, betel nut chewing, alcohol and environmental toxins influence these systems.

A better understanding of the way the cell and the body control their vitamin A supply will allow better definition of vitamin A status, distribution at times of deficiency, and assessment of effects on how distribution is organized. Epidemiologically, the eye has been considered the organ most vulnerable to vitamin A status. However, in the last decade, the importance of vitamin A for immune function has become apparent. Impaired immune function has been identified in populations where ophthalmological signs are rare, and morbidity is reduced by vitamin A supplements. Animal studies have shown that vitamin A deficiency increases susceptibility to chemical carcinogens. Thus, the aspects of vitamin A metabolism that are disrupted during deficiency should be identified, as should the point at which vitamin A depletion occurs. Other questions that still need to be resolved are how adaptation to low vitamin A intake occurs and what pathway is attenuated or blocked so that vulnerability to experimental carcinogenesis is enhanced.

In some situations, different sources of vitamin A (retinol, retinyl palmitate and retinyl acetate) appear to have different effects *in vivo* and comparative experiments should be conducted to investigate such observations in well defined experimental models. Concern was expressed that combinations of other micro-nutrients with vitamin A, as well as foods, might influence retinoid metabolism. These factors should also be studied at the cellular level and include metabolites that might arise under experimental conditions, where large doses are given.

Much current research has been directed to explaining how retinol and other retinoids function at the genetic level. Responses of genes to retinoids controlling cellular differentiation and errors in such control can determine cancer risk. Genetic diversity in human populations means that certain genetic polymorphisms within the population may predispose to cancer. Individuals who respond positively to increased intake of vitamin A or to modifications in retinoid metabolism should be identified.

It is difficult to evaluate and compare results of studies in which protocols differed widely or in which proper controls and differences in the baseline conditions were neglected, omitted or inadequately described. There is an urgent need to develop standard protocols to evaluate the cancer-preventive properties of retinol and retinoids. Standard protocols should specify continuous quality control of supplements and the type of formulation to be used. Such a strategy should be developed in all studies: molecular, cellular, animal and human. Although standardization in human studies is probably the most difficult, these protocols would help to identify, minimize or quantify the variability that undoubtedly exists in human studies.

10. Evaluation

10.1 Cancer-preventive activity

10.1.1 Humans

There is *evidence suggesting lack of cancer-preventive activity* of preformed vitamin A for cancers at the following sites: upper aerodigestive tract, lung, breast (among postmenopausal women), colorectal, bladder, prostate and stomach. There is *inadequate evidence* with respect to possible cancer-preventive activity of preformed vitamin A at all other sites and for second primary cancers of the lung.

10.1.2 Experimental animals

There is *limited evidence* that retinyl esters have cancer-preventive activity in experimental animals. This evaluation is based upon consistent inhibitory effects in rat mammary cancer models, but equivocal effects in mouse mammary cancer models, and the observation that long-term maintenance of rats on a mixture of retinyl acetate and palmitate resulted in an increased incidence of mammary gland carcinomas. In addition, the cancer-preventive activity of retinyl esters in other sites and in other species was inadequate.

10.2 Overall evaluation

Serum retinol concentrations are homeostatically controlled across a wide range of intakes of both provitamin A carotenoids and preformed vitamin A. Research conducted on vitamin A using a wide variety of methods, from cell cultures *in vitro* and experimental models in animals to observational studies and randomized intervention trials in humans needs to be evaluated in terms of the overriding importance of this system of homeostatic control. Some research has been done in the setting of vitamin A deficiency, some in the setting of excess, and some in the wider range of normal intakes.

Observational studies and randomized controlled trials have been carried out within the broad range of intakes which have little or no effect on the levels of retinol in the circultion (although they may well have influenced levels of more active metabolites in other tissues). The results of these studies have been largely negative, supporting the conclusion that for most cancer sites the preponderance of evidence does not support a chemopreventive role for preformed vitamin A. The few randomized, controlled trials conducted to date likewise do not support the idea that preformed vitamin A has a substantial chemopreventive role for cancer. There is a suggestion of a possible benefit of preformed vitamin A against squamous cell skin cancer among those who have had previous skin cancers, and against mesothelioma among asbestos-exposed workers, and against second primary lung cancers among those treated for lung cancer. However, the protective effects for skin cancer and mesothelioma have been seen in only one of the two published studies for each of these end-points, and there has been only one study of preventing second primary cancers by preformed vitamin A following lung cancer, and this study was unusual in that it used very high doses of preformed vitamin A. It is important to note that all the previous trials of vitamin A chemoprevention in humans has been relatively short-term studies, none extending beyond six years. If vitamin A is protective at earlier stages of carcinogenesis, as is suggested by studies which show that vitamin A can protect against genetic effects of other carcinogens *in vitro*, then longer trials would be needed to see preventive effects.

The benefits to health of correcting vitamin A deficiency are clear. Both animal experimental studies and human studies have proven the benefits of correcting vitamin A deficiency for several conditions including total morbidity and mortality. A limited number of animal studies support the hypothesis that vitamin A deficiency might increase cancer risk. Confirmatory studies in vitamin A-deficient populations are lacking. The two cancer chemoprevention trials conducted among populations in China and India with multiple micronutrient insufficiency have shown no apparent effect of preformed vitamin A on cancer incidence.

The suggestion of potential chemopreventive benefits of high doses of preformed vitamin A in rat mammary cancer models are encouraging in that there may be similar benefits for humans, but the fact that these effects are typically seen only at doses that are toxic or teratogenic in humans limits enthusiasm for preformed vitamin A as a widely acceptable cancer chemopreventive agent. Therefore, research is now in progress to discover more effective and less toxic synthetic retinoids. This area of enquiry will be covered in Volume 4 of this *IARC Handbook series*.

In sum, there is little evidence to support the idea that, within the wide range of doses bordered by deficiency and toxicity, modulating preformed vitamin A intake will have any substantial cancer-preventive effect.

References

Abdel Galil, A.M., Wrba, H. & El Mofty, M.M. (1984) Prevention of 3-methylcholanthrene-induced skin tumors in mice by simultaneous application of 13-*cis*-retinoic acid and retinyl palmitate (vitamin A palmitate). *Exp. Pathol.,* **25**, 97–102

Achkar, C.C., Derguini, F., Blumberg, B., Langston, A., Levin, A.A., Speck, J., Evans, R.M., Bolado, J., Jr, Nakanishi, K., Buck, J. & Gudas, L.J. (1996) 4-Oxoretinol, a new natural ligand and transactivator of the retinoic acid receptors. *Proc. Natl. Acad. Sci. USA.,* **93**, 4879–4884

Agarwal, C. & Eckert, R.L. (1990) Immortalization of human keratinocytes by simian virus 40 large T-antigen alters keratin gene response to retinoids. *Cancer Res.,* **50**, 5947–5953

Agnish, N.D. & Kochhar, D.M. (1993) Developmental toxicity of retinoids. In: Koren, G. (ed.), *Retinoids in Clinical Practice. The Risk-Benefit Ratio,* New York, Marcel Dekker, pp. 47–76

Agnish, N.D., Rusin, G. & DiNardo, B. (1990) Taurine failed to protect against the embryotoxic effects of isotretinoin in the rat. *Fundam. Appl. Toxicol.,* **15**, 249–257

Ahmed, F., Ellis, J., Murphy, J., Wootton, S. & Jackson, A.A. (1990) Excessive faecal losses of vitamin A (retinol) in cystic fibrosis. *Arch. Dis. Child.,* **65**, 589–593

Ahmed, F., Mohiduzzaman, M. & Jackson, A.A. (1993) Vitamin A absorption in children with ascariasis. *Br. J. Nutr.,* **69**, 817–825

Alaoui Jamali, M.A., Belanger, P.M., Rossignol, G. & Castonguay, A. (1991a) Metabolism, sister chromatid exchanges, and DNA single-strand breaks induced by 4-(methylnitrosamino)-1-(3-pyridyl)-1-butanone and their modulation by vitamin A *in vitro. Cancer Res.,* **51**, 3946–3950

Alaoui Jamali, M.A., Rossignol, G. & Castonguay, A. (1991b) Protective effects of vitamin A against the genotoxicity of NNK, a nicotine-derived *N*-nitrosamine. *Carcinogenesis,* **12**, 379–384

Alexandrov, V.A., Bespalov, V.G., Boone, C.W., Kelloff, G.J. & Malone, W.F. (1991) Study of postnatal effects of chemopreventive agents on offspring of ethylnitrosourea-induced transplacental carcinogenesis in rats. I. Influence of retinol acetate, α-tocopherol acetate, thiamine chloride, sodium selenite, and α-difluoromethylornithine. *Cancer Lett.,* **60**, 177–184

Allende, L.M., Corell, A., Madrono, A., Gongora, R., Rodriguez Gallego, C., Lopez Goyanes, A., Rosal, M. & Arnaiz Villena, A. (1997) Retinol (vitamin A) is a cofactor in CD3-induced human T-lymphocyte activation. *Immunology,* **90**, 388–396

Althaus, F.R., Lawrence, S.D., Sattler, G.L., Longfellow, D.G. & Pitot, H.C. (1982) Chemical quantification of unscheduled DNA synthesis in cultured hepatocytes as an assay for the rapid screening of potential chemical carcinogens. *Cancer Res.,* **42**, 3010–3015

Alzieu, P., Cassand, P., Colin, C., Grolier, P. & Narbonne, J.F. (1987) Effect of vitamins A, C and glutathione on the mutagenicity of benzo[*a*]-pyrene mediated by S9 from vitamin A-deficient rats. *Mutat. Res.,* **192**, 227–231

Amagase, H., Schaffer, E.M. & Milner, J.A. (1996) Dietary components modify the ability of garlic to suppress 7,12-dimethylbenz(*a*)anthracene-induced mammary DNA adducts. *J. Nutr.,* **126**, 817–824

Amédée-Manesme, O., Mourey, M.S., Therasse, J., Couturier, M., Alvarez, F., Hanck, A. & Bernard, O. (1988) Short- and long-term vitamin A treatment in children with cholestasis. *Am. J. Clin. Nutr.,* **47**, 690–693

An, G., Tesfaigzi, J., Carlson, D.M. & Wu, R. (1993) Expression of a squamous cell marker, the spr1 gene, is post-transcriptionally down-regulated by retinol in airway epithelium. *J. Cell Physiol.,* **157**, 562–568

An, G., Luo, G. & Wu, R. (1994) Expression of MUC2 gene is down-regulated by vitamin A at the transcriptional level *in vitro* in tracheobronchial epithelial cells. *Am. J. Respir. Cell Mol. Biol.,* **10**, 546–551

Andersson, S.O., Wolk, A., Bergstrom, R., Giovannucci, E., Lindgren, C., Baron, J. & Adami, H.O. (1996) Energy, nutrient intake and prostate cancer risk: a population-based case-control study in Sweden. *Int. J. Cancer,* **68**, 716–722

Andreola, F., Fernandez Salguero, P.M., Chiantore, M.V., Petkovich, M.P., Gonzalez, F.J. & De Luca, L.M. (1997) Aryl hydrocarbon receptor knockout mice ($AHR^{-/-}$) exhibit liver retinoid accumulation and reduced retinoic acid metabolism. *Cancer Res.,* **57**, 2835–2838

Ang, H.L., Deltour, L., Hayamizu, T.F., Zgombic-Knight, M. & Duester, G. (1996) Retinoic acid synthesis in mouse embryos during gastrulation and craniofacial development linked to class IV alcohol dehydrogenase gene expression. *J. Biol. Chem.*, **271**, 9526–9534

Arensman, R.M. & Stolar, C.J. (1979) Vitamin A effect on tumor angiogenesis. *J. Pediatr. Surg.*, **14**, 809–813

Armstrong, R.B., Ashenfelter, K.O., Eckhoff, C., Levin, A.A. & Shapiro, S.S. (1994) General and reproductive toxicology of retinoids. In: Sporn, M.B., Roberts, A.B. & Goodman, D.S. (eds), *The Retinoids. Biology, Chemistry, and Medicine,* 2nd edition, New York, Raven Press, pp. 545–572

Arnhold, T., Tzimas, G., Wittfoht, W., Plonait, S. & Nau, H. (1996) Identification of 9-*cis*-retinoic acid, 9,13-di-*cis*-retinoic acid, and 14-hydroxy-4,14-retro-retinol in human plasma after liver consumption. *Life Sci.*, **59**, PL169–PL177

Ascherio, A., Stampfer, M.J., Colditz, G.A., Rimm, E.B., Litin, L. & Willett, W.C. (1992) Correlations of vitamin A and E intakes with the plasma concentrations of carotenoids and tocopherols among American men and women. *J. Nutr.*, **122**, 1792–1801

ATBC Cancer Prevention Study Group (1994) The effect of vitamin E and beta carotene on the incidence of lung cancer and other cancers in male smokers. The Alpha-Tocopherol, Beta-Carotene Cancer Prevention Study Group. *New Engl. J. Med.*, **330**, 1029–1035

Bacon, M.C., White, P.H., Raiten, D.J., Craft, N., Margolis, S., Levander, O.A., Taylor, M.L., Lipnick, R.N. & Sami, S. (1990) Nutritional status and growth in juvenile rheumatoid arthritis. *Semin. Arthritis Rheum.*, **20**, 97–106

Baird, M.B. & Birnbaum, L.S. (1979) Inhibition of 2-fluorenamine-induced mutagenesis in *Salmonella typhimurium* by vitamin A. *J. Natl. Cancer Inst.*, **63**, 1093–1096

Balansky, R., Mircheva, Z. & Blagoeva, P. (1994) Modulation of the mutagenic activity of cigarette smoke, cigarette smoke condensate and benzo[*a*]-pyrene *in vitro* and *in vivo*. *Mutagenesis,* **9**, 107–112

Balbinder, E., Stick, S.M. & Sharma, O.K. (1983) Complex effects of retinol on the metabolic activation of 2-aminofluorene. *Environ. Mutagen.*, **5**, 665–678

Balkan, W., Colbert, M., Bock, C. & Linney, E. (1992) Transgenic indicator mice for studying activated retinoic acid receptors during development. *Proc. Natl. Acad. Sci. USA.*, **89**, 3347–3351

Barclay, A.J., Foster, A. & Sommer, A. (1987) Vitamin A supplements and mortality related to measles: a randomised clinical trial. *Br. Med. J. Clin. Res. Ed.*, **294**, 294–296

Barua, A.B. (1997) Retinoyl β-glucuronide: a biologically active form of vitamin. *Nutr. Rev.*, **55**, 259–267

Barua, A.B. & Olson, J.A. (1986) Retinoyl β-glucuronide: an endogenous compound of human blood. *Am. J. Clin. Nutr.*, **43**, 481–485

Barua, A.B., Furr, H.C., Janick-Buckner, D. & Olson, J.A. (1993) Simultaneous analysis of individual carotenoids, retinol, retinyl esters, and tocopherols in serum by isocratic non-aqueous reversed-phase HPLC. *Food Chem.*, **46**, 419–424

Barua, A.B., Duitsman, P.K., Kostic, D., Barua, M. & Olson, J.A. (1997) Reduction of serum retinol levels following a single oral dose of all-*trans* retinoic acid in humans. *Int. J. Vitam. Nutr. Res.*, **67**, 423–426

Bates, C.J. (1995) Vitamin A. *Lancet,* **345**, 31-35

Batres, R.O. & Olson, J.A. (1987) A marginal vitamin A status alters the distribution of vitamin A among parenchymal and stellate cells in rat liver. *J. Nutr.*, **117**, 874–879

Bayless, J.H., Jablonski, J.E., Roach, S.M. & Sullivan, P.D. (1986) Inhibition of the mutagenicity and metabolism of 6-methyl-benzo[*a*]pyrene and 6-hydroxymethyl-benzo[*a*]pyrene. *Biochem. Pharmacol.*, **35**, 2313–2322

Beck, F. (1976) Comparative placental morphology and function. *Environ. Health Perspect.*, **18**, 5–12

Beisiegel, U., Weber, W. & Bengtsson Olivecrona, G. (1991) Lipoprotein lipase enhances the binding of chylomicrons to low density lipoprotein receptor-related protein. *Proc. Natl. Acad. Sci. USA.*, **88**, 8342–8346

Bell, R.A., Mayer Davis, E.J., Jackson, Y. & Dresser, C. (1997) An epidemiologic review of dietary intake studies among American Indians and Alaska natives: implications for heart disease and cancer risk. *Ann. Epidemiol.*, **7**, 229–240

Bendich, A. & Langseth, L. (1989) Safety of vitamin A. *Am. J. Clin. Nutr.*, **49**, 358–371

Benito, E., Cabeza, E., Moreno, V., Obrador, A. & Bosch, F.X. (1993) Diet and colorectal adenomas: a case-control study in Majorca. *Int. J. Cancer*, **55**, 213–219

Benrabah, R., Lumbroso, L., Limon, S., Hamard, H. & Morin, Y. (1995) [Unexplained bilateral optic disk edema. So-called idiopathic intracranial hypertension of drug origin should be suspected]. *J. Fr. Ophtalmol.*, **18**, 282–285 (in French)

Berberian, I., Chen, L.C., Robinson, F.R., Glauert, H.P., Chow, C.K. & Robertson, L.W. (1995) Effect of dietary retinyl palmitate on the promotion of altered hepatic foci by 3,3′,4,4′-tetrachlorobiphenyl and 2,2′,4,4′,5,5′-hexachlorobiphenyl in rats initiated with diethylnitrosamine. *Carcinogenesis*, **16**, 393–398

Berne, B., Torma, H., Staberg, B., Mikkelsen, S. & Vahlquist, A. (1989) Decreased retinyl ester concentrations in UV-induced murine squamous cell carcinomas. *Acta Derm. Venereol.*, **69**, 503508

Berr, F. (1992) Characterization of chylomicron remnant clearance by retinyl palmitate label in normal humans. *J. Lipid Res.*, **33**, 915–930

Bertram, J.S. (1980) Structure-activity relationships among various retinoids and their ability to inhibit neoplastic transformation and to increase cell adhesion in the C3H/10T1/2 CL8 cell line. *Cancer Res.*, **40**, 3141–3146

Bhat, P.V. (1997) Tissue concentrations of retinol, retinyl esters, and retinoic acid in vitamin A deficient rats administered a single dose of radioactive retinol. *Can. J. Physiol. Pharmacol.*, **75**, 74–77

Bhat, P.V. & Jetten, A.M. (1987) Metabolism of all-*trans*-retinol and all-*trans*-retinoic acid in rabbit tracheal epithelial cells in culture. *Biochim. Biophys. Acta*, **922**, 18–27

Bhat, P.V. & Lacroix, A. (1983) Separation and estimation of retinyl fatty acyl esters in tissues of normal rat by high-performance liquid chromatography. *J. Chromatogr.*, **272**, 269–278

Bhat, P.V., Poissant, L. & Lacroix, A. (1988a) Properties of retinal-oxidizing enzyme activity in rat kidney. *Biochim. Biophys. Acta*, **967**, 211–217

Bhat, P.V., Poissant, L., Falardeau, P. & Lacroix, A. (1988b) Enzymatic oxidation of all-*trans* retinal to retinoic acid in rat tissues. *Biochem. Cell Biol.*, **66**, 735–740

Bhattacharya, R.K., Francis, A.R. & Shetty, T.K. (1987) Modifying role of dietary factors on the mutagenicity of aflatoxin B_1: *in vitro* effect of vitamins. *Mutat. Res.*, **188**, 121–128

Bieri, J.G., Tolliver, T.J. & Catignani, G.L. (1979) Simultaneous determination of α-tocopherol and retinol in plasma or red cells by high pressure liquid chromatography. *Am. J. Clin. Nutr.*, **32**, 2143–2149

Biesalski, H.K. (1990) Separation of retinyl esters and their geometric isomers by isocratic adsorption high-performance liquid chromatography. *Methods Enzymol.*, **189**, 181–189

Bihain, B.E. & Yen, F.T. (1992) Free fatty acids activate a high-affinity saturable pathway for degradation of low-density lipoproteins in fibroblasts from a subject homozygous for familial hypercholesterolemia. *Biochemistry*, **31**, 4628–4636

Binka, F.N., Ross, D.A., Morris, S.S., Kirkwood, B.R., Arthur, P., Dollimore, N., Gyapong, J.O. & Smith, P.G. (1995) Vitamin A supplementation and childhood malaria in northern Ghana. *Am. J. Clin. Nutr.*, **61**, 853–859

Bishop, P.D. & Griswold, M.D. (1987) Uptake and metabolism of retinol in cultured Sertoli cells: evidence for a kinetic model. *Biochemistry*, **26**, 7511-7518

Bisschop, A., Van Rooijen, L.A., Derks, H.J. & Van Wijk, R. (1981) Induction of rat hepatic ornithine decarboxylase by the tumor promotors 12-*O*-tetradecanoylphorbol-13-acetate and phenobarbital *in vivo*; effect of retinyl-acetate. *Carcinogenesis*, **2**, 1283-1287

Biswas, M.G. & Russell, D.W. (1997) Expression cloning and characterization of oxidative 17β- and 3α-hydroxysteroid dehydrogenases from rat and human prostate. *J. Biol. Chem.*, **272**, 15959-15966

Bjelke, E. (1975) Dietary vitamin A and human lung cancer. *Int. J. Cancer*, **15**, 561-565

Blaner, W.S. (1994) Retinoid (vitamin A) metabolism and the liver. In: Arias, I.M., Boyer, J.L., Fausto, N., Jakoby, W.B., Schachter, D. & Shafritz, D.A. (eds), *The Liver: Biology and Pathobiology*, New York, Raven Press, pp. 529-541

Blaner, W.S. & Olson, J.A. (1994) Retinol and retinoic acid metabolism. In: Sporn, M.B., Roberts, A.B. & Goodman, D.S. (eds), *The Retinoids: Biology, Chemistry, and Medicine,* 2nd edition, New York, Raven Press, pp. 229–255

Blaner, W.S., Hendriks, H.F., Brouwer, A., de Leeuw, A.M., Knook, D.L. & Goodman, D.S. (1985) Retinoids, retinoid-binding proteins, and retinyl palmitate hydrolase distributions in different types of rat liver cells. *J. Lipid Res.,* **26**, 1241–1251

Blaner, W.S., Van Bennekum, A.M., Brouwer, A. & Hendriks, H.F. (1990) Distribution of lecithin-retinol acyltransferase activity in different types of rat liver cells and subcellular fractions. *FEBS Lett.,* **274**, 89–92

Blaner, W.S., Hussain, M.M., Talmage, D.A., Wong Yen Kong, L., Piantedosi, R., Mahley, R.W. & Goodman, D.S. (1993) Retinoids are actively metabolized in rabbit bone marrow. In: Livrea, M.A. (ed.), *Retinoids: Progress in Research and Clinical Applications,* New York, Marcel Dekker, pp. 63–72

Blaner, W.S., Obunike, J.C., Kurlandsky, S.B., al Haideri, M., Piantedosi, R., Deckelbaum, R.J. & Goldberg, I.J. (1994) Lipoprotein lipase hydrolysis of retinyl ester. Possible implications for retinoid uptake by cells. *J. Biol. Chem.,* **269**, 16559–16565

Blomhoff, R. R. (1994a) Transport and metabolism of vitamin A. *Nutr. Rev.,* **52**, S13–23

Blomhoff, R. (1994b) *Vitamin A in Health and Disease,* New York, Marcel Dekker

Blomhoff, R., Berg, T. & Norum, K.R. (1988) Transfer of retinol from parenchymal to stellate cells in liver is mediated by retinol-binding protein. *Proc. Natl. Acad. Sci. USA.,* **85**, 3455–3458

Blomhoff, H.K., Smeland, E.B., Erikstein, B., Rasmussen, A.M., Skrede, B., Skjonsberg, C. & Blomhoff, R. (1992) Vitamin A is a key regulator for cell growth, cytokine production, and differentiation in normal B cells. *J. Biol. Chem.,* **267**, 23988–23992

Blot, W.J., Li, J.Y., Taylor, P.R., Guo, W., Dawsey, S., Wang, G.Q., Yang, C.S., Zheng, S.F., Gail, M., Li, G.Y., Yu, Y., Liu, B., Tangrea, J., Sun, Y., Liu, F., Fraumeni, J.F. Jr, Zhang, Y.H. & Li, B. (1993) Nutrition intervention trials in Linxian, China: supplementation with specific vitamin/mineral combinations, cancer incidence, and disease-specific mortality in the general population. *J. Natl. Cancer Inst.,* **85**, 1483–1492

Blot, W.J., Li, J.Y., Taylor, P.R., Guo, W., Dawsey, S.M. & Li, B. (1995) The Linxian trials: mortality rates by vitamin-mineral intervention group. *Am. J. Clin. Nutr.,* **62**, 1424S–1426S

Blumberg, B., Bolado, J., Jr, Derguini, F., Craig, A.G., Moreno, T.A., Chakravarti, D., Heyman, R.A., Buck, J. & Evans, R.M. (1996) Novel retinoic acid receptor ligands in *Xenopus* embryos. *Proc. Natl. Acad. Sci. USA,* **93**, 4873–4878

Boden, S.D., Labropoulos, P.A., Ragsdale, B.D., Gullino, P.M. & Gerber, L.H. (1989) Retinyl acetate-induced arthritis in C3H-A(vy) mice. *Arthritis Rheum.,* **32**, 625–633

Boerman, M.H. & Napoli, J.L. (1995) Characterization of a microsomal retinol dehydrogenase: a short-chain alcohol dehydrogenase with integral and peripheral membrane forms that interacts with holo-CRBP (type I). *Biochemistry,* **34**, 7027–7037

Boit, H.G., ed. (1966) *Beilsteins Handbuch der Organischen Chemie,* Berlin, Springer Verlag, pp. 2787–2797

Boleda, M.D., Saubi, N., Farres, J. & Pares, X. (1993) Physiological substrates for rat alcohol dehydrogenase classes: aldehydes of lipid peroxidation, ω-hydroxyfatty acids, and retinoids. *Arch. Biochem. Biophys.,* **307**, 85–90

Bolognesi, C., Ognio, E., Ferreri Santi, L. & Rossi, L. (1992) Modulation of DNA damage by vitamin A in developing Sprague-Dawley rats. *Anticancer Res.,* **12**, 1587-1591

Bolton-Smith, C., Woodward, M. & Tunstall-Pedoe, H. (1992) The Scottish Heart Health Study. Dietary intake by food frequency questionnaire and odds ratios for coronary heart disease risk. II. The antioxidant vitamins and fibre. *Eur. J. Clin. Nutr.,* **46**, 85–93

Bonewald, L.F., Oreffo, R.O., Lee, C.H., Park Snyder, S., Twardzik, D. & Mundy, G.R. (1997) Effects of retinol on activation of latent transforming growth factor-β by isolated osteoclasts. *Endocrinology,* **138**, 657–666

Bosma, A., Seifert, W.F., Wilson, J.H., Roholl, P.J., Brouwer, A. & Knook, D.L. (1991) Chronic administration of ethanol with high vitamin A supplementation in a liquid diet to rats does not cause liver fibrosis. 1. Morphological observations. *J. Hepatol.,* **13**, 240–248

Boylan, J.F. & Gudas, L.J. (1991) Overexpression of the cellular retinoic acid binding protein-I (CRABP-I) results in a reduction in differentiation-specific gene expression in F9 teratocarcinoma cells. *J. Cell Biol.,* **112**, 965–979

Breitman, T.R., Selonick, S.E. & Collins, S.J. (1980) Induction of differentiation of the human promyelocytic leukemia cell line (HL-60) by retinoic acid. *Proc. Natl. Acad. Sci. USA.,* **77**, 2936–2940

Brent, R.L., Hendrickx, A.G., Holmes, L.B. & Miller, R.K. (1996) Teratogenicity of high vitamin A intake. *New Engl. J. Med.,* **334**, 1196–1196

Bresee, J.S., Fischer, M., Dowell, S.F., Johnston, B.D., Biggs, V.M., Levine, R.S., Lingappa, J.R., Keyserling, H.L., Petersen, K.M., Bak, J.R., Gary, H.E., Jr, Sowell, A.L., Rubens, C.E. & Anderson, L.J. (1996) Vitamin A therapy for children with respiratory syncytial virus infection: a multicenter trial in the United States. *Pediatr. Infect. Dis. J.,* **15**, 777–782

Breslow, R.A., Alberg, A.J., Helzlsouer, K.J., Bush, T.L., Norkus, E.P., Morris, J.S., Spate, V.E. & Comstock, G.W. (1995) Serological precursors of cancer: malignant melanoma, basal and squamous cell skin cancer, and prediagnostic levels of retinol, β-carotene, lycopene, α-tocopherol, and selenium. *Cancer Epidemiol. Biomarkers Prev.,* **4**, 837–842

Brock, K.E., Berry, G., Mock, P.A., MacLennan, R., Truswell, A.S. & Brinton, L.A. (1988) Nutrients in diet and plasma and risk of in situ cervical cancer. *J. Natl. Cancer Inst.,* **80**, 580–585

Brockman, H.E., Stack, H.F. & Waters, M.D. (1992) Antimutagenicity profiles of some natural substances. *Mutat. Res.,* **267**, 157–172

Brooks, H.L., Jr, Driebe, W.T., Jr. & Schemmer, G.G. (1990) Xerophthalmia and cystic fibrosis. *Arch. Ophthalmol.,* **108**, 354–357

Brouwer, A., van den Berg, K.J. & Kukler, A. (1985) Time and dose responses of the reduction in retinoid concentrations in C57BL/Rij and DBA/2 mice induced by 3,4,3′,4′- tetrachlorobiphenyl. *Toxicol. Appl. Pharmacol.,* **78**, 180–189

Brown, R., Gray, R.H. & Bernstein, I.A. (1985) Retinoids alter the direction of differentiation in primary cultures of cutaneous keratinocytes. *Differentiation,* **28**, 268–278

Brown, L.M., Blot, W.J., Schuman, S.H., Smith, V.M., Ershow, A.G., Marks, R.D. & Fraumeni, J.F. (1988) Environmental factors and high risk of esophageal cancer among men in coastal South Carolina. *J. Natl. Cancer Inst.,* **80**, 1620–1625

Bruemmer, B., White, E., Vaughan, T.L. & Cheney, C.L. (1996) Nutrient intake in relation to bladder cancer among middle-aged men and women. *Am. J. Epidemiol.,* **144**, 485–495

Buck, J., Ritter, G., Dannecker, L., Katta, V., Cohen, S.L., Chait, B.T. & Hammerling, U. (1990) Retinol is essential for growth of activated human B cells. *J. Exp. Med.,* **171**, 1613–1624

Buck, J., Myc, A., Garbe, A. & Cathomas, G. (1991a) Differences in the action and metabolism between retinol and retinoic acid in B lymphocytes. *J. Cell. Biol.,* **115**, 851–859

Buck, J., Derguini, F., Levi, E., Nakanishi, K. & Hammerling, U. (1991b) Intracellular signaling by 14-hydroxy-4,14-retro-retinol. *Science,* **254**, 1654–1656

Buck, J., Grun, F., Derguini, F., Chen, Y., Kimura, S., Noy, N. & Hammerling, U. (1993) Anhydroretinol: a naturally occurring inhibitor of lymphocyte physiology. *J. Exp. Med.,* **178**, 675–680

Buckley, D.I., McPherson, R.S., North, C.Q. & Becker, T.M. (1992) Dietary micronutrients and cervical dysplasia in Southwestern American Indian women. *Nutr. Cancer,* **17**, 179–185

Budavari, S. (1996) *The Merck Index,* 12th ed., Whitehouse Station, NJ, Merck & Co.

Budroe, J.D., Shaddock, J.G. & Casciano, D.A. (1987) Modulation of ultraviolet light-, ethyl methanesulfonate-, and 7,12-dimethylbenz[*a*]-anthracene-induced unscheduled DNA synthesis by retinol and retinoic acid in the primary rat hepatocyte. *Environ. Mol. Mutagen.,* **10**, 129–139

Budroe, J.D., Schol, H.M., Shaddock, J.G. & Casciano, D.A. (1988) Inhibition of 7,12 dimethylbenz[*a*]anthracene-induced genotoxicity in Chinese hamster ovary cells by retinol and retinoic acid. *Carcinogenesis,* **9**, 1307–1311

Buiatti, E., Palli, D., Decarli, A., Amadori, D., Avellini, C., Bianchi, S., Bonaguri, C., Cipriani, F., Cocco, P., Giacosa, A., Marubini, E., Minacci, C., Puntoni, R., Russo, A., Vindigni, C., Fraumeni, J.F., Jr & Blot, W.J. (1990) A case-control study of gastric cancer and diet in Italy: II. Association with nutrients. *Int. J. Cancer,* **45**, 896–901

Busk, L. & Ahlborg, U.G. (1980) Retinol (vitamin A) as an inhibitor of the mutagenicity of aflatoxin B. *Toxicol. Lett.*, **6**, 243–249

Busk, L. & Ahlborg, U.G. (1982a) Retinol (vitamin A) as a modifier of 2-aminofluorene and 2-acetylaminofluorene mutagenesis in the *Salmonella*/-microsome assay. *Arch. Toxicol.*, **49**, 169–174

Busk, L. & Ahlborg, U.G. (1982b) Retinoids as inhibitors of *ortho*-aminoazotoluene-induced mutagenesis in the *Salmonella*/liver microsome test. *Mutat. Res.*, **104**, 225–231

Busk, L., Ahlborg, U.G. & Albanus, L. (1982) Inhibition of protein pyrolysate mutagenicity by retinol (vitamin A). *Food Chem. Toxicol.*, **20**, 535–539

Busk, L., Sjostrom, B. & Ahlborg, U.G. (1984) Effects of vitamin A on cyclophosphamide mutagenicity *in vitro* (Ames test) and *in vivo* (mouse micronucleus test). *Food Chem. Toxicol.*, **22**, 725–730

Buss, N.E., Tembe, E.A., Prendergast, B.D., Renwick, A.G. & George, C.F. (1994) The teratogenic metabolites of vitamin A in women following supplements and liver. *Hum. Exp. Toxicol.*, **13**, 33–43

Byers, T., Vena, J., Mettlin, C., Swanson, M. & Graham, S. (1984) Dietary vitamin A and lung cancer risk: an analysis by histologic subtypes. *Am. J. Epidemiol.*, **120**, 769–776

Byers, T.E., Graham, S., Haughey, B.P., Marshall, J.R. & Swanson, M.K. (1987) Diet and lung cancer risk: findings from the Western New York Diet Study. *Am. J. Epidemiol.*, **125**, 351–363

Calhoun, K.H., Stanley, D., Stiernberg, C.M. & Ahmed, A.E. (1989) Vitamins A and E do protect against oral carcinoma. *Arch. Otolaryngol. Head Neck Surg.*, **115**, 484–488

Caliaro, M.J., Vitaux, P., Lafon, C., Lochon, I., Nehme, A., Valette, A., Canal, P., Bugat, R. & Jozan, S. (1997) Multifactorial mechanism for the potentiation of cisplatin (CDDP) cytotoxicity by all-*trans* retinoic acid (ATRA) in human ovarian carcinoma cell lines. *Br. J. Cancer*, **75**, 333–340

Calle, L.M. & Sullivan, P.D. (1982) Screening of antioxidants and other compounds for antimutagenic properties towards benzo[*a*]pyrene-induced mutagenicity in strain TA98 of *Salmonella typhimurium*. *Mutat. Res.*, **101**, 99–114

Camoirano, A., Balansky, R.M., Bennicelli, C., Izzotti, A., D'Agostini, F. & De Flora, S. (1994) Experimental databases on inhibition of the bacterial mutagenicity of 4-nitroquinoline 1-oxide and cigarette smoke. *Mutat. Res.*, **317**, 89–109

Candelora, E.C., Stockwell, H.G., Armstrong, A.W. & Pinkham, P.A. (1992) Dietary intake and risk of lung cancer in women who never smoked. *Nutr. Cancer*, **17**, 263–270

Canfield, L.M., Giuliano, A.R., Neilson, E.M., Yap, H.H., Graver, E.J., Cui, H.A. & Blashill, B.M. (1997) β-Carotene in breast milk and serum is increased after a single β-carotene dose. *Am. J. Clin. Nutr.*, **66**, 52–61

Cardenas, R., Jaime, M.E., Guzman, L. & Granados, H. (1991) Gallstones in the golden hamster. XXXVI. Pigment cholelithiasis produced by retinoic acid. *Arch. Invest. Med. Mex.*, **22**, 209–216

Cassand, P., Maziere, S., Champ, M., Meflah, K., Bornet, F. & Narbonne, J.F. (1997) Effects of resistant starch- and vitamin A-supplemented diets on the promotion of precursor lesions of colon cancer in rats. *Nutr. Cancer*, **27**, 53–59

Catignani, G.L. & Bieri, J.G. (1983) Simultaneous determination of retinol and α-tocopherol in serum or plasma by liquid chromatography. *Clin. Chem.*, **29**, 708–712

Chai, X., Zhai, Y., Popescu, G. & Napoli, J.L. (1995) Cloning of a cDNA for a second retinol dehydrogenase type II. Expression of its mRNA relative to type I. *J. Biol. Chem.*, **270**, 28408–28412

Chai, X., Zhai, Y. & Napoli, J.L. (1996) Cloning of a rat cDNA encoding retinol dehydrogenase isozyme type III. *Gene*, **169**, 219–222

Chai, X., Zhai, Y. & Napoli, J.L. (1997) cDNA cloning and characterization of a *cis*-retinol/3α-hydroxysterol short-chain dehydrogenase. *J. Biol. Chem.*, **272**, 33125–33131

Challem, J.J. (1997) Re: Risk factors for lung cancer and for intervention effects in CARET, the Beta-Carotene and Retinol Efficacy Trial. *J. Natl. Cancer Inst.*, **89**, 325–326

Chambon, P. (1996) A decade of molecular biology of retinoic acid receptors. *FASEB J.*, **10**, 940–954

Chaudhary, L.R. & Nelson, E.C. (1985) The effect of retinol deficiency on the metabolism of all-*trans*- retinyl acetate in rat testes. *Int. J. Vitam. Nutr. Res.*, **55**, 383–390

Chaudhary, L.R. & Nelson, E.C. (1986) Metabolism of all-*trans*-[11-^{3}H]retinyl acetate in the testes of young rats. *Ann. Nutr. Metab.,* **30**, 1–8

Chen, L.C., Berberian, I., Koch, B., Mercier, M., Azais Braesco, V., Glauert, H.P., Chow, C.K. & Robertson, L.W. (1992a) Polychlorinated and polybrominated biphenyl congeners and retinoid levels in rat tissues: structure-activity relationships. *Toxicol. Appl. Pharmacol.,* **114**, 47–55

Chen, Y., Huang, L., Russo, A.F. & Solursh, M. (1992b) Retinoic acid is enriched in Hensen's node and is developmentally regulated in the early chicken embryo. *Proc. Natl. Acad. Sci. USA.,* **89**, 10056–10059

Chen, Y., Huang, L. & Solursh, M. (1994) A concentration gradient of retinoids in the early *Xenopus laevis* embryo. *Dev. Biol.,* **161**, 70–76

Chen, H., Namkung, M.J. & Juchau, M.R. (1996a) Effects of ethanol on biotransformation of all-*trans*-retinol and all-*trans*-retinal to all-*trans*-retinoic acid in rat conceptal cytosol. *Alcohol Clin. Exp. Res.,* **20**, 942–947

Chen, C., Mistry, G., Jensen, B., Heizmann, P., Timm, U., van Brummelen, P. & Rakhit, A.K. (1996b) Pharmacokinetics of retinoids in women after meal consumption or vitamin A supplementation. *J. Clin. Pharmacol.,* **36**, 799–808

Chen, X., Harrison, E.H. & Fisher, E.A. (1997a) Molecular cloning of the cDNA for rat hepatic, bile salt-dependent cholesteryl ester/retinyl ester hydrolase demonstrates identity with pancreatic carboxylester lipase. *Proc. Soc. Exp. Biol. Med.,* **215**, 186–191

Chen, A.C., Guo, X., Derguini, F. & Gudas, L.J. (1997b) Human breast cancer cells and normal mammary epithelial cells: retinol metabolism and growth inhibition by the retinol metabolite 4-oxoretinol. *Cancer Res.,* **57**, 4642–4651

Cheng, L.L. & Wilkie, D. (1991) Mitochondrial activity and cytotoxicity of vitamin A (retinol) in yeast and human cell cultures. Protective effect of antioxidants. *Biochem. Pharmacol.,* **42**, 1237–1240

Chiesa, F., Tradati, N., Marazza, M., Rossi, N., Boracchi, P., Mariani, L., Clerici, M., Formelli, F., Barzan, L., Carrassi, A., Pastorini, A., Camerini, T., Giardini, R., Zurrida, S., Minn, F.L., Costa, A., De Palo, G. & Veronesi, U. (1992) Prevention of local relapses and new localisations of oral leukoplakias with the synthetic retinoid fenretinide (4-HPR). Preliminary results. *Eur. J. Cancer B. Oral Oncol.,* **28B**, 97–102

Chiesa, F., Tradati, N., Marazza, M., Rossi, N., Boracchi, P., Mariani, L., Formelli, F., Giardini, R., Costa, A., De Palo, G. & Veronesi, U. (1993) Fenretinide (4-HPR) in chemoprevention of oral leukoplakia. *J. Cell Biochem. Suppl.,* **17F**, 255–261

Chopra, D.P. & Flaxman, B.A. (1975) The effect of vitamin A on growth and differentiation of human keratinocytes *in vitro*. *J. Invest. Dermatol.,* **64**, 19–22

Chustecka, Z. (1998) New generations of retinoid compounds. *Pharmaprojects,* **3**, 24-27

Clamon, G.H., Sporn, M.B., Smith, J.M. & Saffiotti, U. (1974) α- and β-Retinyl acetate reverse metaplasias of vitamin A deficiency in hamster trachea in organ culture. *Nature,* **250**, 64-66

Clark, J.N. & Marchok, A.C. (1979) The effect of vitamin A on cellular differentiation and mucous glycoprotein synthesis in long-term rat tracheal organ cultures. *Differentiation,* **14**, 175-183

Clark, J.N., Klein Szanto, A.J., Pine, A.H., Stephenson, K.B. & Marchok, A.C. (1980) Reestablishment of a mucociliary epithelium in tracheal organ cultures exposed to retinyl acetate: a biochemical and morphometric study. *Eur. J. Cell Biol.,* **21**, 261–268

Cline, P.R. & Rice, R.H. (1983) Modulation of involucrin and envelope competence in human keratinocytes by hydrocortisone, retinyl acetate, and growth arrest. *Cancer Res.,* **43**, 3203–3207

Cohen, S.M., Wittenberg, J.F. & Bryan, G.T. (1976) Effect of avitaminosis A and hypervitaminosis A on urinary bladder carcinogenicity of *N*-(4-(5-nitro-2-furyl)-2-thiazolyl)formamide. *Cancer Res.,* **36**, 2334–2339

Cohlan, S.Q. (1953) Excessive intake of vitamin A as a cause of congenital anomalies in the rat. *Science,* **117**, 535–536

Colin, C., Narbonne, J.F., Migaud, M.L., Grolier, P., Cassand, P. & Pellissier, M.A. (1991) Lipid peroxidation and benzo[*a*]pyrene activation to mutagenic metabolites: *in vivo* influence of vitamins A, E and C and glutathione in both dietary vitamin A sufficiency and deficiency. *Mutat. Res.,* **246**, 159–168

Collins, M.D., Eckhoff, C., Chahoud, I., Bochert, G. & Nau, H. (1992) 4-Methylpyrazole partially ameliorated the teratogenicity of retinol and reduced the metabolic formation of all-*trans*-retinoic acid in the mouse. *Arch. Toxicol.*, **66**, 652–659

Collins, M.D., Tzimas, G., Hummler, H., Burgin, H. & Nau, H. (1994) Comparative teratology and transplacental pharmacokinetics of all-*trans*-retinoic acid, 13-*cis*-retinoic acid, and retinyl palmitate following daily administrations in rats. *Toxicol. Appl. Pharmacol.*, **127**, 132–144

Comstock, G. W., Burke, A. E., Hoffman, S. C., Helzlsouer, K. J., Bendich, A., Masi, A. T., Norkus, E. P., Malamet, R. L. & Gershwin, M. E. (1997) Serum concentrations of α-tocopherol, β-carotene, and retinol preceding the diagnosis of rheumatoid arthritis and systemic lupus erythematosus. *Ann. Rheum. Dis.*, **56**, 323–325

Connor, M.J. (1988) Oxidation of retinol to retinoic acid as a requirement for biological activity in mouse epidermis. *Cancer Res.*, **48**, 7038–7040

Connor, M.J., Ashton, R.E. & Lowe, N.J. (1986) A comparative study of the induction of epidermal hyperplasia by natural and synthetic retinoids. *J. Pharmacol. Exp. Ther.*, **237**, 31–35

Cooper, A.D. (1997) Hepatic uptake of chylomicron remnants. *J. Lipid Res.*, **38**, 2173–2192

Cope, F.O. & Wille, J.J. (1989) Retinoid receptor antisense DNAs inhibit alkaline phosphatase induction and clonogenicity in malignant keratinocytes. *Proc. Natl. Acad. Sci. USA.*, **86**, 5590–5594

Copper, M. P., Klaassen, I., Teerlink, T., Snow, G. B. & Braakhuis, B.J.M. (1998) Plasma retinoids levels in head and neck cancer patients: a comparison with healthy controls and the effect of retinyl-palmitate treatment. In: Biomarkers in chemoprevention of second primary tumours in head and neck cancer patients (thesis), University of Amsterdam, pp. 77–84

Corrocher, R., Ferrari, S., de Gironcoli, M., Bassi, A., Olivieri, O., Guarini, P., Stanzial, A., Barba, A.L. & Gregolini, L. (1989) Effect of fish oil supplementation on erythrocyte lipid pattern, malondialdehyde production and glutathione-peroxidase activity in psoriasis. *Clin. Chim. Acta,* **179**, 121–131

Cosmetic Ingredient Review Expert Panel of the American College of Toxicology (1987) Final report on the safety assessment of retinyl palmitate and retinol. *J. Am. Coll. Toxicol.*, **6**, 279–320

Costaridis, P., Horton, C., Zeitlinger, J., Holder, N. & Maden, M. (1996) Endogenous retinoids in the zebrafish embryo and adult. *Dev. Dyn.*, **205**, 41–51

Coutsoudis, A., Coovadia, H.M., Broughton, M., Salisbury, R.T. & Elson, I. (1991) Micronutrient utilisation during measles treated with vitamin A or placebo. *Int. J. Vitam. Nutr. Res.*, **61**, 199–204

Cozzi, R., Bona, R., Polani, S. & De Salvia, R. (1990) Retinoids as modulators of metabolism: their inhibitory effect on cyclophosphamide and 7,12-dimethylbenz[*a*]anthracene induced sister chromatid exchanges in a metabolically competent cell line. *Mutagenesis,* **5**, 397–401

Creech Kraft, J. (1992) Pharmacokinetics, placental transfer, and teratogenicity of 13-*cis*-retinoic acid, its isomer and metabolites. In: Morriss-Kay, G. (ed.), *Retinoids in Normal Development and Teratogenesis,* Oxford, Oxford University Press, pp. 267–280

Creech Kraft, J., Lofberg, B., Chahoud, I., Bochert, G. & Nau, H. (1989) Teratogenicity and placental transfer of all-*trans*-, 13-*cis*-, 4- oxo-all-*trans*-, and 4-oxo-13-*cis*-retinoic acid after administration of a low oral dose during organogenesis in mice. *Toxicol. Appl. Pharmacol.*, **100**, 162–176

Creek, K.E., Jenkins, G.R., Khan, M.A., Batova, A., Hodam, J.R., Tolleson, W.H. & Pirisi, L. (1994) Retinoic acid suppresses human papillomavirus type 16 (HPV16)- mediated transformation of human keratinocytes and inhibits the expression of the HPV16 oncogenes. *Adv. Exp. Med. Biol.*, **354**, 19–35

Crettaz, M., Baron, A., Siegenthaler, G. & Hunziker, W. (1990) Ligand specificities of recombinant retinoic acid receptors RARα and RARβ. *Biochem. J.*, **272**, 391–397

Cullum, M.E. & Zile, M.H. (1985) Metabolism of all-*trans*-retinoic acid and all-*trans*-retinyl acetate. Demonstration of common physiological metabolites in rat small intestinal mucosa and circulation. *J. Biol. Chem.*, **260**, 10590–10596

Curtale, F., Vaidya, Y., Muhilal & Tilden, R.L. (1994) Ascariasis, hookworm infection and serum retinol amongst children in Nepal. *Panminerva Med.*, **36**, 19–21

Cuzick, J., De Stavola, B.L., Russell, M.J. & Thomas, B.S. (1990) Vitamin A, vitamin E and the risk of cervical intraepithelial neoplasia. *Br. J. Cancer,* **62**, 651–652

Czeizel, A.E. & Dudas, I. (1992) Prevention of the first occurrence of neural-tube defects by periconceptional vitamin supplementation. *New Engl. J. Med.,* **327**, 1832–1835

Dai, S., Morre, D.J., Geilen, C.C., Almond-Roesler, B., Orfanos, C.E. & Morre, D.M. (1997) Inhibition of plasma membrane NADH oxidase activity and growth of HeLa cells by natural and synthetic retinoids. *Mol. Cell Biochem.,* **166**, 101–109

Dartigues, J.F., Dabis, F., Gros, N., Moise, A., Bois, G., Salamon, R., Dilhuydy, J.M. & Courty, G. (1990) Dietary vitamin A, β-carotene and risk of epidermoid lung cancer in south-western France. *Eur. J. Epidemiol.,* **6**, 261–265

Darwiche, N., Celli, G., Tennenbaum, T., Glick, A.B., Yuspa, S.H. & De Luca, L.M. (1995) Mouse skin tumor progression results in differential expression of retinoic acid and retinoid X receptors. *Cancer Res.,* **55**, 2774–2782

Das, B.S., Thurnham, D.I. & Das, D.B. (1996) Plasma α-tocopherol, retinol, and carotenoids in children with falciparum malaria. *Am. J. Clin. Nutr.,* **64**, 94–100

Dawson, M.I. & Hobbs, P.D. (1994) The synthetic chemistry of retinoids. In: Sporn, M.B., Roberts, A.B. & Goodman, D.S. (eds), *The Retinoids: Biology, Chemistry, and Medicine,* 2nd edition, New York, Raven Press, pp. 5–178

Day, G.L., Shore, R.E., Blot, W.J., McLaughlin, J.K., Austin, D.F., Greenberg, R.S., Liff, J.M., Preston Martin, S., Sarkar, S., Schoenberg, J.B. & Fraumeni, J.F., Jr (1994) Dietary factors and second primary cancers: a follow-up of oral and pharyngeal cancer patients. *Nutr. Cancer,* **21**, 223–232

de Bruijn, D.R., Oerlemans, F., Hendriks, W., Baats, E., Ploemacher, R., Wieringa, B. & Geurts van Kessel, A. (1994) Normal development, growth and reproduction in cellular retinoic acid binding protein-I (CRABPI) null mutant mice. *Differentiation,* **58**, 141–148

De Coster, R., Wouters, W. & Bruynseels, J. (1996) P450-dependent enzymes as targets for prostate cancer therapy. *J. Steroid Biochem. Mol. Biol.,* **56**, 133–143

de Faria, E., Fong, L.G., Komaromy, M. & Cooper, A.D. (1996) Relative roles of the LDL receptor, the LDL receptor-like protein, and hepatic lipase in chylomicron remnant removal by the liver. *J. Lipid Res.,* **37**, 197–209

De Flora, S., Bennicelli, C., Rovida, A., Scatolini, L. & Camoirano, A. (1994) Inhibition of the 'spontaneous' mutagenicity in *Salmonella typhimurium* TA102 and TA104. *Mutat. Res.,* **307**, 157–167

de Klerk, N.H., Musk, A.W., Ambrosini, G.L., Eccles, J.L., Hansen, J., Olsen, N., Watts, V.L., Lund, H.G., Pang, S.C., Beilby, J. & Hobbs, M.S. (1998) Vitamin A and cancer prevention II: Comparison of the effects of retinol and β-carotene. *Int. J. Cancer,* **75**, 362–367

De Leenheer, A.P., Lambert, W.E. & Claeys, I. (1982) All-*trans*-retinoic acid: measurement of reference values in human serum by high performance liquid chromatography. *J. Lipid Res.,* **23**, 1362–1367

De Luca, L.M. (1991) Retinoids and their receptors in differentiation, embryogenesis, and neoplasia. *FASEB J.,* **5**, 2924–2933

De Luca, L.M., Sly, L., Jones, C.S. & Chen, L.C. (1992) Dietary retinoids are essential for skin papilloma formation induced by either the two-stage or the complete tumorigenesis model in female SENCAR mice. *Cancer Lett.,* **66**, 233–239

de Pee, S. & West, C.E. (1996) Dietary carotenoids and their role in combating vitamin A deficiency: a review of the literature. *Eur. J. Clin. Nutr.,* **50 Suppl. 3**, S38–S53

de Vet, H.C., Knipschild, P.G., Grol, M.E., Schouten, H.J. & Sturmans, F. (1991) The role of β-carotene and other dietary factors in the aetiology of cervical dysplasia: results of a case-control study. *Int. J. Epidemiol.,* **20**, 603–610

de Vries, N., van Zandwijk, N. & Pastorino, U. (1991) The EUROSCAN Study. EUROSCAN Steering Committee. *Br. J. Cancer,* **64**, 985–989

de Vries, N., van Zandwijk, N. & Pastorino, U. (1993) The EUROSCAN study: a progress report. *Am. J. Otolaryngol.,* **14**, 62–66

Decarli, A., Liati, P., Negri, E., Franceschi, S. & La Vecchia, C. (1987) Vitamin A and other dietary factors in the etiology of esophageal cancer. *Nutr. Cancer,* **10**, 29–37

Decoudu, S., Cassand, P., Daubeze, M., Frayssinet, C. & Narbonne, J.F. (1992) Effect of vitamin A dietary intake on *in vitro* and *in vivo* activation of aflatoxin B_1. *Mutat. Res.*, **269**, 269–278

Devery, J. & Milborrow, B.V. (1994) β-Carotene-15,15'-dioxygenase (EC 1.13.11.21) isolation reaction mechanism and an improved assay procedure. *Br. J. Nutr.*, **72**, 397–414

Dew, S.E. & Ong, D.E. (1994) Specificity of the retinol transporter of the rat small intestine brush border. *Biochemistry,* **33**, 12340–12345

Dockx, P., Decree, J. & Degreef, H. (1995) Inhibition of the metabolism of endogenous retinoic acid as treatment for severe psoriasis: an open study with oral liarozole. *Br. J. Dermatol.*, **133**, 426–432

Doireau, V., Macher, M.A., Brun, P., Bernard, O. & Loirat, C. (1996) [Vitamin A poisoning revealed by hypercalcaemia in a child with kidney failure]. *Arch. Pediatr.*, **3**, 888–890 (in French)

Dong, D. & Zile, M.H. (1995) Endogenous retinoids in the early avian embryo. *Biochem. Biophys. Res. Commun.*, **217**, 1026–1031

Douer, D. & Koeffler, H.P. (1982) Retinoic acid enhances colony-stimulating factor-induced clonal growth of normal human myeloid progenitor cells *in vitro*. *Exp. Cell Res.*, **138**, 193–198

Dowell, S.F., Papic, Z., Bresee, J.S., Larranaga, C., Mendez, M., Sowell, A.L., Gary, H.E., Jr, Anderson, L.J. & Avendano, L.F. (1996) Treatment of respiratory syncytial virus infection with vitamin A: a randomized, placebo-controlled trial in Santiago, Chile. *Pediatr. Infect. Dis. J.*, **15**, 782–786

Dozi-Vassiliades, J., Myrtsiotis, A., Granitsas, A. & Mourelatos, D. (1985) Induction of sister-chromatid exchanges and cell-cycle delays in human lymphocytes by vitamin A alone or in combination with melphalan and caffeine. *Eur. J. Cancer Clin. Oncol.*, **21**, 1089–1092

Driessen, C.A., Janssen, B.P., Winkens, H.J., van Vugt, A.H., de Leeuw, T.L. & Janssen, J.J. (1995) Cloning and expression of a cDNA encoding bovine retinal pigment epithelial 11-*cis* retinol dehydrogenase. *Invest. Ophthalmol. Vis. Sci.*, **36**, 1988–1996

Dubois, A., Balducchi, J.P., Barbuat, C., Fabre, J., Flaisler, F., Joujoux, J.M., Pignodel, C., Jourdan, J. & Fourcade, J. (1991) [Portal hypertension and hypervitaminosis A. Apropos of 2 cases and review of the literature]. *Rev. Méd. Interne,* **12**, 295–298 (in French)

Duester, G. (1996) Involvement of alcohol dehydrogenase, short-chain dehydrogenase/reductase, aldehyde dehydrogenase, and cytochrome P450 in the control of retinoid signaling by activation of retinoic acid synthesis. *Biochemistry,* **35**, 12221–12227

Durston, A.J., Timmermans, J.P., Hage, W.J., Hendriks, H.F., de Vries, N.J., Heideveld, M. & Nieuwkoop, P.D. (1989) Retinoic acid causes an anteroposterior transformation in the developing central nervous system. *Nature,* **340**, 140–144

Duszka, C., Grolier, P., Azim, E.M., Alexandre Gouabau, M.C., Borel, P. & Azais Braesco, V. (1996) Rat intestinal β-carotene dioxygenase activity is located primarily in the cytosol of mature jejunal enterocytes. *J. Nutr.*, **126**, 2550–2556

Eckhoff, C. (1991) Untersuchungen zur Bedeutung des Metabolismus von Retinol für den Mechanismus der terategenen Wirkung von hochdosiertem Vitamin bei Maus, Affe, und Mensch, (thesis), Freie Universitat Berlin

Eckhoff, C. & Nau, H. (1990a) Identification and quantitation of all-*trans*- and 13-*cis*-retinoic acid and 13-*cis*-4-oxoretinoic acid in human plasma. *J. Lipid Res.*, **31**, 1445–1454

Eckhoff, C. & Nau, H. (1990b) Vitamin A supplementation increases levels of retinoic acid compounds in human plasma: possible implications for teratogenesis. *Arch. Toxicol.*, **64**, 502–503

Eckhoff, C., Lofberg, B., Chahoud, I., Bochert, G. & Nau, H. (1989) Transplacental pharmacokinetics and teratogenicity of a single dose of retinol (vitamin A) during organogenesis in the mouse. *Toxicol. Lett.*, **48**, 171–184

Eckhoff, C., Wittfoht, W., Nau, H. & Slikker, W.J. (1990) Characterization of oxidized and glucuronidated metabolites of retinol in monkey plasma by thermospray liquid chromatography/mass spectrometry. *Biomed. Environ. Mass. Spectrom.*, **19**, 428–433

Eckhoff, C., Collins, M.D. & Nau, H. (1991a) Human plasma all-*trans*-, 13-*cis*- and 13-*cis*-4-oxoretinoic acid profiles during subchronic vitamin A supplementation: comparison to retinol and retinyl ester plasma levels. *J. Nutr.*, **121**, 1016–1025

Eckhoff, C., Bailey, J.R., Collins, M.D., Slikker, W., Jr. & Nau, H. (1991b) Influence of dose and pharmaceutical formulation of vitamin A on plasma levels of retinyl esters and retinol and metabolic generation of retinoic acid compounds and β-glucuronides in the cynomolgus monkey. *Toxicol. Appl. Pharmacol.,* **111**, 116–127

Edmondson, S.W. & Mossman, B.T. (1991) Alterations in keratin expression in hamster tracheal epithelial cells exposed to benzo[*a*]pyrene. *Carcinogenesis,* **12**, 679–684

Edmondson, S.W., Wu, R. & Mossman, B.T. (1990) Regulation of differentiation and keratin protein expression by vitamin A in primary cultures of hamster tracheal epithelial cells. *J. Cell Physiol.,* **142**, 21–30

Edwards, R.B., Adler, A.J., Dev, S. & Claycomb, R.C. (1992) Synthesis of retinoic acid from retinol by cultured rabbit Müller cells. *Exp. Eye Res.,* **54**, 481–490

Eglitis, M.A. & Sherman, M.I. (1983) Murine embryonal carcinoma cells differentiate *in vitro* in response to retinol. *Exp. Cell Res.,* **146**, 289–296

Eichholzer, M., Stahelin, H.B., Gey, K.F., Ludin, E. & Bernasconi, F. (1996) Prediction of male cancer mortality by plasma levels of interacting vitamins: 17-year follow-up of the prospective Basel study. *Int. J. Cancer,* **66**, 145–150

El Akawi, Z. & Napoli, J.L. (1994) Rat liver cytosolic retinal dehydrogenase: comparison of 13-*cis*-, 9-*cis*-, and all-*trans*-retinal as substrates and effects of cellular retinoid-binding proteins and retinoic acid on activity. *Biochemistry,* **33**, 1938–1943

ElAttar, T.M. & Lin, H.S. (1991) Effect of retinoids and carotenoids on prostaglandin formation by oral squamous carcinoma cells. *Prostaglandins Leukot. Essent. Fatty Acids,* **43**, 175–178

Elmazar, M.M.A., Ruhl, R., Reichert, U., Shroot, B. & Nau, H. (1997) RARα-mediated teratogenicity in mice is potentiated by an RXR agonist and reduced by an RAR antagonist: dissection of retinoid receptor-induced pathways. *Toxicol. Appl. Pharmacol.,* **146**, 21–28

elSisi, A.E., Hall, P., Sim, W.L., Earnest, D.L. & Sipes, I.G. (1993a) Characterization of vitamin A potentiation of carbon tetrachloride-induced liver injury. *Toxicol. Appl. Pharmacol.,* **119**, 280–288

elSisi, A.E., Earnest, D.L. & Sipes, I.G. (1993b) Vitamin A potentiation of carbon tetrachloride hepatotoxicity: role of liver macrophages and active oxygen species. *Toxicol. Appl. Pharmacol.,* **119**, 295–301

elSisi, A.E., Earnest, D.L. & Sipes, I.G. (1993c) Vitamin A potentiation of carbon tetrachloride hepatotoxicity: enhanced lipid peroxidation without enhanced biotransformation. *Toxicol. Appl. Pharmacol.,* **119**, 289–294

Emura, M., Mohr, U., Riebe, M., Aufderheide, M. & Dungworth, D.L. (1988) Regulation of growth and differentiation by vitamin A in a cloned fetal lung epithelial cell line cultured on collagen gel in hormone-supplemented medium. *In vitro Cell Dev. Biol.,* **24**, 639–648

Eppinger, T.M., Buck, J. & Hammerling, U. (1993) Growth control or terminal differentiation: endogenous production and differential activities of vitamin A metabolites in HL-60 cells. *J. Exp. Med.,* **178**, 1995–2005

Estève, J., Riboli, E., Pequignot, G., Terracini, B., Merletti, F., Crosignani, P., Ascunce, N., Zubiri, L., Blanchet, F., Raymond, L., Repetto, F. & Tuyns, A.J. (1996) Diet and cancers of the larynx and hypopharynx: the IARC multi-center study in southwestern Europe. *Cancer Causes Control,* **7**, 240–252

FAO/WHO (1988) Requirements of vitamin A, iron, folate and vitamin B_{12}. Report of a Joint FAO/WHO Expert Consultation. *FAO Food and Nutrition Series No. 23,* Rome, FAO Press, pp. 1–107

Fawcett, D., Pasceri, P., Fraser, R., Colbert, M., Rossant, J. & Giguere, V. (1995) Postaxial polydactyly in forelimbs of CRABP-II mutant mice. *Development,* **121**, 671–679

Fazely, F., Ledinko, N. & Smith, D.J. (1988) Inhibition by retinoids of *in vitro* invasive ability of human lung carcinoma cells. *Anticancer Res.,* **8**, 1387–1391

Ferrari, N., Agradi, E. & Vidali, G. (1983) Effect of retinol on macromolecular synthesis in cultured cell lines. *Acta Vitaminol. Enzymol.,* **5**, 119–124

Ferrari, N., Rocco, M., Aprile, A., Fassina, G. & Vidali, G. (1989) Interaction retinol-chromatin: an analysis of DNA from vitamin A-treated V79 Chinese hamster cells. *Biochim. Biophys. Acta,* **1007**, 30–35

Ferraroni, M., La Vecchia, C., D'Avanzo, B., Negri, E., Franceschi, S. & Decarli, A. (1994) Selected micronutrient intake and the risk of colorectal cancer. *Br. J. Cancer,* **70**, 1150–1155

Ferreri, A.M., Grilli, M.P., Capucci, A., Prodi, G., Rocchi, P. & Bianucci, F. (1986) Effect of antioxidants on mutagenesis induced by DMBA in human cells. *Nutr. Cancer,* **8**, 267–272

Filteau, S.M., Morris, S.S., Abbott, R.A., Tomkins, A.M., Kirkwood, B.R., Arthur, P., Ross, D.A., Gyapong, J.O. & Raynes, J.G. (1993) Influence of morbidity on serum retinol of children in a community-based study in northern Ghana. *Am. J. Clin. Nutr.,* **58**, 192–197

Fiorella, P.D. & Napoli, J.L. (1991) Expression of cellular retinoic acid binding protein (CRABP) in *Escherichia coli*. Characterization and evidence that holo-CRABP is a substrate in retinoic acid metabolism. *J. Biol. Chem.,* **266**, 16572–16579

Flood, M.T., Bridges, C.D., Alvarez, R.A., Blaner, W.S. & Gouras, P. (1983) Vitamin A utilization in human retinal pigment epithelial cells *in vitro*. *Invest. Ophthalmol. Vis. Sci.,* **24**, 1227–1235

Florentino, R.F., Tanchoco, C.C., Ramos, A.C., Mendoza, T.S., Natividad, E.P., Tangco, J.B. & Sommer, A. (1990) Tolerance of preschoolers to two dosage strengths of vitamin A preparation. *Am. J. Clin. Nutr.,* **52**, 694–700

Folman, Y., Russell, R.M., Tang, G.W. & Wolf, D.G. (1989) Rabbits fed on β-carotene have higher serum levels of all-*trans* retinoic acid than those receiving no β-carotene. *Br. J. Nutr.,* **62**, 195–201

Fontham, E.T., Pickle, L.W., Haenszel, W., Correa, P., Lin, Y.P. & Falk, R.T. (1988) Dietary vitamins A and C and lung cancer risk in Louisiana. *Cancer,* **62**, 2267–2273

Formelli, F., Barua, A.B. & Olson, J.A. (1996) Bioactivities of *N*-(4-hydroxyphenyl) retinamide and retinoyl β-glucuronide. *FASEB J.,* **10**, 1014-1024

Forni, G., Cerruti Sola, S., Giovarelli, M., Santoni, A., Martinetto, P. & Vietti, D. (1986) Effect of prolonged administration of low doses of dietary retinoids on cell-mediated immunity and the growth of transplantable tumors in mice. *J. Natl. Cancer Inst.,* **76**, 527–533

Forsyth, K.S., Watson, R.R. & Gensler, H.L. (1989) Osteotoxicity after chronic dietary administration of 13-*cis*-retinoic acid, retinyl palmitate or selenium in mice exposed to tumor initiation and promotion. *Life Sci.,* **45**, 2149–2156

Fortes, C., Forastiere, F., Agabiti, N., Fano, V., Pacifici, R., Virgili, F., Piras, G., Guidi, L., Bartoloni, C., Tricerri, A., Zuccaro, P., Ebrahim, S. & Perucci, C.A. (1998) The effect of zinc and vitamin A supplementation on immune response in an older population. *J. Am. Geriatr. Soc.,* **46**, 19–26

Frame, B., Jackson, C.E., Reynolds, W.A. & Umphrey, J.E. (1974) Hypercalcemia and skeletal effects in chronic hypervitaminosis A. *Ann. Intern. Med.,* **80**, 44–48

Freudenheim, J.L., Graham, S., Byers, T.E., Marshall, J.R.,`Haughey, B.P., Swanson, M.K. & Wilkinson, G. (1992) Diet, smoking, and alcohol in cancer of the larynx: a case-control study. *Nutr. Cancer,* **17**, 33–45

Frickel, F. (1984) Chemistry and physical properties of retinoids. In: Sporn, M.B., Roberts, A.B. & Goodman, D.S. (eds), *The Retinoids*, Orlando, Academic Press, pp. 7–145

Friedman, S.L. (1993) Seminars in medicine of the Beth Israel Hospital, Boston. The cellular basis of hepatic fibrosis. Mechanisms and treatment strategies. *New Engl. J. Med.,* **328**, 1828–1835

Friedman, G.D., Blaner, W.S., Goodman, D.S., Vogelman, J.H., Brind, J.L., Hoover, R., Fireman, B.H. & Orentreich, N. (1986) Serum retinol and retinol-binding protein levels do not predict subsequent lung cancer. *Am. J. Epidemiol.,* **123**, 781–789

Friedman, S.L., Wei, S. & Blaner, W.S. (1993) Retinol release by activated rat hepatic lipocytes: regulation by Kupffer cell-conditioned medium and PDGF. *Am. J. Physiol.,* **264**, G947–952

Frolik, C.A. & Olson, J.A. (1984) Extraction, separation, and chemical analysis of retinoids. In: Sporn, M.B., Roberts, A.B. & Goodman, D.S. (eds), *The Retinoids*, Orlando, Academic Press, pp. 181–233

Fuchs, E. & Green, H. (1981) Regulation of terminal differentiation of cultured human keratinocytes by vitamin A. *Cell,* **25**, 617–625

Fujii, H., Sato, T., Kaneko, S., Gotoh, O., Fujii Kuriyama, Y., Osawa, K., Kato, S. & Hamada, H. (1997) Metabolic inactivation of retinoic acid by a novel P450 differentially expressed in developing mouse embryos. *EMBO J.,* **16**, 4163–4173

Furr, H.C., Amédée Manesme, O., Clifford, A.J., Bergen, H.R.3, Jones, A.D., Anderson, D.P. & Olson, J.A. (1989) Vitamin A concentrations in liver determined by isotope dilution assay with tetradeuterated vitamin A and by biopsy in generally healthy adult humans. *Am. J. Clin. Nutr.*, **49**, 713–716

Furr, H.C., Barua, A.B. & Olson, J.A. (1992) Retinoids and carotenoids. In: De Leenheer, A.P., Lambert, W.E. & Nelis, H.J. (eds), *Modern Chromatographic Analysis of Vitamins*, New York, Marcel Dekker, pp. 1-71

Furr, H.C., Barua, A.B. & Olson, J.A. (1994) Analytical methods. In: Sporn, M.B., Roberts, A.B. & Goodman, D.S. (eds), *The Retinoids: Biology, Chemistry, and Medicine*, 2nd edition, New York, Raven Press, pp. 179-209

Gao, Y.T., McLaughlin, J.K., Gridley, G., Blot, W.J., Ji, B.T., Dai, Q. & Fraumeni, J.F. (1994) Risk factors for esophageal cancer in Shanghai, China. II. Role of diet and nutrients. *Int. J. Cancer*, **58**, 197-202

Garbis-Berkvens, J.M. & Peters, P.W.J. (1987) Comparative morphology and physiology of embryonic and fetal membranes. In: Nau, H. & Scott, W.J.J. (eds), *Pharmacokinetics in Teratogenesis*, Boca Raton, CRC Press, pp. 13–44

Garewal, H.S., Meyskens, F.L., Jr, Killen, D., Reeves, D., Kiersch, T.A., Elletson, H., Strosberg, A., King, D. & Steinbronn, K. (1990) Response of oral leukoplakia to β-carotene. *J. Clin. Oncol.*, **8**, 1715–1720

Geelen, J.A. (1979) Hypervitaminosis A induced teratogenesis. *CRC Crit. Rev. Toxicol.*, **6**, 351–375

Geerts, A., Bleser, P.D., Hautekeete, M.L., Niki, T. & Wisse, E. (1994) Fat-storing (Ito) cell biology. In: Arias, I.M., Boyer, J.L., Fausto, N., Jakoby, W.B., Schachter, D. & Shafritz, D.A. (eds), *The Liver: Biology and Pathobiology*, New York, Raven Press, pp. 819–838

Genchi, G., Wang, W., Barua, A., Bidlack, W.R. & Olson, J.A. (1996) Formation of β-glucuronides and of β-galacturonides of various retinoids catalyzed by induced and noninduced microsomal UDP-glucuronosyltransferases of rat liver. *Biochim. Biophys. Acta*, **1289**, 284–290

Genchi, G., Barua, A.B., Wang, W., Bidlack, W.R. & Olson, J.A. (1998) The effects of pH on the enzymatic formation of β-glucuronides of various retinoids by induced and noninduced microsomal UDPGA-glucuronosyltransferases of several rat tissues *in vitro*. *J. Nutr. Biochem.* (in press)

Gensler, H.L., Watson, R.R., Moriguchi, S. & Bowden, G.T. (1987) Effects of dietary retinyl palmitate or 13-*cis*-retinoic acid on the promotion of tumors in mouse skin. *Cancer Res.*, **47**, 967–970

Gensler, H.L., Aickin, M. & Peng, Y.M. (1990) Cumulative reduction of primary skin tumor growth in UV-irradiated mice by the combination of retinyl palmitate and canthaxanthin. *Cancer Lett.*, **53**, 27–31

Geradts, J., Chen, J.Y., Russell, E.K., Yankaskas, J.R., Nieves, L. & Minna, J.D. (1993) Human lung cancer cell lines exhibit resistance to retinoic acid treatment. *Cell Growth Differ.*, **4**, 799–809

Gergely, P., Gonzalez Cabello, R., Jakab, I., Vien, C.V. & Bodo, I. (1988) Effect of vitamin A treatment on cellular immune reactivity in patients with CLL. *Acta Med. Hung.*, **45**, 307–311

Gerlach, T.H. & Zile, M.H. (1990) Upregulation of serum retinol in experimental acute renal failure. *FASEB J.*, **4**, 2511–2517

Gerlach, T.H. & Zile, M.H. (1991) Metabolism and secretion of retinol transport complex in acute renal failure. *J. Lipid Res.*, **32**, 515-520

Gerlach, T., Biesalski, H.K., Weiser, H., Haeussermann, B. & Baessler, K.H. (1989) Vitamin A in parenteral nutrition: uptake and distribution of retinyl esters after intravenous application. *Am. J. Clin. Nutr.*, **50**, 1029–1038

Gerster, H. (1997) Vitamin A — functions, dietary requirements and safety in humans. *Int. J. Vitam. Nutr. Res.*, **67**, 71–90

Geubel, A.P., De Galocsy, C., Alves, N., Rahier, J. & Dive, C. (1991) Liver damage caused by therapeutic vitamin A administration: estimate of dose-related toxicity in 41 cases. *Gastroenterology*, **100**, 1701–1709

Ghadirian, P., Lacroix, A., Maisonneuve, P., Perret, C., Drouin, G., Perrault, J.P., Beland, G., Rohan, T.E. & Howe, G.R. (1996) Nutritional factors and prostate cancer: a case-control study of French Canadians in Montreal, Canada. *Cancer Causes Control*, **7**, 428–436

Ghana VAST Study Team (1993) Vitamin A supplementation in northern Ghana: effects on clinic attendances, hospital admissions, and child mortality. *Lancet,* **342**, 7–12

Giguere, V. (1994) Retinoic acid receptors and cellular retinoid binding proteins: complex interplay in retinoid signaling. *Endocr. Rev.,* **15**, 61–79

Giovannucci, E., Ascherio, A., Rimm, E.B., Stampfer, M.J., Colditz, G.A. & Willett, W.C. (1995) Intake of carotenoids and retinol in relation to risk of prostate cancer. *J. Natl. Cancer Inst.,* **87**, 1767–1776

Glasziou, P.P. & Mackerras, D.E.M. (1993) Vitamin A supplementation in infectious diseases: a meta-analysis. *Br. Med. J.,* **306**, 366–370

Glick, A.B., McCune, B.K., Abdulkarem, N., Flanders, K.C., Lumadue, J.A., Smith, J.M. & Sporn, M.B. (1991) Complex regulation of TGFβ expression by retinoic acid in the vitamin A-deficient rat. *Development,* **111**, 1081–1086

Godel, J.C., Basu, T.K., Pabst, H.F., Hodges, R.S., Hodges, P.E. & Ng, M.L. (1996) Perinatal vitamin A (retinol) status of northern Canadian mothers and their infants. *Biol. Neonate,* **69**, 133–139

Gonzalez, C.A., Riboli, E., Badosa, J., Batiste, E., Cardona, T., Pita, S., Sanz, J.M., Torrent, M. & Agudo, A. (1994) Nutritional factors and gastric cancer in Spain. *Am. J. Epidemiol.,* **139**, 466–473

Goodman, D.S. (1984) Plasma retinol-binding protein. In: Sporn, M.B., Roberts, A.B. & Goodman, D.S. (eds), *The Retinoids,* Orlando, Academic Press, pp. 41–88

Goodman, D.S. & Blaner, W.S. (1984) Biosynthesis, absorption, and hepatic metabolism of retinol. In: Sporn, M.B., Roberts, A.B. & Goodman, D.S. (eds), *The Retinoids,* Orlando, Academic Press, pp. 1–39

Goodman, D.S. & Huang, H.S. (1965) Biosynthesis of vitamin A with rat intestinal enzymes. *Science,* **149**, 879–880

Goodman, D.G., Huang, H.S. & Shiratori, T. (1965) Tissue distribution and metabolism of newly absorbed vitamin A in the rat. *J. Lipid Res.,* **6**, 390–396

Goodman, G.E., Omenn, G.S., Thornquist, M.D., Lund, B., Metch, B. & Gylys Colwell, I. (1993) The Carotene and Retinol Efficacy Trial (CARET) to prevent lung cancer in high-risk populations: pilot study with cigarette smokers. *Cancer Epidemiol. Biomarkers. Prev.,* **2**, 389–396

Goodman, G.E., Metch, B.J. & Omenn, G.S. (1994) The effect of long-term β-carotene and vitamin A administration on serum concentrations of α-tocopherol. *Cancer Epidemiol. Biomarkers. Prev.,* **3**, 429–432

Goodman, G.E., Thornquist, M., Kestin, M., Metch, B., Anderson, G. & Omenn, G.S. (1996) The association between participant characteristics and serum concentrations of β-carotene, retinol, retinyl palmitate, and α-tocopherol among participants in the Carotene and Retinol Efficacy Trial (CARET) for prevention of lung cancer. *Cancer Epidemiol. Biomarkers. Prev.,* **5**, 815–821

Gorry, P., Lufkin, T., Dierich, A., Rochette Egly, C., Decimo, D., Dolle, P., Mark, M., Durand, B. & Chambon, P. (1994) The cellular retinoic acid binding protein I is dispensable. *Proc. Natl. Acad. Sci. USA.,* **91**, 9032–9036

Goss, G.D. & McBurney, M.W. (1992) Physiological and clinical aspects of vitamin A and its metabolites. *Crit. Rev. Clin. Lab. Sci.,* **29**, 185–215

Gossel, T.A. & Bricker, J.D. (1994) Vitamins. In: Gossel, T.A. & Bricker, J.D. (eds), *Principles of Clinical Toxicology,* New York, Raven Press, pp. 403–417

Graham, S., Marshall, J., Mettlin, C., Rzepka, T., Nemoto, T. & Byers, T. (1982) Diet in the epidemiology of breast cancer. *Am. J. Epidemiol.,* **116**, 68–75

Graham, S., Haughey, B., Marshall, J., Priore, R., Byers, T., Rzepka, T., Mettlin, C. & Pontes, J.E. (1983) Diet in the epidemiology of carcinoma of the prostate gland. *J. Natl. Cancer Inst.,* **70**, 687–692

Graham, V., Surwit, E.S., Weiner, S. & Meyskens, F.L.J. (1986) Phase II trial of β-all-*trans*-retinoic acid for cervical intraepithelial neoplasia delivered via a collagen sponge and cervical cap. *West. J. Med.,* **145**, 192–195

Graham, S., Marshall, J., Haughey, B., Mittelman, A., Swanson, M., Zielezny, M., Byers, T., Wilkinson, G. & West, D. (1988) Dietary epidemiology of cancer of the colon in western New York. *Am. J. Epidemiol.,* **128**, 490–503

Graham, S., Marshall, J., Haughey, B., Brasure, J., Freudenheim, J., Zielezny, M., Wilkinson, G. & Nolan, J. (1990a) Nutritional epidemiology of cancer of the esophagus. *Am. J. Epidemiol.,* **131**, 454–467

Graham, S., Haughey, B., Marshall, J., Brasure, J., Zielezny, M., Freudenheim, J., West, D., Nolan, J. & Wilkinson, G. (1990b) Diet in the epidemiology of gastric cancer. *Nutr. Cancer,* **13**, 19–34

Graham, S., Zielezny, M., Marshall, J., Priore, R., Freudenheim, J., Brasure, J., Haughey, B., Nasca, P. & Zdeb, M. (1992) Diet in the epidemiology of postmenopausal breast cancer in the New York State Cohort. *Am. J. Epidemiol.,* **136**, 1327–1337

Green, M.H. & Green, J.B. (1994) Dynamics and control of plasma retinol. In: Blomhoff, R. (ed.), *Vitamin A in Health and Disease,* New York, Marcel Dekker, pp. 119–133

Green, H. & Watt, F.M. (1982) Regulation by vitamin A of envelope cross-linking in cultured keratinocytes derived from different human epithelia. *Mol. Cell Biol.,* **2**, 1115–1117

Green, M.H., Uhl, L. & Green, J.B. (1985) A multicompartmental model of vitamin A kinetics in rats with marginal liver vitamin A stores. *J. Lipid Res.,* **26**, 806–818

Green, M.H., Green, J.B. & Lewis, K.C. (1987) Variation in retinol utilization rate with vitamin A status in the rat. *J. Nutr.,* **117**, 694–703

Gregor, A., Lee, P.N., Roe, F.J., Wilson, M.J. & Melton, A. (1980) Comparison of dietary histories in lung cancer cases and controls with special reference to vitamin A. *Nutr. Cancer,* **2**, 93–97

Gregory, J.R., Foster, K., Tyler, H. & Wiseman, M. (1990) *The Dietary and Nutritional Survey of British Adults,* London, Her Majesty's Stationery Office

Gridley, G., McLaughlin, J.K., Block, G., Blot, W.J., Winn, D.M., Greenberg, R.S., Schoenberg, J.B., Preston Martin, S., Austin, D.F. & Fraumeni, J.F. (1990) Diet and oral and pharyngeal cancer among blacks. *Nutr. Cancer,* **14**, 219–225

Gridley, G., McLaughlin, J.K., Block, G., Blot, W.J., Gluch, M. & Fraumeni, J.F., Jr (1992) Vitamin supplement use and reduced risk of oral and pharyngeal cancer. *Am. J. Epidemiol.,* **135**, 1083–1092

Grosse, Y., Chekir Ghedira, L., Huc, A., Obrecht Pflumio, S., Dirheimer, G., Bacha, H. & Pfohl Leszkowicz, A. (1997) Retinol, ascorbic acid and α-tocopherol prevent DNA adduct formation in mice treated with the mycotoxins ochratoxin A and zearalenone. *Cancer Lett.,* **114**, 225–229

Grubbs, C.J., Eto, I., Juliana, M.M., Hardin, J.M. & Whitaker, L.M. (1990) Effect of retinyl acetate and 4-hydroxyphenylretinamide on initiation of chemically-induced mammary tumors. *Anticancer Res.,* **10**, 661–666

Gudas, L.J. (1994) Retinoids and vertebrate development. *J. Biol. Chem.,* **269**, 15399–15402

Gudas, L.J., Sporn, M.B. & Roberts, A.B. (1994) Cellular biology and biochemistry of the retinoids. In: Sporn, M.B., Roberts, A.B. & Goodman, D.S. (eds), *The Retinoids: Biology, Chemistry, and Medicine,* 2nd edition, New York, Raven Press, pp. 443–520

Gustafson, A.L., Dencker, L. & Eriksson, U. (1993) Non-overlapping expression of CRBP I and CRABP I during pattern formation of limbs and craniofacial structures in the early mouse embryo. *Development,* **117**, 451–460

Gustafson, A.L., Donovan, M., Annerwall, E., Dencker, L. & Eriksson, U. (1996) Nuclear import of cellular retinoic acid-binding protein type I in mouse embryonic cells. *Mech. Dev.,* **58**, 27–38

Haenszel, W., Correa, P., Lopez, A., Cuello, C., Zarama, G., Zavala, D. & Fontham, E. (1985) Serum micronutrient levels in relation to gastric pathology. *Int. J. Cancer,* **36**, 43–48

Hale, F. (1933) Pigs born without eye balls. *J. Hered.,* **24**, 105–106

Halevy, O. & Sklan, D. (1987) Inhibition of arachidonic acid oxidation by β-carotene, retinol and α-tocopherol. *Biochim. Biophys. Acta,* **918**, 30–307

Halter, S.A., Fraker, L.D., Parl, F., Bradley, R. & Briggs, R. (1990) Selective isolation of human breast carcinoma cells resistant to the growth-inhibitory effects of retinol. *Nutr. Cancer,* **14**, 43–56

Halter, S.A., Winnier, A.R. & Arteaga, C.L. (1993) Pretreatment with vitamin A inhibits transforming growth factor alpha stimulation of human mammary carcinoma cells. *J. Cell Physiol.,* **156**, 80–87

Hamilton, R.L., Wong, J.S., Guo, L.S., Krisans, S. & Havel, R.J. (1990) Apolipoprotein E localization in rat hepatocytes by immunogold labeling of cryothin sections. *J. Lipid Res.,* **31**, 1589–1603

Han, J.S. (1992) Effects of various chemical compounds on spontaneous and hydrogen peroxide-induced reversion in strain TA104 of *Salmonella typhimurium. Mutat. Res.,* **266**, 77–84

Handelman, G.J., Packer, L. & Cross, C.E. (1996) Destruction of tocopherols, carotenoids, and retinol in human plasma by cigarette smoke. *Am. J. Clin. Nutr.*, **63**, 559–565

Hansson, L.E., Nyren, O., Bergstrom, R., Wolk, A., Lindgren, A., Baron, J. & Adami, H.O. (1994) Nutrients and gastric cancer risk. A population-based case-control study in Sweden. *Int. J. Cancer*, **57**, 638–644

Haq, R., Pfahl, M. & Chytil, F. (1991) Retinoic acid affects the expression of nuclear retinoic acid receptors in tissues of retinol-deficient rats. *Proc. Natl. Acad. Sci. USA.*, **88**, 8272–8276

Harnish, D.C., Barua, A.B., Soprano, K.J. & Soprano, D.R. (1990) Induction of β-retinoic acid receptor mRNA by teratogenic doses of retinoids in murine fetuses. *Differentiation*, **45**, 103–108

Harrison, E.H. (1993) Enzymes catalyzing the hydrolysis of retinyl esters. *Biochim. Biophys. Acta*, **1170**, 99–108

Harrison, E.H., Blaner, W.S., Goodman, D.S. & Ross, A.C. (1987) Subcellular localization of retinoids, retinoid-binding proteins, and acyl-CoA:retinol acyltransferase in rat liver. *J. Lipid Res.*, **28**, 973–981

Harrison, E.H., Gad, M.Z. & Ross, A.C. (1995) Hepatic uptake and metabolism of chylomicron retinyl esters: probable role of plasma membrane/endosomal retinyl ester hydrolases. *J. Lipid Res.*, **36**, 1498–1506

Haskell, M.J., Handelman, G.J., Peerson, J.M., Jones, A.D., Rabbi, M.A., Awal, M.A., Wahed, M.A., Mahalanabis, D. & Brown, K.H. (1997) Assessment of vitamin A status by the deuterated-retinol-dilution technique and comparison with hepatic vitamin A concentration in Bangladeshi surgical patients. *Am. J. Clin. Nutr.*, **66**, 67–74

Hathcock, J.N., Hattan, D.G., Jenkins, M.Y., McDonald, J.T., Sundaresan, P.R. & Wilkening, V.L. (1990) Evaluation of vitamin A toxicity. *Am. J. Clin. Nutr.*, **52**, 183–202

Hazuka, M.B., Edwards-Prasad, J., Newman, F., Kinzie, J.J. & Prasad, K.N. (1990) β-Carotene induces morphological differentiation and decreases adenylate cyclase activity in melanoma cells in culture. *J. Am. Coll. Nutr.*, **9**, 143–149

Hébuterne, X., Wang, X.D., Johnson, E.J., Krinsky, N.I. & Russell, R.M. (1995) Intestinal absorption and metabolism of 9-*cis*-β-carotene *in vivo*: biosynthesis of 9-*cis*-retinoic acid. *J. Lipid Res.*, **36**, 1264–1273

Heilbrun, L.K., Nomura, A., Hankin, J.H. & Stemmermann, G.N. (1989) Diet and colorectal cancer with special reference to fiber intake. *Int. J. Cancer*, **44**, 1–6

Heller, E.H. & Shiffman, N.J. (1985) Synthetic retinoids in dermatology. *Can. Med. Assoc. J.*, **132**, 1129–1136

Helzlsouer, K.J., Comstock, G.W. & Morris, J.S. (1989) Selenium, lycopene, α-tocopherol, β-carotene, retinol, and subsequent bladder cancer. *Cancer Res.*, **49**, 6144–6148

Hendrickx, A.G. & Hummler, H. (1992) Teratogenicity of all-*trans* retinoic acid during early embryonic development in the cynomolgus monkey (*Macaca fascicularis*). *Teratology*, **45**, 65–74

Hendrickx, A.G., Hummler, H. & Oneda, S. (1997) Vitamin A teratogenicity and risk assessment in the cynomolgus monkey. *Teratology*, **55**, 68–68

Herrero, R., Potischman, N., Brinton, L.A., Reeves, W.C., Brenes, M.M., Tenorio, F., de Britton, R.C. & Gaitan, E. (1991) A case-control study of nutrient status and invasive cervical cancer. I. Dietary indicators. *Am. J. Epidemiol.*, **134**, 1335–1346

Herz, J., Qiu, S.Q., Oesterle, A., DeSilva, H.V., Shafi, S. & Havel, R.J. (1995) Initial hepatic removal of chylomicron remnants is unaffected but endocytosis is delayed in mice lacking the low density lipoprotein receptor. *Proc. Natl. Acad. Sci. USA.*, **92**, 4611–4615

Heshmat, M.Y., Kaul, L., Kovi, J., Jackson, M.A., Jackson, A.G., Jones, G.W., Edson, M., Enterline, J.P., Worrell, R.G. & Perry, S.L. (1985) Nutrition and prostate cancer: a case-control study. *Prostate*, **6**, 7–17

Heyman, R.A., Mangelsdorf, D.J., Dyck, J.A., Stein, R.B., Eichele, G., Evans, R.M. & Thaller, C. (1992) 9-*cis* Retinoic acid is a high affinity ligand for the retinoid X receptor. *Cell*, **68**, 397–406

Higuchi, C.M. & Wang, W. (1995) Comodulation of cellular polyamines and proliferation: biomarker application to colorectal mucosa. *J. Cell Biochem.*, **57**, 256–261

Hinds, M.W., Kolonel, L.N., Hankin, J.H. & Lee, J. (1984) Dietary vitamin A, carotene, vitamin C and risk of lung cancer in Hawaii. *Am. J. Epidemiol.*, **119**, 227–237

Ho, S.C., Donnan, S.P., Martin, C.W. & Tsao, S.Y. (1988) Dietary vitamin A, β-carotene and risk of epidermoid lung cancer among Chinese males. *Sing. Med. J.*, **29**, 213–218

Hofmann, C. & Eichele, G. (1994) Retinoids in development. In: Sporn, M.B., Roberts, A.B. & Goodman, D.S. (eds), *The Retinoids. Biology, Chemistry and Medicine*, 2nd edition, New York, Raven Press, pp. 387–441

Hogan, B.L., Thaller, C. & Eichele, G. (1992) Evidence that Hensen's node is a site of retinoic acid synthesis. *Nature*, **359**, 237–241

Hoglen, N.C., Abril, E.A., Sauer, J.M., Earnest, D.L., McCuskey, R.S., Lantz, R.C., Mobley, S.A. & Sipes, I.G. (1997) Modulation of Kupffer cell and peripheral blood monocyte activity by *in vivo* treatment of rats with all-*trans*-retinol. *Liver*, **17**, 157–165

Holder, N. & Hill, J. (1991) Retinoic acid modifies development of the midbrain-hindbrain border and affects cranial ganglion formation in zebrafish embryos. *Development*, **113**, 1159–1170

Holmberg, L., Ohlander, E.M., Byers, T., Zack, M., Wolk, A., Bergstrom, R., Bergkvist, L., Thurfjell, E., Bruce, A. & Adami, H.O. (1994) Diet and breast cancer risk. Results from a population-based, case-control study in Sweden. *Arch. Intern. Med.*, **154**, 1805–1811

Holtzman, S. (1988) Retinyl acetate inhibits estrogen-induced mammary carcinogenesis in female ACI rats. *Carcinogenesis*, **9**, 305–307

Hong, W.K., Endicott, J., Itri, L.M., Doos, W., Batsakis, J.G., Bell, R., Fofonoff, S., Byers, R., Atkinson, E.N., Vaughan, C., Toth, B.B., Kramer, A., Dimery, I.W., Skipper, P. & Strong, S. (1986) 13-*cis*-Retinoic acid in the treatment of oral leukoplakia. *New Engl. J. Med.*, **315**, 1501–1505

Hong, W.K., Lippman, S.M., Hittelman, W.N. & Lotan, R. (1995) Retinoid chemoprevention of aerodigestive cancer: from basic research to the clinic. *Clin. Cancer Res.*, **1**, 677–686

Honkanen, V., Konttinen, Y.T. & Mussalo Rauhamaa, H. (1989) Vitamins A and E, retinol binding protein and zinc in rheumatoid arthritis. *Clin. Exp. Rheumatol.*, **7**, 465–469

Horton, C. & Maden, M. (1995) Endogenous distribution of retinoids during normal development and teratogenesis in the mouse embryo. *Dev. Dyn.*, **202**, 312–323

Hossain, M.Z., Wilkens, L.R., Mehta, P.P., Loewenstein, W. & Bertram, J.S. (1989) Enhancement of gap junctional communication by retinoids correlates with their ability to inhibit neoplastic transformation. *Carcinogenesis*, **10**, 1743–1748

Howe, G.R., Hirohata, T., Hislop, T.G., Iscovich, J.M., Yuan, J.M., Katsouyanni, K., Lubin, F., Marubini, E., Modan, B., Rohan, T., Toniolo, P. & Yu, S.Z. (1990) Dietary factors and risk of breast cancer: combined analysis of 12 case-control studies. *J. Natl. Cancer Inst.*, **82**, 561–569

Hsing, A.W., McLaughlin, J.K., Schuman, L.M., Bjelke, E., Gridley, G., Wacholder, S., Chien, H.T. & Blot, W.J. (1990a) Diet, tobacco use, and fatal prostate cancer: results from the Lutheran Brotherhood Cohort Study. *Cancer Res.*, **50**, 6836–6840

Hsing, A.W., Comstock, G.W., Abbey, H. & Polk, B.F. (1990b) Serologic precursors of cancer. Retinol, carotenoids, and tocopherol and risk of prostate cancer. *J. Natl. Cancer Inst.*, **82**, 941–946

Hu, J., Nyren, O., Wolk, A., Bergstrom, R., Yuen, J., Adami, H.O., Guo, L., Li, H., Huang, G., Xu, X., Zhao, F., Chen, Y., Wang, C., Qin, H., Hu, C. & Li, Y. (1994) Risk factors for oesophageal cancer in northeast China. *Int. J. Cancer*, **57**, 38–46

Huang, C.C. (1987) Retinol (vitamin A) inhibition of dimethylnitrosamine (DMN) and diethylnitrosamine (DEN) induced sister-chromatid exchanges in V79 cells and mutations in *Salmo-nella*/microsome assays. *Mutat. Res.*, **187**, 133–140

Huang, C.C., Hsueh, J.L., Chen, H.H. & Batt, T.R. (1982) Retinol (vitamin A) inhibits sister chromatid exchanges and cell cycle delay induced by cyclophosphamide and aflatoxin B_1 in Chinese hamster V79 cells. *Carcinogenesis*, **3**, 1–5

Huang, C., Zhang, X., Qiao, Z., Guan, L., Peng, S., Liu, J., Xie, R. & Zheng, L. (1992) A case-control study of dietary factors in patients with lung cancer. *Biomed. Environ. Sci.*, **5**, 257–265

Huang, T.H., Ann, D.K., Zhang, Y.J., Chang, A.T., Crabb, J.W. & Wu, R. (1994) Control of keratin gene expression by vitamin A in tracheobronchial epithelial cells. *Am. J. Respir. Cell Mol. Biol.*, **10**, 192–201

Hubbard, R., Brown, P.K. & Brownds, D. (1971) Methodology of vitamin A and visual pigments. *Methods Enzymol.*, **18C**, 615–653

Hummler, H., Korte, R. & Hendrickx, A.G. (1990) Induction of malformations in the cynomolgus monkey with 13-*cis* retinoic acid. *Teratology*, **42**, 263–272

Hummler, H., Hendrickx, A.G. & Nau, H. (1994) Maternal toxicokinetics, metabolism, and embryo exposure following a teratogenic dosing regimen with 13-*cis*-retinoic acid (isotretinoin) in the cynomolgus monkey. *Teratology*, **50**, 184–193

Hunter, D.J., Colditz, G.A., Stampfer, M.J., Rosner, B., Willett, W.C. & Speizer, F.E. (1992) Diet and risk of basal cell carcinoma of the skin in a prospective cohort of women. *Ann. Epidemiol.*, **2**, 231–239

Hunter, D.J., Manson, J.E., Colditz, G.A., Stampfer, M.J., Rosner, B., Hennekens, C.H., Speizer, F.E. & Willett, W.C. (1993) A prospective study of the intake of vitamins C, E, and A and the risk of breast cancer. *New Engl. J. Med.*, **329**, 234–240

Hupert, J., Mobarhan, S., Layden, T.J., Papa, V.M. & Lucchesi, D.J. (1991) *In vitro* formation of retinoic acid from retinal in rat liver. *Biochem. Cell Biol.*, **69**, 509–514

Hussain, M.M., Goldberg, I.J., Weisgraber, K.H., Mahley, R.W. & Innerarity, T.L. (1997) Uptake of chylomicrons by the liver, but not by the bone marrow, is modulated by lipoprotein lipase activity. *Arterioscler. Thromb. Vasc. Biol.*, **17**, 1407–1413

Hussey, G.D. & Klein, M. (1990) A randomized, controlled trial of vitamin A in children with severe measles. *New Engl. J. Med.*, **323**, 160–164

IARC (1998) *IARC Handbooks of Cancer Prevention*, Vol. 2, *Carotenoids*, Lyon

Infante, M., Pastorino, U., Chiesa, G., Bera, E., Pisani, P., Valente, M. & Ravasi, G. (1991) Laboratory evaluation during high-dose vitamin A administration: a randomized study on lung cancer patients after surgical resection. *J. Cancer Res. Clin. Oncol.*, **117**, 156–162

Ingram, D.M., Nottage, E. & Roberts, T. (1991) The role of diet in the development of breast cancer: a case-control study of patients with breast cancer, benign epithelial hyperplasia and fibrocystic disease of the breast. *Br. J. Cancer*, **64**, 187–191

Inoue, I., Yamamoto, Y., Ito, T. & Takahashi, H. (1993) Chemoprevention of tongue carcinogenesis in rats. *Oral Surg. Oral Med. Oral Pathol.*, **76**, 608–615

Inoue, I., Yamamoto, Y., Takasaki, T. & Takahashi, H. (1995) Inhibitory effects of selenium, vitamin A and butylated hydroxytoluene on *in vitro* growth of human tongue cancer cells. *Eur. Arch. Otorhinolaryngol.*, **252**, 509–512

Ioannides, C., Ayrton, A.D., Keele, A., Lewis, D.F., Flatt, P.R. & Walker, R. (1990) Mechanism of the *in vitro* antimutagenic action of retinol. *Mutagenesis*, **5**, 257–262

Ishibashi, S., Herz, J., Maeda, N., Goldstein, J.L. & Brown, M.S. (1994) The two-receptor model of lipoprotein clearance: tests of the hypothesis in "knockout" mice lacking the low density lipoprotein receptor, apolipoprotein E, or both proteins. *Proc. Natl. Acad. Sci. USA.*, **91**, 4431–4435

Ishibashi, S., Perrey, S., Chen, Z., Osuga Ji, Shimada, M., Ohashi, K., Harada, K., Yazaki, Y. & Yamada, N. (1996) Role of the low density lipoprotein (LDL) receptor pathway in the metabolism of chylomicron remnants. A quantitative study in knockout mice lacking the LDL receptor, apolipoprotein E, or both. *J. Biol. Chem.*, **271**, 22422–22427

Isler, O., Ronco, A., Guex, W., Hindley, N.C., Huber, W., Dialer, K. & Kofler, M. (1949) Uber die Ester und Ather des synthetischen Vitamins A. *Helv. Chim. Acta*, **32**, 489–505

Isler, O., Gutmann, H. & Solms, U. (1971) *Carotenoids*, Basel, Birkhäuser Verlag

Isono, T. & Seto, A. (1991) Antitumor effects of vitamin A against Shope carcinoma cells. *Cancer Lett.*, **59**, 25–29

Issing, W.J., Struck, R. & Naumann, A. (1997) Positive impact of retinyl palmitate in leukoplakia of the larynx. *Eur. Arch. Otorhinolaryngol. Suppl.*, **254**, S105–S109

Jain, M., Burch, J.D., Howe, G.R., Risch, H.A. & Miller, A.B. (1990) Dietary factors and risk of lung cancer: results from a case-control study, Toronto, 1981-1985. *Int. J. Cancer*, **45**, 287–293

Janowski, B.A., Willy, P.J., Devi, T.R., Falck, J.R. & Mangelsdorf, D.J. (1996) An oxysterol signalling pathway mediated by the nuclear receptor LXRα. *Nature*, **383**, 728–731

Jendryczko, A. & Drozdz, M. (1989) Plasma retinol, β-carotene and vitamin E levels in relation to the future risk of pre-eclampsia. *Zentralbl. Gynakol.*, **111**, 1121–1123

Jetten, A.M., Nervi, C., Saunders, N.A., Vollberg, T.M., Fujimoto, W. & Noji, S. (1993) Role of nuclear retinoic acid receptors in the control of differentiation of epidermal keratinocytes. In: Hong, W.K. & Lotan, R. (eds), *Retinoids in Oncology*, New York, Marcel Dekker, pp. 73–88

Ji, Z.S., Fazio, S., Lee, Y.L. & Mahley, R.W. (1994) Secretion-capture role for apolipoprotein E in remnant lipoprotein metabolism involving cell surface heparan sulfate proteoglycans. *J. Biol. Chem.*, **269**, 2764–2772

Ji, Z.S., Sanan, D.A. & Mahley, R.W. (1995) Intravenous heparinase inhibits remnant lipoprotein clearance from the plasma and uptake by the liver: *in vivo* role of heparan sulfate proteoglycans. *J. Lipid Res.*, **36**, 583–592

Jollie, W.P. (1990) Development, morphology, and function of the yolk-sac placenta of laboratory rodents. *Teratology*, **41**, 361–381

Jyothirmayi, R., Ramadas, K., Varghese, C., Jacob, R., Nair, M.K. & Sankaranarayanan, R. (1996) Efficacy of vitamin A in the prevention of loco-regional recurrence and second primaries in head and neck cancer. *Eur. J. Cancer B. Oral Oncol.*, **32B**, 373–376

Kalandidi, A., Katsouyanni, K., Voropoulou, N., Bastas, G., Saracci, R. & Trichopoulos, D. (1990) Passive smoking and diet in the etiology of lung cancer among non-smokers. *Cancer Causes Control*, **1**, 15–21

Kalter, H. & Warkany, J. (1959) Experimental production of congenital malformations in mammals by metabolic procedure. *Physiol. Rev.*, **39**, 69–115

Kalter, H. & Warkany, J. (1961) Experimental production of congenital anomalies in strains of inbred mice by maternal treatment with hypervitaminosis A. *Am. J. Pathol.*, **38**, 1–15

Kamm, J.J., Ashenfelter, K.O. & Ehmann, C.W. (1984) Preclinical and clinical toxicology of selected retinoids. In: Sporn, M.B., Roberts, A.B. & Goodman, D.S. (eds), *The Retinoids*, Orlando, Academic Press, pp. 287–326

Kanamaru, H., Hashimura, T. & Yoshida, O. (1988) Effects of retinoids and inhibitors of arachidonic acid metabolism on tumor-promoter-induced soft agar colony formation of mouse epidermal cells and rat urinary bladder cells. *Jpn. J. Cancer Res.*, **79**, 1043–1047

Karagas, M.R., Greenberg, E.R., Nierenberg, D., Stukel, T.A., Morris, J.S., Stevens, M.M. & Baron, J.A. (1997) Risk of squamous cell carcinoma of the skin in relation to plasma selenium, α-tocopherol, β-carotene, and retinol: a nested case-control study. *Cancer Epidemiol. Biomarkers Prev.*, **6**, 25–29

Karpe, F., Olivecrona, T., Hamsten, A. & Hultin, M. (1997) Chylomicron/chylomicron remnant turnover in humans: evidence for margination of chylomicrons and poor conversion of larger to smaller chylomicron remnants. *J. Lipid Res.*, **38**, 949–961

Kastner, P., Grondona, J.M., Mark, M., Gansmuller, A., LeMeur, M., Decimo, D., Vonesch, J.L., Dolle, P. & Chambon, P. (1994) Genetic analysis of RXRα developmental function: convergence of RXR and RAR signaling pathways in heart and eye morphogenesis. *Cell*, **78**, 987–1003

Kastner, P., Mark, M., Leid, M., Gansmuller, A., Chin, W., Grondona, J.M., Decimo, D., Krezel, W., Dierich, A. & Chambon, P. (1996) Abnormal spermatogenesis in RXRβ mutant mice. *Genes Dev.*, **10**, 80–92

Kastner, P., Mark, M., Ghyselinck, N., Krezel, W., Dupe, V., Grondona, J.M. & Chambon, P. (1997) Genetic evidence that the retinoid signal is transduced by heterodimeric RXR/RAR functional units during mouse development. *Development*, **124**, 313–326

Katsouyanni, K., Willett, W., Trichopoulos, D., Boyle, P., Trichopoulou, A., Vasilaros, S., Papadiamantis, J. & MacMahon, B. (1988) Risk of breast cancer among Greek women in relation to nutrient intake. *Cancer*, **61**, 181–185

Kaul, S. & Olson, J.A. (1998) Effect of vitamin A deficiency on the hydrolysis of retinoyl β-glucuronide to retinoic acid by rat tissue organelles *in vitro*. *Int. J. Vitam. Nutr. Res.*, **68**, 232–236

Kawamura, H. & Hashimoto, Y. (1980) Vitamin A receptor in cancers and *in vitro*-transformed epithelial cells of the rat urinary bladder: its implication in the preventive effect of vitamin A on *in vitro* keratinization. *Gann.*, **71**, 507–513

Keidel, S., Rupp, E. & Szardenings, M. (1992) Recombinant human retinoic acid receptor a. Binding of DNA and synthetic retinoids to the protein expressed in *Escherichia coli*. *Eur. J. Biochem.*, **204**, 1141–1148

Keilson, B., Underwood, B.A. & Loerch, J.D. (1979) Effects of retinoic acid on the mobilization of vitamin A from the liver in rats. *J. Nutr.*, **109**, 787–795

Kelloff, G.J., Crowell, J.A., Boone, C.W., Steele, V.E., Lubet, R.A., Greenwald, P., Alberts, D.S., Covey, J.M., Doody, L.A., Knapp, G.G., Nayfield, S., Parkinson, D.R., Prasad, V.K., Prorok, P.C., Sausville, E.A. & Sigman, C.C. (1994) Strategy and planning for chemopreventive drug development: clinical development plans. Chemoprevention Branch and Agent Development Committee. National Cancer Institute. *J. Cell Biochem.*, **Suppl. 20**, 55–62

Kelloff, G.J., Crowell, J.A., Hawk, E.T., Steele, V.E., Lubet, R.A., Boone, C.W., Covey, J.M., Doody, L.A., Omenn, G.S., Greenwald, P., Hong, W.K., Parkinson, D.R., Bagheri, D., Baxter, G.T., Blunden, M., Doeltz, M.K., Eisenhauer, K.M., Johnson, K., Knapp, G.G., Longfellow, D.G., Malone, W.F., Nayfield, S.G., Seifried, H.E., Swall, L.M. & Sigman, C.C. (1996) Clinical development plans for cancer chemopreventive agents: Vitamin A. *J. Cell Biochem.*, **Suppl. 26**, 269–306

Kelly, G.E., Meikle, W.D. & Sheil, A.G. (1989) Effects of oral retinoid (vitamin A and etretinate) therapy on photocarcinogenesis in hairless mice. *Photochem. Photobiol.*, **50**, 213–215

Key, T., Oakes, S., Davey, G., Moore, J., Edmond, L.M., McLoone, U.J. & Thurnham, D.I. (1996) Stability of vitamins A, C, and E, carotenoids, lipids, and testosterone in whole blood stored at 4°C for 6 and 24 hours before separation of serum and plasma. *Cancer Epidemiol. Biomarkers. Prev.*, **5**, 811–814

Khachik, F., Spangler, C.J., Smith, J.C. Jr, Canfield, L.M., Steck, A. & Pfander, H. (1997) Identification, quantification, and relative concentrations of carotenoids and their metabolites in human milk and serum. *Anal. Chem.*, **69**, 1873–1881

Khoury, M.J., Moore, C.A. & Mulinare, J. (1996) Vitamin A and birth defects. *Lancet*, **347**, 322–322

Kim, K.H., Schwartz, F. & Fuchs, E. (1984) Differences in keratin synthesis between normal epithelial cells and squamous cell carcinomas are mediated by vitamin A. *Proc. Natl. Acad. Sci. USA*, **81**, 4280–4284

Kirkpatrick, C.S., White, E. & Lee, J.A. (1994) Case-control study of malignant melanoma in Washington State. II. Diet, alcohol, and obesity. *Am. J. Epidemiol.*, **139**, 869–880

Kistler, A. (1981) Teratogenesis of retinoic acid in rats: susceptible stages and suppression of retinoic acid-induced limb malformations by cycloheximide. *Teratology*, **23**, 25–31

Kistler, A. (1987) Limb bud cell cultures for estimating the teratogenic potential of compounds. Validation of the test system with retinoids. *Arch. Toxicol.*, **60**, 403–414

Kitamura, H., Shibagaki, T., Inayama, Y., Ito, T. & Kanisawa, M. (1990) Growth and differentiation of human distal airway epithelial cells in culture. Effects of small amounts of serum in defined medium. *Lab. Invest.*, **63**, 420–428

Kitamura, Y., Tanaka, K., Kiyohara, C., Hirohata, T., Tomita, Y., Ishibashi, M. & Kido, K. (1997) Relationship of alcohol use, physical activity and dietary habits with serum carotenoids, retinol and α-tocopherol among male Japanese smokers. *Int. J. Epidemiol.*, **26**, 307–314

Knasmüller, S., Huber, W.W., Kienzl, H. & Schulte-Hermann, R. (1992) Inhibition of repairable DNA-damage in *Escherichia coli* K-12 cells recovered from various organs of nitrosamine-treated mice by vitamin A, phenethylisothiocyanate, oleic acid and triolein. *Carcinogenesis*, **13**, 1643–1650

Knekt, P., Aromaa, A., Maatela, J., Aaran, R.K., Nikkari, T., Hakama, M., Hakulinen, T., Peto, R. & Teppo, L. (1990) Serum vitamin A and subsequent risk of cancer: cancer incidence follow-up of the Finnish Mobile Clinic Health Examination Survey. *Am. J. Epidemiol.*, **132**, 857–870

Knekt, P., Järvinen, R., Seppänen, R., Rissanen, A., Aromaa, A., Heinonen, O.P., Albanes, D., Heinonen, M., Pukkala, E. & Teppo, L. (1991a) Dietary antioxidants and the risk of lung cancer. *Am. J. Epidemiol.*, **134**, 471–479

Knekt, P., Aromaa, A., Maatela, J., Alfthan, G., Aaran, R.K., Nikkari, T., Hakama, M., Hakulinen, T. & Teppo, L. (1991b) Serum micronutrients and risk of cancers of low incidence in Finland. *Am. J. Epidemiol.*, **134**, 356–361

Knook, D.L., Bosma, A. & Seifert, W.F. (1995) Role of vitamin A in liver fibrosis. *J. Gastroenterol. Hepatol.*, **10 Suppl. 1**, S47–49

Koch, H.F. (1978) Biochemical treatment of precancerous oral lesions: the effectiveness of various analogues of retinoic acid. *J. Maxillofac. Surg.*, **6**, 59–63

Koch, H.F. (1981) Effect of retinoids on precancerous lesions in oral mucosa. In: Orfanos, C.E. (ed.), *Retinoids. Advances in Basic Research and Therapy*, Berlin, Springer Verlag, pp. 307–312

Kochhar, D.M., Penner, J.D. & Satre, M.A. (1988) Derivation of retinoic acid and metabolites from a teratogenic dose of retinol (vitamin A) in mice. *Toxicol. Appl. Pharmacol.*, **96**, 429–441

Kolonel, L.N., Hankin, J.H. & Yoshizawa, C.N. (1987) Vitamin A and prostate cancer in elderly men: enhancement of risk. *Cancer Res.*, **47**, 2982–2985

Kolonel, L.N., Yoshizawa, C.N. & Hankin, J.H. (1988) Diet and prostatic cancer: a case-control study in Hawaii. *Am. J. Epidemiol.*, **127**, 999–1012

Koo, L.C. (1988) Dietary habits and lung cancer risk among Chinese females in Hong Kong who never smoked. *Nutr. Cancer*, **11**, 155–172

Kowalski, T.E., Falestiny, M., Furth, E. & Malet, P.F. (1994) Vitamin A hepatotoxicity: a cautionary note regarding 25,000 IU supplements. *Am. J. Med.*, **97**, 523–528

Kraft, J.C., Kochhar, D.M., Scott, W.J. & Nau, H. (1987) Low teratogenicity of 13-*cis*-retinoic acid (isotretinoin) in the mouse corresponds to low embryo concentrations during organogenesis: comparison to the all-*trans* isomer. *Toxicol. Appl. Pharmacol.*, **87**, 474–482

Kraft, J.C., Shepard, T. & Juchau, M.R. (1993) Tissue levels of retinoids in human embryos/fetuses. *Reprod. Toxicol.*, **7**, 11–15

Kraft, J.C., Schuh, T., Juchau, M. & Kimelman, D. (1994) The retinoid X receptor ligand, 9-*cis*-retinoic acid, is a potential regulator of early *Xenopus* development. *Proc. Natl. Acad. Sci. USA*, **91**, 3067–3071

Krasinski, S.D., Cohn, J.S., Schaefer, E.J. & Russell, R.M. (1990a) Postprandial plasma retinyl ester response is greater in older subjects compared with younger subjects. Evidence for delayed plasma clearance of intestinal lipoproteins. *J. Clin. Invest.*, **85**, 883–892

Krasinski, S.D., Cohn, J.S., Russell, R.M. & Schaefer, E.J. (1990b) Postprandial plasma vitamin A metabolism in humans: a reassessment of the use of plasma retinyl esters as markers for intestinally derived chylomicrons and their remnants. *Metabolism*, **39**, 357–365

Krinsky, N.I., Wang, X.D., Tang, G. & Russell, R.M. (1993) Mechanism of carotenoid cleavage to retinoids. *Ann. N. Y. Acad. Sci.*, **691**, 167–176

Kroschwitz, I. (1998) *Kirk-Othmer Encyclopedia of Chemical Technology*, New York, John Wiley

Kudo, S. (1989) Morphology of the release of vitamin A-containing lipid droplets by perisinusoidal lipocytes in the rat liver. *Acta Anat. Basel.*, **135**, 261–268

Kumar, R., Shoemaker, A.R. & Verma, A.K. (1994) Retinoic acid nuclear receptors and tumor promotion: decreased expression of retinoic acid nuclear receptors by the tumor promoter 12-O-tetradecanoylphorbol-13-acetate. *Carcinogenesis*, **15**, 701–705

Kumari, D. & Sinha, S.P. (1994) Effect of retinol on ochratoxin-produced genotoxicity in mice. *Food Chem. Toxicol.*, **32**, 471–475

Kune, G.A., Kune, S., Watson, L.F., Pierce, R., Field, B., Vitetta, L., Merenstein, D., Hayes, A. & Irving, L. (1989) Serum levels of β-carotene, vitamin A, and zinc in male lung cancer cases and controls. *Nutr. Cancer*, **12**, 169–176

Kune, G.A., Bannerman, S., Field, B., Watson, L.F., Cleland, H., Merenstein, D. & Vitetta, L. (1992) Diet, alcohol, smoking, serum β-carotene, and vitamin A in male nonmelanocytic skin cancer patients and controls. *Nutr. Cancer*, **18**, 237–244

Kune, G.A., Kune, S., Field, B., Watson, L.F., Cleland, H., Merenstein, D. & Vitetta, L. (1993) Oral and pharyngeal cancer, diet, smoking, alcohol, and serum vitamin A and β-carotene levels: a case-control study in men. *Nutr. Cancer*, **20**, 61–70

Kurlandsky, S.B., Xiao, J.H., Duell, E.A., Voorhees, J.J. & Fisher, G.J. (1994) Biological activity of all-*trans* retinol requires metabolic conversion to all-*trans* retinoic acid and is mediated through activation of nuclear retinoid receptors in human keratinocytes. *J. Biol. Chem.*, **269**, 32821–32827

Kurlandsky, S.B., Gamble, M.V., Ramakrishnan, R. & Blaner, W.S. (1995) Plasma delivery of retinoic acid to tissues in the rat. *J. Biol. Chem.,* **270,** 17850–17857

Kuroda, Y. (1990) Antimutagenic activity of vitamins in cultured mammalian cells. In: Kuroda, Y., Shankel, D.M. & Waters, M.D. (eds), *Anti-mutagenesis and Anticarcinogenesis Mechanisms II,* New York, Plenum Press, pp. 233–256

Kurokawa, Y., Hayashi, Y., Maekawa, A., Takahashi, M. & Kukubo, T. (1985) High incidences of pheochromocytomas after long-term administration of retinol acetate to F344/DuCrj rats. *J. Natl. Cancer Inst.,* **74,** 715–723

Kushi, L.H., Fee, R.M., Sellers, T.A., Zheng, W. & Folsom, A.R. (1996a) Intake of vitamins A, C, and E and postmenopausal breast cancer. The Iowa Women's Health Study. *Am. J. Epidemiol.,* **144,** 165–174

Kushi, L.H., Folsom, A.R., Prineas, R.J., Mink, P.J., Wu, Y. & Bostick, R.M. (1996b) Dietary antioxidant vitamins and death from coronary heart disease in postmenopausal women. *New Engl. J. Med.,* **334,** 1156–1162

Kvåle, G., Bjelke, E. & Gart, J.J. (1983) Dietary habits and lung cancer risk. *Int. J. Cancer,* **31,** 397–405

La Vecchia, C., Negri, E., Decarli, A., D'Avanzo, B. & Franceschi, S. (1987a) A case-control study of diet and gastric cancer in northern Italy. *Int. J. Cancer,* **40,** 484–489

La Vecchia, C., Decarli, A., Franceschi, S., Gentile, A., Negri, E. & Parazzini, F. (1987b) Dietary factors and the risk of breast cancer. *Nutr. Cancer,* **10,** 205–214

La Vecchia, C., Decarli, A., Fasoli, M., Parazzini, F., Franceschi, S., Gentile, A. & Negri, E. (1988) Dietary vitamin A and the risk of intraepithelial and invasive cervical neoplasia. *Gynecol. Oncol.,* **30,** 187–195

La Vecchia, C., Negri, E., Decarli, A., D'Avanzo, B., Liberati, C. & Franceschi, S. (1989) Dietary factors in the risk of bladder cancer. *Nutr. Cancer,* **12,** 93–101

La Vecchia, C., Ferraroni, M., D'Avanzo, B., Decarli, A. & Franceschi, S. (1994) Selected micronutrient intake and the risk of gastric cancer. *Cancer Epidemiol. Biomarkers Prev.,* **3,** 393–398

La Vecchia, C., Braga, C., Negri, E., Franceschi, S., Russo, A., Conti, E., Falcini, F., Giacosa, A., Montella, M. & Decarli, A. (1997) Intake of selected micronutrients and risk of colorectal cancer. *Int. J. Cancer,* **73,** 525–530

Labrecque, J., Bhat, P.V. & Lacroix, A. (1993) Purification and partial characterization of a rat kidney aldehyde dehydrogenase that oxidizes retinal to retinoic acid. *Biochem. Cell Biol.,* **71,** 85–89

Labrecque, J., Dumas, F., Lacroix, A. & Bhat, P.V. (1995) A novel isoenzyme of aldehyde dehydrogenase specifically involved in the biosynthesis of 9-*cis* and all-*trans* retinoic acid. *Biochem. J.,* **305,** 681–684

Lambert, B., Brisson, G. & Bielmann, P. (1981) Plasma vitamin A and precancerous lesions of cervix uteri: a preliminary report. *Gynecol. Oncol.,* **11,** 136–139

Lamm, D.L., Riggs, D.R., Shriver, J.S., vanGilder, P.F., Rach, J.F. & DeHaven, J.I. (1994) Megadose vitamins in bladder cancer: a double-blind clinical trial. *J. Urol.,* **151,** 21–26

Lammer, E.J., Chen, D.T., Hoar, R.M., Agnish, N.D., Benke, P.J., Braun, J.T., Curry, C.J., Fernhoff, P.M., Grix, A.W., Jr, Lott, I.T., Richard, J.M. & Sun, S.C. (1985) Retinoic acid embryopathy. *New Engl. J. Med.,* **313,** 837–841

Lampron, C., Rochette Egly, C., Gorry, P., Dolle, P., Mark, M., Lufkin, T., LeMeur, M. & Chambon, P. (1995) Mice deficient in cellular retinoic acid binding protein II (CRABPII) or in both CRABPI and CRABPII are essentially normal. *Development,* **121,** 539–548

Lasnitzki, I. (1955) The influence of A-hypervitaminosis on the effect of 20-methylcholanthrene on mouse prostate gland *in vitro. Br. J. Cancer,* **9,** 434–441

Lasnitzki, I. (1962) Hypovitaminosis A in the mouse prostate gland cultured in chemically defined medium. *Exp. Cell Res.,* **28,** 40–51

Lasnitzki, I. & Goodman, D.S. (1974) Inhibition of the effects of methylcholanthrene on mouse prostate in organ culture by vitamin A and its analogs. *Cancer Res.,* **34,** 1564–1571

Le Marchand, L., Yoshizawa, C.N., Kolonel, L.N., Hankin, J.H. & Goodman, M.T. (1989) Vegetable consumption and lung cancer risk: a population-based case-control study in Hawaii. *J. Natl. Cancer Inst.,* **81,** 1158–1164

Le Marchand, L., Hankin, J.H., Kolonel, L.N. & Wilkens, L.R. (1991) Vegetable and fruit consumption in relation to prostate cancer risk in Hawaii: a reevaluation of the effect of dietary β-carotene. *Am. J. Epidemiol.,* **133**, 215–219

Lederman, J.D., Overton, K.M., Hofmann, N.E., Moore, B.J., Thornton, J. & Erdman, J.W. (1998) Ferrets (*Mustela putoius furo*) inefficiently convert β-carotene to vitamin A. *J. Nutr.,* **128**, 271–279

Lee, M.O., Manthey, C.L. & Sladek, N.E. (1991) Identification of mouse liver aldehyde dehydrogenases that catalyze the oxidation of retinaldehyde to retinoic acid. *Biochem. Pharmacol.,* **42**, 1279–1285

Leo, M.A. & Lieber, C.S. (1983) Hepatic fibrosis after long-term administration of ethanol and moderate vitamin A supplementation in the rat. *Hepatology,* **3**, 1–11

Leo, M.A., Iida, S. & Lieber, C.S. (1984) Retinoic acid metabolism by a system reconstituted with cytochrome P-450. *Arch. Biochem. Biophys.,* **234**, 305–312

Leo, M.A., Lasker, J.M., Raucy, J.L., Kim, C.I., Black, M. & Lieber, C.S. (1989) Metabolism of retinol and retinoic acid by human liver cytochrome P450IIC8. *Arch. Biochem. Biophys.,* **269**, 305–312

Lettinga, K.D., Gutter, W., Van Noorden, C.J., Schellens, J.P. & Frederiks, W.M. (1996) Early effects of high doses of retinol (vitamin A) on the *in situ* cellular metabolism in rat liver. *Liver,* **16**, 1–11

Levin, A.A., Sturzenbecker, L.J., Kazmer, S., Bosakowski, T., Huselton, C., Allenby, G., Speck, J., Kratzeisen, C., Rosenberger, M., Lovey, A. & Grippo, J.F. (1992) 9-cis retinoic acid stereoisomer binds and activates the nuclear receptor RXRα. *Nature,* **355**, 359–361

Levine, N., Moon, T.E., Cartmel, B., Bangert, J.L., Rodney, S., Dong, Q., Peng, Y.M. & Alberts, D.S. (1997) Trial of retinol and isotretinoin in skin cancer prevention: a randomized, double-blind, controlled trial. Southwest Skin Cancer Prevention Study Group. *Cancer Epidemiol. Biomarkers. Prev.,* **6**, 957–961

Lewis, K.C., Green, M.H. & Underwood, B.A. (1981) Vitamin A turnover in rats as influenced by vitamin A status. *J. Nutr.,* **111**, 1135–1144

Lewis, K.C., Green, M.H., Green, J.B. & Zech, L.A. (1990) Retinol metabolism in rats with low vitamin A status: a compartmental model. *J. Lipid Res.,* **31**, 1535–1548

Li, E. & Norris, A.W. (1996) Structure/function of cytoplasmic vitamin A-binding proteins. *Annu. Rev. Nutr.,* **16**, 205–234

Li, J.Y., Taylor, P.R., Li, B., Dawsey, S., Wang, G.Q., Ershow, A.G., Guo, W., Liu, S.F., Yang, C.S., Shen, Q., Wang, W., Mark, S.D., Zou, X.N., Greenwald, P., Wu, Y.P. & Blot, W.J. (1993) Nutrition intervention trials in Linxian, China: multiple vitamin/ mineral supplementation, cancer incidence, and disease-specific mortality among adults with esophageal dysplasia. *J. Natl. Cancer Inst.,* **85**, 1492–1498

Lingen, M.W., Polverini, P.J. & Bouck, N.P. (1996) Inhibition of squamous cell carcinoma angiogenesis by direct interaction of retinoic acid with endothelial cells. *Lab. Invest.,* **74**, 476–483

Lippman, S.M., Batsakis, J.G., Toth, B.B., Weber, R.S., Lee, J.J., Martin, J.W., Hays, G.L., Goepfert, H. & Hong, W.K. (1993) Comparison of low-dose isotretinoin with β-carotene to prevent oral carcinogenesis. *New Engl. J. Med.,* **328**, 15–20

Liu, T., Soong, S.J., Alvarez, R.D. & Butterworth, C.E. Jr (1995) A longitudinal analysis of human papillomavirus 16 infection, nutritional status, and cervical dysplasia progression. *Cancer Epidemiol. Biomarkers Prev.,* **4**, 373–380

Livrea, M.A., Tesoriere, L., Bongiorno, A., Pintaudi, A.M., Ciaccio, M. & Riccio, A. (1995) Contribution of vitamin A to the oxidation resistance of human low density lipoproteins. *Free Radic. Biol. Med.,* **18**, 401–409

Lohnes, D., Kastner, P., Dierich, A., Mark, M., LeMeur, M. & Chambon, P. (1993) Function of retinoic acid receptor γ in the mouse. *Cell,* **73**, 643–658

Lohnes, D., Mark, M., Mendelsohn, C., Dolle, P., Decimo, D., LeMeur, M., Dierich, A., Gorry, P. & Chambon, P. (1995) Developmental roles of the retinoic acid receptors. *J. Steroid Biochem. Mol. Biol.,* **53**, 475–486

London, S.J., Stein, E.A., Henderson, I.C., Stampfer, M.J., Wood, W.C., Remine, S., Dmochowski, J.R., Robert, N.J. & Willett, W.C. (1992) Carotenoids, retinol, and vitamin E and risk of proliferative benign breast disease and breast cancer. *Cancer Causes Control,* **3**, 503–512

Long, C. (1961) Table of vital statistics. *Biochem. Handbook,* Cleveland, CRC Press, pp. 639

Longnecker, M.P., Newcomb, P.A., Mittendorf, R., Greenberg, E.R. & Willett, W.C. (1997) Intake of carrots, spinach, and supplements containing vitamin A in relation to risk of breast cancer. *Cancer Epidemiol. Biomarkers Prev.,* **6**, 887–892

Look, J., Landwehr, J., Bauer, F., Hoffmann, A.S., Bluethmann, H. & LeMotte, P. (1995) Marked resistance of RARγ-deficient mice to the toxic effects of retinoic acid. *Am. J. Physiol.,* **269**, E91–E98

Lotan, R. (1996) Retinoids in cancer chemoprevention. *FASEB J.,* **10**, 1031–1039

Lotan, R. & Nicolson, G.L. (1977) Inhibitory effects of retinoic acid or retinyl acetate on the growth of untransformed, transformed, and tumor cells *in vitro. J. Natl. Cancer Inst.,* **59**, 1717–1722

Lotan, R., Giotta, G., Nork, E. & Nicolson, G.L. (1978) Characterization of the inhibitory effects of retinoids on the *in vitro* growth of two malignant murine melanomas. *J. Natl. Cancer Inst.,* **60**, 1035–1041

Lotan, R., Xu, X.C., Lippman, S.M., Ro, J.Y., Lee, J.S., Lee, J.J. & Hong, W.K. (1995) Suppression of retinoic acid receptor-β in premalignant oral lesions and its up-regulation by isotretinoin. *New Engl. J. Med.,* **332**, 1405–1410

Lufkin, T., Lohnes, D., Mark, M., Dierich, A., Gorry, P., Gaub, M.P., LeMeur, M. & Chambon, P. (1993) High postnatal lethality and testis degeneration in retinoic acid receptor α mutant mice. *Proc. Natl. Acad. Sci. USA.,* **90**, 7225–7229

Lupulescu, A. (1986) Inhibition of DNA synthesis and neoplastic cell growth by vitamin A (retinol). *J. Natl. Cancer Inst.,* **77**, 149–156

Lyn, S. & Giguere, V. (1994) Localization of CRABP-I and CRABP-II mRNA in the early mouse embryo by whole-mount *in situ* hybridization: implications for teratogenesis and neural development. *Dev. Dyn.,* **199**, 280–291

Lyon, J.L., Mahoney, A.W., West, D.W., Gardner, J.W., Smith, K.R., Sorenson, A.W. & Stanish, W. (1987) Energy intake: its relationship to colon cancer risk. *J. Natl. Cancer Inst.,* **78**, 853–861

Mackerras, D., Buffler, P.A., Randall, D.E., Nichaman, M.Z., Pickle, L.W. & Mason, T.J. (1988) Carotene intake and the risk of laryngeal cancer in coastal Texas. *Am. J. Epidemiol.,* **128**, 980–988

Maden, M. (1994) Distribution of cellular retinoic acid-binding proteins I and II in the chick embryo and their relationship to teratogenesis. *Teratology,* **50**, 294–301

Mahley, R.W. & Hussain, M.M. (1991) Chylomicron and chylomicron remnant catabolism. *Curr. Opin. Lipidol.,* **2**, 170–176

Maiorana, A. & Gullino, P.M. (1980) Effect of retinyl acetate on the incidence of mammary carcinomas and hepatomas in mice. *J. Natl. Cancer Inst.,* **64**, 655–663

Malkovsky, M., Dore, C., Hunt, R., Palmer, L., Chandler, P. & Medawar, P.B. (1983) Enhancement of specific antitumor immunity in mice fed a diet enriched in vitamin A acetate. *Proc. Natl. Acad. Sci. USA.,* **80**, 6322–6326

Malkovsky, M., Hunt, R., Palmer, L., Dore, C. & Medawar, P.B. (1984) Retinyl acetate-mediated augmentation of resistance to a transplantable 3-methylcholanthrene-induced fibrosarcoma. The dose response and time course. *Transplantation,* **38**, 158–161

Mangelsdorf, D.J. & Evans, R.M. (1995) The RXR heterodimers and orphan receptors. *Cell,* **83**, 841–850

Mangelsdorf, D.J., Borgmeyer, U., Heyman, R.A., Zhou, J.Y., Ong, E.S., Oro, A.E., Kakizuka, A. & Evans, R.M. (1992) Characterization of three RXR genes that mediate the action of 9-*cis* retinoic acid. *Genes Dev.,* **6**, 329–344

Mangelsdorf, D.J., Umesono, K. & Evans, R.M. (1994) The retinoid receptors. In: Sporn, M.B., Roberts, A.B. & Goodman, D.S. (eds), *The Retinoids: Biology, Chemistry, and Medicine,* 2nd edition, New York, Raven Press, pp. 319–350

Mann, C.J., Khallou, J., Chevreuil, O., Troussard, A.A., Guermani, L.M., Launay, K., Delplanque, B., Yen, F.T. & Bihain, B.E. (1995) Mechanism of activation and functional significance of the lipolysis-stimulated receptor. Evidence for a role as chylomicron remnant receptor. *Biochemistry,* **34**, 10421–10431

Manson, J.E., Stampfer, M.J., Willett, W.C., Colditz, G.A., Rosner, B., Speizer, F.E. & Hennekens, C.H. (1991) A prospective study of antioxidant vitamins and incidence of coronary heart disease in women. *Circulation,* **84, Suppl. II**, 2168

Marchok, A.C., Clark, J.N. & Klein Szanto, A. (1981) Modulation of growth, differentiation, and mucous glycoprotein synthesis by retinyl acetate in cloned carcinoma cell lines. *J. Natl. Cancer Inst.*, **66**, 1165–1174

Marnett, L.J. & Ji, C. (1994) Modulation of oxidant formation in mouse skin *in vivo* by tumor-promoting phorbol esters. *Cancer Res.*, **54**, 1886s–1889s

Marsden, J.R. (1989) Lipid metabolism and retinoid therapy. *Pharmacol. Ther.*, **40**, 55–65

Marshall, J., Graham, S., Mettlin, C., Shedd, D. & Swanson, M. (1982) Diet in the epidemiology of oral cancer. *Nutr. Cancer*, **3**, 145–149

Marshall, J.R., Graham, S., Byers, T., Swanson, M. & Brasure, J. (1983) Diet and smoking in the epidemiology of cancer of the cervix. *J. Natl. Cancer Inst.*, **70**, 847–851

Martinez Frias, M.L. & Salvador, J. (1990) Epidemiological aspects of prenatal exposure to high doses of vitamin A in Spain. *Eur. J. Epidemiol.*, **6**, 118–123

Marubini, E., Decarli, A., Costa, A., Mazzoleni, C., Andreoli, C., Barbieri, A., Capitelli, E., Carlucci, M., Cavallo, F., Monferroni, N., Pastorino, U. & Salvini, S. (1988) The relationship of dietary intake and serum levels of retinol and β-carotene with breast cancer. Results of a case-control study. *Cancer*, **61**, 173–180

Matsuno, T. (1991) Xanthophylls as precursors of retinoids. *Pure Appl. Chem.*, **63**, 81–88

Matsuura, T. & Ross, A.C. (1993) Regulation of hepatic lecithin: retinol acyltransferase activity by retinoic acid. *Arch. Biochem. Biophys.*, **301**, 221–227

Matsuura, T., Nagamori, S., Hasumura, S., Sujino, H., Shimizu, K., Niiya, M. & Hirosawa, K. (1993a) Retinol transport in cultured stellate cells of rat liver: studies by light and electron microscope autoradiography. *Exp. Cell Res.*, **206**, 111–118

Matsuura, T., Nagamori, S., Hasumura, S., Sujino, H., Niiya, M. & Shimizu, K. (1993b) Regulation of vitamin A transport into cultured stellate cells of rat liver: studies by anchored cell analysis and sorting system. *Exp. Cell Res.*, **209**, 33–37

Matsuura, T., Gad, M.Z., Harrison, E.H. & Ross, A.C. (1997) Lecithin:retinol acyltransferase and retinyl ester hydrolase activities are differentially regulated by retinoids and have distinct distributions between hepatocyte and non-parenchymal cell fractions of rat liver. *J. Nutr.*, **127**, 218–224

Mayne, S.T. & Lippman, S.M. (1997) Cancer prevention: chemopreventive agents. In: DeVita, V.T., Hellman, S. & Rosenberg, S.A. (eds), *Cancer Principles and Practice of Oncology*, Philadelphia, Lippincott-Raven, pp. 585–599

Maziere, S., Cassand, P., Narbonne, J.F. & Meflah, K. (1997) Vitamin A and apoptosis in colonic tumor cells. *Int. J. Vitam. Nutr. Res.*, **67**, 237–241

McCaffery, P. & Dräger, U.C. (1995) Retinoic acid synthesizing enzymes in the embryonic and adult vertebrate. *Adv. Exp. Med. Biol.*, **372**, 173–183

McCarthy, D.J., Lindamood, C.3 & Hill, D.L. (1987) Effects of retinoids on metabolizing enzymes and on binding of benzo(a)pyrene to rat tissue DNA. *Cancer Res.*, **47**, 5014–5020

McCarthy, D.J., Lindamood, C.3, Gundberg, C.M. & Hill, D.L. (1989) Retinoid-induced hemorrhaging and bone toxicity in rats fed diets deficient in vitamin K. *Toxicol. Appl. Pharmacol.*, **97**, 300–310

McCormick, D.L. & Moon, R.C. (1982) Influence of delayed administration of retinyl acetate on mammary carcinogenesis. *Cancer Res.*, **42**, 2639–2643

McCormick, D.L., Burns, F.J. & Albert, R.E. (1980) Inhibition of rat mammary carcinogenesis by short dietary exposure to retinyl acetate. *Cancer Res.*, **40**, 1140–1143

McCormick, D.L., Burns, F.J. & Albert, R.E. (1981) Inhibition of benz[*a*]pyrene-induced mammary carcinogenesis by retinyl acetate. *J. Natl. Cancer Inst.*, **66**, 559–564

McCormick, D.L., Sowell, Z.L., Thompson, C.A. & Moon, R.C. (1983) Inhibition by retinoid and ovariectomy of additional primary malignancies in rats following surgical removal of the first mammary cancer. *Cancer*, **51**, 594–599

McCormick, D.L., May, C.M., Thomas, C.F. & Detrisac, C.J. (1986) Anticarcinogenic and hepatotoxic interactions between retinyl acetate and butylated hydroxytoluene in rats. *Cancer Res.*, **46**, 5264–5269

McKeown Eyssen, G.E. & Bright See, E. (1984) Dietary factors in colon cancer: international relationships. *Nutr. Cancer*, **6**, 160–170

McLaren, D.S. (1994) Dietary vitamin A requirements. In: Blomhoff, R. (ed.), *Vitamin A in Health and Disease*, Marcel Dekker, New York, pp. 665–670

McLaren, D.S. & Frigg, M. (1997) *Sight and Life Manual on Vitamin A Deficiency Disorders (VADD).* Basel, Task Force Sight and Life

McLarty, J.W., Holiday, D.B., Girard, W.M., Yanagihara, R.H., Kummet, T.D. & Greenberg, S.D. (1995) β-Carotene, vitamin A, and lung cancer chemoprevention: results of an intermediate endpoint study. *Am. J. Clin. Nutr.*, **62**, 1431S–1438S

McLaughlin, J.K., Gridley, G., Block, G., Winn, D.M., Preston-Martin, S., Schoenberg, J.B., Greenberg, R.S., Stemhagen, A., Austin, D.F., Ershow, A.G., Blot, W.J. & Fraumeni, J.F., Jr (1988) Dietary factors in oral and pharyngeal cancer. *J. Natl. Cancer Inst.*, **80**, 1237–1243

MDL Information Systems (1998) *Directory of Chemical Producers CD-ROM Service*, San Leandro, CA

Means, A.L. & Gudas, L.J. (1995) The roles of retinoids in vertebrate development. *Annu. Rev. Biochem.*, **64**, 201–233

Mehta, R.G. & Moon, R.C. (1980) Inhibition of DNA synthesis by retinyl acetate during chemically induced mammary carcinogenesis. *Cancer Res.*, **40**, 1109–1111

Mejia, L.A. & Arroyave, G. (1982) The effect of vitamin A fortification of sugar on iron metabolism in preschool children in Guatemala. *Am. J. Clin. Nutr.*, **36**, 87–93

Mendelsohn, C., Ruberte, E., LeMeur, M., Morriss Kay, G. & Chambon, P. (1991) Developmental analysis of the retinoic acid-inducible RAR-β 2 promoter in transgenic animals. *Development*, **113**, 723–734

Mendelsohn, C., Ruberte, E. & Chambon, P. (1992) Retinoid receptors in vertebrate limb development. *Dev. Biol.*, **152**, 50–61

Menkes, M.S., Comstock, G.W., Vuilleumier, J.P., Helsing, K.J., Rider, A.A. & Brookmeyer, R. (1986) Serum β-carotene, vitamins A and E, selenium, and the risk of lung cancer. *New Engl. J. Med.*, **315**, 1250–1254

Merriman, R.L. & Bertram, J.S. (1979) Reversible inhibition by retinoids of 3-methylcholanthrene-induced neoplastic transformation in C3H/10T1/2 clone 8 cells. *Cancer Res.*, **39**, 1661–1666

Mertz, J.R., Shang, E., Piantedosi, R., Wei, S., Wolgemuth, D.J. & Blaner, W.S. (1997) Identification and characterization of a stereo-specific human enzyme that catalyzes 9-*cis*-retinol oxidation. A possible role in 9-*cis*-retinoic acid formation. *J. Biol. Chem.*, **272**, 11744–11749

Mestre, J.R., Subbaramaiah, K., Sacks, P.G., Schantz, S.P., Tanabe, T., Inoue, H. & Dannenberg, A.J. (1997) Retinoids suppress epidermal growth factor-induced transcription of cyclooxygenase-2 in human oral squamous carcinoma cells. *Cancer Res.*, **57**, 2890–2895

Mettlin, C. & Graham, S. (1979) Dietary risk factors in human bladder cancer. *Am. J. Epidemiol.*, **110**, 255–263

Mettlin, C., Graham, S. & Swanson, M. (1979) Vitamin A and lung cancer. *J. Natl. Cancer Inst.*, **62**, 1435–1438

Mettlin, C., Selenskas, S., Natarajan, N. & Huben, R. (1989) Beta-carotene and animal fats and their relationship to prostate cancer risk. A case-control study. *Cancer*, **64**, 605–612

Meyers, D.G., Maloley, P.A. & Weeks, D. (1996) Safety of antioxidant vitamins. *Arch. Intern. Med.*, **156**, 925–935

Meyskens, F.L., Jr, Graham, V., Chvapil, M., Dorr, R.T., Alberts, D.S. & Surwit, E.A. (1983) A phase I trial of β-all-*trans*-retinoic acid delivered via a collagen sponge and a cervical cap for mild or moderate intraepithelial cervical neoplasia. *J. Natl. Cancer Inst.*, **71**, 921–925

Meyskens, F.L., Jr, Liu, P.Y., Tuthill, R.J., Sondak, V.K., Fletcher, W.S., Jewell, W.R., Samlowski, W., Balcerzak, S.P., Rector, D.J., Noyes, R.D. & Costanzi, J.J. (1994) Randomized trial of vitamin A versus observation as adjuvant therapy in high-risk primary malignant melanoma: a Southwest Oncology Group study. *J. Clin. Oncol.*, **12**, 2060–2065

Mezes, M., Bartosiewicz, G. & Nemeth, J. (1986) Comparative investigations on vitamin A level of plasma in some rheumatic diseases. *Clin. Rheumatol.*, **5**, 221–224

Michalek, A.M., Cummings, K.M. & Phelan, J. (1987) Vitamin A and tumor recurrence in bladder cancer. *Nutr. Cancer*, **9**, 143–146

Micksche, M., Cerni, C., Kokron, O., Titscher, R. & Wrba, H. (1977) Stimulation of immune response in lung cancer patients by vitamin A therapy. *Oncology*, **34**, 234-238

Middleton, B., Byers, T., Marshall, J. & Graham, S. (1986) Dietary vitamin A and cancer — a multisite case-control study. *Nutr. Cancer,* **8**, 107–116

Mierauskienè, J., Lekevicius, R. & Lazutka, J.R. (1993) Anticlastogenic effects of Aevitum intake in a group of chemical industry workers. *Hereditas,* **118**, 201–204

Mikkelsen, S., Berne, B., Staberg, B. & Vahlquist, A. (1998) Potentiating effect of dietary vitamin A on photocarcinogenesis in hairless mice. *Carcinogenesis,* **19**, 663–666

Miller, L.A., Cheng, L.Z. & Wu, R. (1993) Inhibition of epidermal growth factor-like growth factor secretion in tracheobronchial epithelial cells by vitamin A. *Cancer Res.,* **53**, 2527–2533

Miller, R.K., Hendrickx, A.G., Mills, J.L., Hummler, H. & Wiegand, U.W. (1998) Periconceptional vitamin A use: how much is teratogenic? *Reprod. Toxicol.,* **12**, 75–88

Mills, J.L., Simpson, J.L., Cunningham, G.C., Conley, M.R. & Rhoads, G.G. (1997) Vitamin A and birth defects. *Am. J. Obstet. Gynecol.,* **177**, 31–36

Mitchell, M.F., Hittelman, W.K., Lotan, R., Nishioka, K., Tortolero Luna, G., Richards Kortum, R., Wharton, J.T. & Hong, W.K. (1995) Chemoprevention trials and surrogate end point biomarkers in the cervix. *Cancer,* **76**, 1956–1977

Mitsumori, K., Onodera, H., Takahashi, M., Shimo, T., Yasuhara, K., Takegawa, K. & Hayashi, Y. (1996) Promoting effect of large amounts of vitamin A on cell proliferation of thyroid pro-liferative lesions induced by simultaneous treatment with thiourea. *Cancer Lett.,* **103**, 19–31

Miyata, Y., Tsuda, H., Matayoshi Miyasato, K., Fukushima, S., Murasaki, G., Ogiso, T. & Ito, N. (1978) Effect of vitamin A acetate on urinary bladder carcinogenesis induced by *N*-butyl-*N*-(4-hydroxybutyl)nitrosamine in rats. *Gann.,* **69**, 845–848

Monga, M. (1997) Vitamin A and its congeners. *Semin. Perinatol.,* **21**, 135–142

Moon, R.C., Grubbs, C.J. & Sporn, M.B. (1976) Inhibition of 7,12-dimethylbenz(*a*)anthracene-induced mammary carcinogenesis by retinyl acetate. *Cancer Res.,* **36**, 2626–2630

Moon, R.C., Grubbs, C.J., Sporn, M.B. & Goodman, D.G. (1977) Retinyl acetate inhibits mammary carcinogenesis induced by *N*-methyl-*N*-nitrosourea. *Nature,* **267**, 620–621

Moon, R.C., McCormick, D.L. & Mehta, R.G. (1983) Inhibition of carcinogenesis by retinoids. *Cancer Res.,* **43**, 2469s–2475s

Moon, T.E., Levine, N., Cartmel, B., Bangert, J.L., Rodney, S., Dong, Q., Peng, Y.M. & Alberts, D.S. (1997) Effect of retinol in preventing squamous cell skin cancer in moderate-risk subjects: a randomized, double-blind, controlled trial. Southwest Skin Cancer Prevention Study Group. *Cancer Epidemiol. Biomarkers Prev.,* **6**, 949–956

Mooney, L.A., Bell, D.A., Santella, R.M., Van Bennekum, A.M., Ottman, R., Paik, M., Blaner, W.S., Lucier, G.W., Covey, L., Young, T.L., Cooper, T.B., Glassman, A.H. & Perera, F.P. (1997) Contribution of genetic and nutritional factors to DNA damage in heavy smokers. *Carcinogenesis,* **18**, 503–509

Moore, T. (1957) *Vitamin A*, Amsterdam, Elsevier

Moore, P.S., Allen, S., Sowell, A.L., Van de Perre, P., Huff, D.L., Serufilira, A., Nsengumuremyi, F. & Hulley, S.B. (1993) Role of nutritional status and weight loss in HIV seroconversion among Rwandan women. *J. Acquir. Immune. Defic. Syndr.,* **6**, 611–616

Mordan, L.J. (1989) Inhibition by retinoids of platelet growth factor-dependent stimulation of DNA synthesis and cell division in density-arrested C3H 10T1/2 fibroblasts. *Cancer Res.,* **49**, 906–909

Mordan, L.J., Bergin, L.M., Budnick, J.E., Meegan, R.R. & Bertram, J.S. (1982) Isolation of methylcholanthrene-"initiated" C3H/10T1/2 cells by inhibiting neoplastic progression with retinyl acetate. *Carcinogenesis,* **3**, 279–285

Moreno, F.S., Wu, T.S., Penteado, M.V., Rizzi, M.B., Jordao Junior, A.A., Almeida Muradian, L.B. & Dagli, M.L. (1995) A comparison of β-carotene and vitamin A effects on a hepatocarcinogenesis model. *Int. J. Vitam. Nutr. Res.,* **65**, 87-94

Moriguchi, S., Werner, L. & Watson, R.R. (1985) High dietary vitamin A (retinyl palmitate) and cellular immune functions in mice. *Immunology,* **56**, 169–177

Morkeberg, J.C., Edmund, C., Prause, J.U., Lanng, S., Koch, C. & Michaelsen, K.F. (1995) Ocular findings in cystic fibrosis patients receiving vitamin A supplementation. *Graefes. Arch. Clin. Exp. Ophthalmol.,* **233**, 709–713

Mortimer, B.C., Beveridge, D.J., Martins, I.J. & Redgrave, T.G. (1995) Intracellular localization and metabolism of chylomicron remnants in the livers of low density lipoprotein receptor-deficient mice and apoE-deficient mice. Evidence for slow metabolism via an alternative apoE-dependent pathway. *J. Biol. Chem.*, **270**, 28767–28776

Moskowitz, Y., Leibowitz, E., Ronen, M. & Aviel, E. (1993) Pseudotumor cerebri induced by vitamin A combined with minocycline. *Ann. Ophthalmol.*, **25**, 306–308

Muhilal, Murdiana, A., Azis, I., Saidin, S., Jahari, A.B. & Karyadi, D. (1988) Vitamin A-fortified monosodium glutamate and vitamin A status: a controlled field trial. *Am. J. Clin. Nutr.*, **48**, 1265–1270

Muñoz, N., Wahrendorf, J., Bang, L.J., Crespi, M., Thurnham, D.I., Day, N.E., Ji, Z.H., Grassi, A., Yan, L.W., Lin, L.G., Quan, L.Y., Yun, Z.C., Fang, Z.S., Yao, L.J., Correa, P., O'Conor, G.T. & Bosch, X. (1985) No effect of riboflavine, retinol, and zinc on prevalence of precancerous lesions of oesophagus. Randomised double-blind intervention study in high-risk population of China. *Lancet*, **2**, 111–114

Muñoz, N., Hayashi, M., Bang, L.J., Wahrendorf, J., Crespi, M. & Bosch, F.X. (1987) Effect of riboflavin, retinol, and zinc on micronuclei of buccal mucosa and of esophagus: a randomized double-blind intervention study in China. *J. Natl. Cancer Inst.*, **79**, 687–691

Musk, A.W., de Klerk, N.H., Ambrosini, G.L., Eccles, J.L., Hansen, J., Olsen, N.J., Watts, V.L., Lund, H.G., Pang, S.C., Beilby, J. & Hobbs, M.S. (1998) Vitamin A and cancer prevention I: observations in workers previously exposed to asbestos at Wittenoom, Western Australia. *Int. J. Cancer*, **75**, 355–361

Nagao, A. & Olson, J.A. (1994) Enzymatic formation of 9-*cis*, 13-*cis*, and all-*trans* retinals from isomers of β-carotene. *FASEB J.*, **8**, 968–972

Nagao, A., During, A., Hoshino, C., Terao, J. & Olson, J.A. (1996) Stoichiometric conversion of all *trans*-β-carotene to retinal by pig intestinal extract. *Arch. Biochem. Biophys.*, **328**, 57–63

Nagy, N.E., Holven, K.B., Roos, N., Senoo, H., Kojima, N., Norum, K.R. & Blomhoff, R. (1997) Storage of vitamin A in extrahepatic stellate cells in normal rats. *J. Lipid Res.*, **38**, 645–658

Nair, P.P., Lohani, A., Norkus, E.P., Feagins, H. & Bhagavan, H.N. (1996) Uptake and distribution of carotenoids, retinol, and tocopherols in human colonic epithelial cells *in vivo*. *Cancer Epidemiol. Biomarkers. Prev.*, **5**, 913–916

Nakajima, M., Lotan, D., Baig, M.M., Carralero, R.M., Wood, W.R., Hendrix, M.J. & Lotan, R. (1989) Inhibition by retinoic acid of type IV collagenolysis and invasion through reconstituted basement membrane by metastatic rat mammary adenocarcinoma cells. *Cancer Res.*, **49**, 1698–1706

Napoli, J.L. (1994) Retinoic acid homeostatis. Prospective roles of β-carotene, retinol, CRBP and CRABP. In: Blomhoff, R. (ed.), *Vitamin A in Health and Disease*, New York, Marcel Dekker, pp. 135–188

Napoli, J.L. (1996) Retinoic acid biosynthesis and metabolism. *FASEB J.*, **10**, 993–1001

Napoli, J.L. & Beck, C.D. (1984) α-Tocopherol and phylloquinone as non-competitive inhibitors of retinyl ester hydrolysis. *Biochem. J.*, **223**, 267–270

Napoli, J.L. & Race, K.R. (1988) Biogenesis of retinoic acid from β-carotene. Differences between the metabolism of β-carotene and retinal. *J. Biol. Chem.*, **263**, 17372–17377

Napoli, J.L., McCormick, A.M., O'Meara, B. & Dratz, E.A. (1984) Vitamin A metabolism: α-tocopherol modulates tissue retinol levels *in vivo*, and retinyl palmitate hydrolysis *in vitro*. *Arch. Biochem. Biophys.*, **230**, 194–202

Napoli, J.L., Pramanik, B.C., Williams, J.B., Dawson, M.I. & Hobbs, P.D. (1985) Quantification of retinoic acid by gas-liquid chromatography-mass spectrometry: total versus all-*trans*-retinoic acid in human plasma. *J. Lipid Res.*, **26**, 387–392

Napoli, J.L., Pacia, E.B. & Salerno, G.J. (1989) Cholate effects on all-*trans*-retinyl palmitate hydrolysis in tissue homogenates: solubilization of multiple kidney membrane hydrolases. *Arch. Biochem. Biophys.*, **274**, 192–199

National Research Council (1989) *Recommended Dietary Allowances*. Food and Nutrition Board, 10th edition, Washington, DC, National Academy Press, pp. 1–284

Nau, H. (1986) Species differences in pharmacokinetics and drug teratogenesis. *Environ. Health Perspect.*, **70**, 113–129

Nau, H. (1990) Correlation of transplacental and maternal pharmacokinetics of retinoids during organogenesis with teratogenicity. *Methods Enzymol.*, **190**, 437–448

Nauss, K.M., Bueche, D. & Newberne, P.M. (1987) Effect of vitamin A nutriture on experimental esophageal carcinogenesis. *J. Natl. Cancer Inst.*, **79**, 145–147

Negri, E., La Vecchia, C., Franceschi, S., D'Avanzo, B., Talamini, R., Parpinel, M., Ferraroni, M., Filiberti, R., Montella, M., Falcini, F., Conti, E. & Decarli, A. (1996) Intake of selected micronutrients and the risk of breast cancer. *Int. J. Cancer*, **65**, 140–144

Nettesheim, P., Snyder, C. & Kim, J.C. (1979) Vitamin A and the susceptibility of respiratory tract tissues to carcinogenic insult. *Environ. Health Perspect.*, **29**, 89–93

Newberne, P.M. & Rogers, A.E. (1973) Rat colon carcinomas associated with aflatoxin and marginal vitamin A. *J. Natl. Cancer Inst.*, **50**, 439–448

Newcomer, M.E. (1995) Retinoid-binding proteins: structural determinants important for function. *FASEB J.*, **9**, 229–239

Newton, D.L., Henderson, W.R. & Sporn, M.B. (1980) Structure-activity relationships of retinoids in hamster tracheal organ culture. *Cancer Res.*, **40**, 3413–3425

Nicholson, R.C., Mader, S., Nagpal, S., Leid, M., Rochette Egly, C. & Chambon, P. (1990) Negative regulation of the rat stromelysin gene promoter by retinoic acid is mediated by an AP1 binding site. *EMBO J.*, **9**, 4443–4454

Niederreither, K., McCaffery, P., Drager, U.C., Chambon, P. & Dolle, P. (1997) Restricted expression and retinoic acid-induced downregulation of the retinaldehyde dehydrogenase type 2 (RALDH-2) gene during mouse development. *Mech. Dev.*, **62**, 67–78

Noji, S., Nohno, T., Koyama, E., Muto, K., Ohyama, K., Aoki, Y., Tamura, K., Ohsugi, K., Ide, H., Taniguchi, S. & Saito, T. (1991) Retinoic acid induces polarizing activity but is unlikely to be a morphogen in the chick limb bud. *Nature*, **350**, 83–86

Nomura, A.M., Stemmermann, G.N., Heilbrun, L.K., Salkeld, R.M. & Vuilleumier, J.P. (1985) Serum vitamin levels and the risk of cancer of specific sites in men of Japanese ancestry in Hawaii. *Cancer Res.*, **45**, 2369–2372

Nomura, A.M., Kolonel, L.N., Hankin, J.H. & Yoshizawa, C.N. (1991) Dietary factors in cancer of the lower urinary tract. *Int. J. Cancer*, **48**, 199–205

Nomura, A.M., Stemmermann, G.N. & Chyou, P.H. (1995) Gastric cancer among the Japanese in Hawaii. *Jpn. J. Cancer Res.*, **86**, 916–923

Nomura, A.M., Ziegler, R.G., Stemmermann, G.N., Chyou, P.H. & Craft, N.E. (1997a) Serum micronutrients and upper aerodigestive tract cancer. *Cancer Epidemiol. Biomarkers Prev.*, **6**, 407–412

Nomura, A.M., Stemmermann, G.N., Lee, J. & Craft, N.E. (1997b) Serum micronutrients and prostate cancer in Japanese Americans in Hawaii. *Cancer Epidemiol. Biomarkers Prev.*, **6**, 487–491

Noy, N. (1992a) The ionization behavior of retinoic acid in aqueous environments and bound to serum albumin. *Biochim. Biophys. Acta*, **1106**, 151–158

Noy, N. (1992b) The ionization behavior of retinoic acid in lipid bilayers and in membranes. *Biochim. Biophys. Acta*, **1106**, 159–164

O'Connell, M.J., Chua, R., Hoyos, B., Buck, J., Chen, Y., Derguini, F. & Hammerling, U. (1996) Retro-retinoids in regulated cell growth and death. *J. Exp. Med.*, **184**, 549–555

Odetti, P., Cheli, V., Carta, G., Maiello, M. & Viviani, G.L. (1984) Effect of nicotinic acid associated with retinol and tocopherols on plasma lipids in hyperlipoproteinaemic patients. *Pharmatherapeutica.*, **4**, 21–24

Odin, A.P. (1997) Vitamins as antimutagens: advantages and some possible mechanisms of antimutagenic action. *Mutat. Res.*, **386**, 39–67

Ogura, T., Alvarez, I.S., Vogel, A., Rodriguez, C., Evans, R.M. & Izpisua Belmonte, J.C. (1996) Evidence that Shh cooperates with a retinoic acid inducible co-factor to establish ZPA-like activity. *Development*, **122**, 537–542

Ohashi, Y., Watanabe, H., Kinoshita, S., Hosotani, H., Umemoto, M. & Manabe, R. (1988) Vitamin A eyedrops for superior limbic keratoconjunctivitis. *Am. J. Ophthalmol.*, **105**, 523–527

Ohno, Y., Yoshida, O., Oishi, K., Okada, K., Yamabe, H. & Schroeder, F.H. (1988) Dietary β-carotene and cancer of the prostate: a case-control study in Kyoto, Japan. *Cancer Res.*, **48**, 1331–1336

Oikawa, T., Hirotani, K., Nakamura, O., Shudo, K., Hiragun, A. & Iwaguchi, T. (1989) A highly potent antiangiogenic activity of retinoids. *Cancer Lett.*, **48**, 157–162

Okabe, T., Yorifuji, H., Yamada, E. & Takaku, F. (1984) Isolation and characterization of vitamin-A-storing lung cells. *Exp. Cell Res.*, **154**, 125–135

Okai, Y., Higashi Okai, K., Nakamura, S., Yano, Y. & Otani, S. (1996) Suppressive effects of retinoids, carotenoids and antioxidant vitamins on heterocyclic amine-induced umu C gene expression in *Salmonella typhimurium* (TA 1535/pSK 1002). *Mutat. Res.*, **368**, 133–140

Okuno, M., Moriwaki, H., Imai, S., Muto, Y., Kawada, N., Suzuki, Y. & Kojima, S. (1997) Retinoids exacerbate rat liver fibrosis by inducing the activation of latent TGF-β in liver stellate cells. *Hepatology*, **26**, 913–921

Oliveira, J.A., Silva Netto, C.R., Sala, M.A., Lopes, R.A. & Maia Campos, G. (1990) [Experimental hypervitaminosis A in the rat. 14. Morphological and morphometric study of changes in the esophageal epithelium]. *Rev. Odontol. Univ. Sao. Paulo*, **4**, 200–205 (in Portuguese)

Olmedilla, B., Granado, F., Blanco, I. & Rojas Hidalgo, E. (1996) Evaluation of retinol, α-tocopherol, and carotenoids in serum of men with cancer of the larynx before and after commercial enteral formula feeding. *J. Parenter. Enteral. Nutr.*, **20**, 145–149

Olsen, J., Kronborg, O., Lynggaard, J. & Ewertz, M. (1994) Dietary risk factors for cancer and adenomas of the large intestine. A case-control study within a screening trial in Denmark. *Eur. J. Cancer*, **30A**, 53–60

Olson, J.A. (1987) Recommended dietary intakes (RDI) of vitamin A in humans. *Am. J. Clin. Nutr.*, **45**, 704–716

Olson, J.A. (1990) Vitamin A. In: Machlin, L.J. (ed.), *Handbook of Vitamins*, New York, Marcel Dekker, pp. 1–57

Olson, J.A. (1994a) Needs and sources of carotenoids and vitamin A. *Nutr. Rev.*, **52**, S67–S73

Olson, J.A. (1994b) Vitamin A, retinoids, and carotenoids. In: Shils, M.E., Olson, J.A. & Shike, M. (eds), *Modern Nutrition in Health and Disease*, 8th edition, Philadelphia, Lea & Febiger, pp. 287–307

Olson, J.A. (1995) Vitamin A metabolism during infection. *J. Nutr. Immunol.*, **4**, 17–34

Olson, J.A. (1998) Carotenoids. In: Shils, M.E., Olson, J.A., Shike, M. & Ross, A.C. (eds), *Modern Nutrition in Health and Disease*, 9th edition, Baltimore, Williams & Wilkins, pp. 525–542

Olson, J.A. & Hayaishi, O. (1965) The enzymatic cleavage of β-carotene into vitamin A by soluble enzymes of rat liver and intestine. *Proc. Natl. Acad. Sci. USA*, **54**, 1364–1370

Omenn, G.S., Goodman, G.E., Thornquist, M.D., Rosenstock, L., Barnhart, S., Gylys Colwell, I., Metch, B. & Lund, B. (1993a) The Carotene and Retinol Efficacy Trial (CARET) to prevent lung cancer in high-risk populations: pilot study with asbestos-exposed workers. *Cancer Epidemiol. Biomarkers. Prev.*, **2**, 381–387

Omenn, G.S. & and CARET co-investigators (1993b) CARET, the beta-carotene and retinol efficacy trial to prevent lung cancer in asbestos-exposed workers and in smokers. In: *Sourcebook on Asbestos Diseases: Medical, Legal, and Engineering Aspects*, Vol. 7, Charlottesville, VA, Lexis, pp. 219–241

Omenn, G.S., Goodman, G., Thornquist, M., Grizzle, J., Rosenstock, L., Barnhart, S., Balmes, J., Cherniack, M.G., Cullen, M.R., Glass, A., Keogh, J., Meyskens, F. Jr, Valanis, B. & Williams, J., Jr. (1994a) The β-carotene and retinol efficacy trial (CARET) for chemoprevention of lung cancer in high risk populations: smokers and asbestos-exposed workers. *Cancer Res.*, **54**, 2038s–2043s

Omenn, G.S., Goodman, G.E., Thornquist, M. & Brunzell, J.D. (1994b) Long-term vitamin A does not produce clinically significant hypertriglyceridemia: results from CARET, the β-carotene and retinol efficacy trial. *Cancer Epidemiol. Biomarkers. Prev.*, **3**, 711–713

Omenn, G.S., Goodman, G.E., Thornquist, M.D., Balmes, J., Cullen, M.R., Glass, A., Keogh, J.P., Meyskens, F.L., Valanis, B., Williams, J.H., Barnhart, S. & Hammar, S. (1996a) Effects of a combination of beta carotene and vitamin A on lung cancer and cardiovascular disease. *New Engl. J. Med.*, **334**, 1150–1155

Omenn, G.S., Goodman, G.E., Thornquist, M.D., Balmes, J., Cullen, M.R., Glass, A., Keogh, J.P., Meyskens, F.L., Jr, Valanis, B., Williams, J.H., Jr, Barnhart, S., Cherniack, M.G., Brodkin, C.A. & Hammar, S. (1996b) Risk factors for lung cancer and for intervention effects in CARET, the beta-Carotene and Retinol Efficacy Trial. *J. Natl. Cancer Inst.*, **88**, 1550–1559

Omenn, G.S., Goodman, G., Thornquist, M., Barnhart, S., Balmes, J., Cherniack, M., Cullen, M., Glass, A., Keogh, J., Liu, D., Meyskens, F., Jr, Perloff, M., Valanis, B. & Williams, J.J. (1996c) Chemoprevention of lung cancer: the β-Carotene and Retinol Efficacy Trial (CARET) in high-risk smokers and asbestos-exposed workers. In: Hakama, M., Beral, V., Buiatti, E., Faivre, J. & Parkin, D.M. (eds), *Chemoprevention in Cancer Control*, (IARC Scientific Publications No. 136), Lyon, IARC, pp. 67–85

Ong, D.E. (1994) Absorption of vitamin A. In: Blomhoff, R. (ed.), *Vitamin A in Health and Disease*, New York, Marcel Dekker, pp. 37–72

Ong, T., Whong, W.Z., Stewart, J.D. & Brockman, H.E. (1989) Comparative antimutagenicity of 5 compounds against 5 mutagenic complex mixtures in *Salmonella typhimurium* strain TA98. *Mutat. Res.*, **222**, 19–25

Ong, D.E., Newcomer, M.E. & Chytil, F. (1994) Cellular retinoid-binding proteins. In: Sporn, M.B., Roberts, A.B. & Goodman, D.S. (eds), *The Retinoids: Biology, Chemistry, and Medicine*, 2nd edition, New York, Raven Press, pp. 283–312

Paganini-Hill, A., Chao, A., Ross, R.K. & Henderson, B.E. (1987) Vitamin A, β-carotene, and the risk of cancer: a prospective study. *J. Natl. Cancer Inst.*, **79**, 443–448

Palan, P.R., Mikhail, M.S., Goldberg, G.L., Basu, J., Runowicz, C.D. & Romney, S.L. (1996) Plasma levels of β-carotene, lycopene, canthaxanthin, retinol, and α- and τ-tocopherol in cervical intraepithelial neoplasia and cancer. *Clin. Cancer Res.*, **2**, 181–185

Palmer, H.J., Maher, V.M. & McCormick, J.J. (1989) Effect of retinoids on growth factor-induced anchorage independent growth of human fibroblasts. *In vitro Cell Dev. Biol.*, **25**, 1009–1015

Pamuk, E.R., Byers, T., Coates, R.J., Vann, J.W., Sowell, A.L., Gunter, E.W. & Glass, D. (1994) Effect of smoking on serum nutrient concentrations in African-American women. *Am. J. Clin. Nutr.*, **59**, 891–895

Parker, R.S. (1996) Absorption, metabolism, and transport of carotenoids. *FASEB J.*, **10**, 542–551

Pasquali, D., Thaller, C. & Eichele, G. (1996) Abnormal level of retinoic acid in prostate cancer tissues. *J. Clin. Endocrinol. Metab.*, **81**, 2186–2191

Pastorino, U., Pisani, P., Berrino, F., Andreoli, C., Barbieri, A., Costa, A., Mazzoleni, C., Gramegna, G. & Marubini, E. (1987) Vitamin A and female lung cancer: a case-control study on plasma and diet. *Nutr. Cancer*, **10**, 171–179

Pastorino, U., Chiesa, G., Infante, M., Soresi, E., Clerici, M., Valente, M., Belloni, P.A. & Ravasi, G. (1991) Safety of high-dose vitamin A. Randomized trial on lung cancer chemoprevention. *Oncology*, **48**, 131–137

Pastorino, U., Infante, M., Maioli, M., Chiesa, G., Buyse, M., Firket, P., Rosmentz, N., Clerici, M., Soresi, E., Valente, M., Belloni, P.A. & Ravasi, G. (1993) Adjuvant treatment of stage I lung cancer with high-dose vitamin A. *J. Clin. Oncol.*, **11**, 1216–1222

Patel, D.J. (1969) 220 MHz proton nuclear magnetic resonance spectra of retinals. *Nature*, **221**, 825–828

Patterson, R.E., White, E., Kristal, A.R., Neuhouser, M.L. & Potter, J.D. (1997) Vitamin supplements and cancer risk: the epidemiologic evidence. *Cancer Causes Control*, **8**, 786–802

Peck, G.L. & DiGiovanna, J.J. (1994) Synthetic retinoids in dermatology. In: Sporn, M.B., Roberts, A.B. & Goodman, D.S. (eds), *The Retinoids: Biology, Chemistry, and Medicine*, 2nd edition, New York, Raven Press, pp. 631–658

Peiker, G., Eckhoff, C. & Nau, H. (1991) [Plasma level and metabolism of vitamin A (Vitadral) in women of reproductive age]. *Zentralbl. Gynakol.*, **113**, 1100–1106 (in German)

Peng, Y.M., Alberts, D.S., Graham, V., Surwit, E.A., Weiner, S. & Meyskens, F.L.J. (1986) Cervical tissue uptake of all-*trans*-retinoic acid delivered via a collagen sponge-cervical cap delivery device in patients with cervical dysplasia. *Invest. New Drugs*, **4**, 245–249

Periquet, B.A., Jammes, N.M., Lambert, W.E., Tricoire, J., Moussa, M.M., Garcia, J., Ghisolfi, J. & Thouvenot, J. (1995) Micronutrient levels in HIV-1-infected children. *AIDS*, **9**, 887–893

Pfander, H. (1987) *Key to Carotenoids*, Basel, Birkhäuser Verlag

Physicians' Desk Reference (1997) Montvale, NJ, Medical Economics Co.

Piersma, A.H., Bode, W., Verhoef, A. & Olling, M. (1996) Teratogenicity of a single oral dose of retinyl palmitate in the rat, and the role of dietary vitamin A status. *Pharmacol. Toxicol.,* **79**, 131–135

Pijnappel, W.W., Hendriks, H.F., Folkers, G.E., van den Brink, C.E., Dekker, E.J., Edelenbosch, C., van der Saag, P.T. & Durston, A.J. (1993) The retinoid ligand 4-oxo-retinoic acid is a highly active modulator of positional specification. *Nature,* **366**, 340–344

Pilch, S.M. (1985) *Assessment of the Vitamin A Nutritional Status of the US Population Based on Data Collected in the Health and Nutrition Examination Surveys* (FDA 223-84-2059), Bethesda, Life Sciences Research Office, pp. 1–49

Pinnock, C.B., Douglas, R.M. & Badcock, N.R. (1986) Vitamin A status in children who are prone to respiratory tract infections. *Aust. Paediatr. J.,* **22**, 95–99

Pirisi, L., Batova, A., Jenkins, G.R., Hodam, J.R. & Creek, K.E. (1992) Increased sensitivity of human keratinocytes immortalized by human papillomavirus type 16 DNA to growth control by retinoids. *Cancer Res.,* **52**, 187–193

Poddar, S., Hong, W.K., Thacher, S.M. & Lotan, R. (1991) Retinoic acid suppression of squamous differentiation in human head-and-neck squamous carcinoma cells. *Int. J. Cancer,* **48**, 239–247

Posch, K.C., Boerman, M.H., Burns, R.D. & Napoli, J.L. (1991) Holocellular retinol binding protein as a substrate for microsomal retinal synthesis. *Biochemistry,* **30**, 6224–6230

Potischman, N., McCulloch, C.E., Byers, T., Nemoto, T., Stubbe, N., Milch, R., Parker, R., Rasmussen, K.M., Root, M., Graham, S. & Campbell, T.C. (1990) Breast cancer and dietary and plasma concentrations of carotenoids and vitamin A. *Am. J. Clin. Nutr.,* **52**, 909–915

Potischman, N., Herrero, R., Brinton, L.A., Reeves, W.C., Stacewicz Sapuntzakis, M., Jones, C.J., Brenes, M.M., Tenorio, F., de Britton, R.C. & Gaitan, E. (1991) A case-control study of nutrient status and invasive cervical cancer. II. Serologic indicators. *Am. J. Epidemiol.,* **134**, 1347–1355

Potter, J.D. (1996) Nutrition and colorectal cancer. *Cancer Causes Control,* **7**, 127–146

Potter, J.D. & McMichael, A.J. (1986) Diet and cancer of the colon and rectum: a case-control study. *J. Natl. Cancer Inst.,* **76**, 557–569

Pouchert, C.J. (1985) *The Aldrich Library of Infrared Spectra,* Milwaukee, WI, Aldrich Chemical Co.

Pouchert, C.J. & Behnke, J. (1993) *The Aldrich Library of* ^{13}*C and* ^{1}*H FT NMR Spectra,* Milwaukee, WI, Aldrich Chemical Co.

Prasad, M.P., Mukundan, M.A. & Krishnaswamy, K. (1995) Micronuclei and carcinogen DNA adducts as intermediate end points in nutrient intervention trial of precancerous lesions in the oral cavity. *Eur. J. Cancer, B. Oral Oncol.,* **31B**, 155–159

Qin, S. & Huang, C.C. (1985) Effect of retinoids on carcinogen-induced mutagenesis in *Salmonella* tester strains. *Mutat. Res.,* **142**, 115–120

Qin, S. & Huang, C.C. (1986) Influence of mouse liver stored vitamin A on the induction of mutations (Ames tests) and SCE of bone marrow cells by aflatoxin B_1, benzo(*a*)pyrene, or cyclophosphamide. *Environ. Mutagen.,* **8**, 839–847

Qin, S., Batt, T. & Huang, C.C. (1985) Influence of retinol on carcinogen-induced sister chromatid exchanges and chromosome aberrations in V79 cells. *Environ. Mutagen.,* **7**, 137–146

Rabl, H., Khoschsorur, G. & Petek, W. (1995) Antioxidative vitamin treatment: effect on lipid peroxidation and limb swelling after revascularization operations. *World J. Surg.,* **19**, 738–744

Rahman, M.M., Mahalanabis, D., Wahed, M.A., Islam, M.A. & Habte, D. (1995) Administration of 25,000 IU vitamin A doses at routine immunisation in young infants. *Eur. J. Clin. Nutr.,* **49**, 439–445

Raica, N., Jr, Scott, J., Lowry, L. & Sauberlich, H.E. (1972) Vitamin A concentration in human tissues collected from five areas in the United States. *Am. J. Clin. Nutr.,* **25**, 291–296

Raina, V. & Gurtoo, H.L. (1985) Effects of vitamins A, C, and E on aflatoxin B_1-induced mutagenesis in *Salmonella typhimurium* TA-98 and TA-100. *Teratog. Carcinog. Mutagen.,* **5**, 29–40

Rajguru, S.U., Kang, Y.H. & Ahluwalia, B.S. (1982) Localization of retinol (vitamin A) in rat testes. *J. Nutr.,* **112**, 1881–1891

Ramaswamy, G., Rao, V.R., Kumaraswamy, S.V. & Anantha, N. (1996) Serum vitamins' status in oral leucoplakias — a preliminary study. *Eur. J. Cancer, B. Oral Oncol.,* **32B**, 120–122

Ramesha, A., Rao, N., Rao, A.R., Jannu, L.N. & Hussain, S.P. (1990) Chemoprevention of 7,12-dimethylbenz[*a*]anthracene-induced mammary carcinogenesis in rat by the combined actions of selenium, magnesium, ascorbic acid and retinyl acetate. *Jpn. J. Cancer Res.*, **81**, 1239–1246

Rando, R.R. (1994) Retinoid isomerization reactions in the visual system. In: Blomhoff, R. (ed.), *Vitamin A in Health and Disease*, New York, Marcel Dekker, pp. 503–529

Randolph, R.K. & Ross, A.C. (1991) Vitamin A status regulates hepatic lecithin: retinol acyltransferase activity in rats. *J. Biol. Chem.*, **266**, 16453–16457

Rao, K.P., Ramadevi, G. & Das, U.N. (1986) Vitamin A can prevent genetic damage induced by benzo(*a*)pyrene to the bone marrow cells of mice. *Int. J. Tissue React.*, **8**, 219–223

Rao, A.R., Hussain, S.P., Jannu, L.N., Kumari, M.V. & Aradhana (1990) Modulatory influences of tamoxifen, tocopherol, retinyl acetate, aminoglutethimide, ergocryptine and selenium on DMBA-induced initiation of mammary carcinogenesis in rats. *Indian J. Exp. Biol.*, **28**, 409–416

Raque, C.J., Biondo, R.V., Keeran, M.G., Honeycutt, W.M. & Jansen, G.T. (1975) Snuff dippers keratosis (snuff-induced leukoplakia). *South. Med. J.*, **68**, 565–568

Rasmussen, M., Michalsen, H., Lie, S.O., Nilsson, A., Petersen, L.B. & Norum, K.R. (1986) Intestinal retinol esterification and serum retinol in children with cystic fibrosis. *J. Pediatr. Gastroenterol. Nutr.*, **5**, 397–403

Rayner, R.J., Tyrrell, J.C., Hiller, E.J., Marenah, C., Neugebauer, M.A., Vernon, S.A. & Brimlow, G. (1989) Night blindness and conjunctival xerosis caused by vitamin A deficiency in patients with cystic fibrosis. *Arch. Dis. Child.*, **64**, 1151–1156

Redlich, C.A., Grauer, J.N., Van Bennekum, A.M., Clever, S.L., Ponn, R.B. & Blaner, W.S. (1996) Characterization of carotenoid, vitamin A, and α-tocopheral levels in human lung tissue and pulmonary macrophages. *Am. J. Respir. Crit. Care Med.*, **154**, 1436–1443

Reese, D.H. & Politano, V.A. (1981) Evidence for the retinoid control of urothelial alkaline phosphatase. *Biochem. Biophys. Res. Commun.*, **102**, 322–327

Reichman, M.E., Hayes, R.B., Ziegler, R.G., Schatzkin, A., Taylor, P.R., Kahle, L.L. & Fraumeni, J.F., Jr (1990) Serum vitamin A and subsequent development of prostate cancer in the first National Health and Nutrition Examination Survey Epidemiologic Follow-up Study. *Cancer Res.*, **50**, 2311–2315

Reinersdorff, D.V., Bush, E. & Liberato, D.J. (1996) Plasma kinetics of vitamin A in humans after a single oral dose of [8,9,19-^{13}C]retinyl palmitate. *J. Lipid Res.*, **37**, 1875–1885

Renner, H.W. (1985) Anticlastogenic effect of β-carotene in Chinese hamsters. Time and dose response studies with different mutagens. *Mutat. Res.*, **144**, 251-256

Repa, J.J., Hanson, K.K. & Clagett Dame, M. (1993) All-*trans*-retinol is a ligand for the retinoic acid receptors. *Proc. Natl. Acad. Sci. USA.*, **90**, 7293–7297

Reynolds, J.E.F. (1989) *Martindale. The Extra Pharmacopoeia*, London, Pharmaceutical Press

Rezabek, M.S., Sleight, S.D., Jensen, R.K. & Aust, S.D. (1989) Effects of dietary retinyl acetate on the promotion of hepatic enzyme-altered foci by polybrominated biphenyls in initiated rats. *Food Chem. Toxicol.*, **27**, 539–544

Ribaya-Mercado, J.D., Fox, J.G., Rosenblad, W.D., Blanco, M.C. & Russell, R.M. (1992) β-Carotene, retinol and retinyl ester concentrations in serum and selected tissues of ferrets fed β-carotene. *J. Nutr.*, **122**, 1898–1903

Ribaya-Mercado, J.D., Blanco, M.C., Fox, J.G. & Russell, R.M. (1994) High concentrations of vitamin A esters circulate primarily as retinyl stearate and are stored primarily as retinyl palmitate in ferret tissues. *J. Am. Coll. Nutr.*, **13**, 83–86

Riboli, E., Gonzalez, C.A., Lopez Abente, G., Errezola, M., Izarzugaza, I., Escolar, A., Nebot, M., Hemon, B. & Agudo, A. (1991) Diet and bladder cancer in Spain: a multi-centre case-control study. *Int. J. Cancer*, **49**, 214–219

Richardson, S., Gerber, M. & Cenee, S. (1991) The role of fat, animal protein and some vitamin consumption in breast cancer: a case control study in southern France. *Int. J. Cancer*, **48**, 1–9

Riddle, R.D., Johnson, R.L., Laufer, E. & Tabin, C. (1993) Sonic hedgehog mediates the polarizing activity of the ZPA. *Cell*, **75**, 1401–1416

Rigas, J.R., Miller, V.A., Zhang, Z.F., Klimstra, D.S., Tong, W.P., Kris, M.G. & Warrell, R.P.J. (1996) Metabolic phenotypes of retinoic acid and the risk of lung cancer. *Cancer Res.,* **56**, 2692–2696

Rigtrup, K.M. & Ong, D.E. (1992) A retinyl ester hydrolase activity intrinsic to the brush border membrane of rat small intestine. *Biochemistry,* **31**, 2920–2926

Rigtrup, K.M., Kakkad, B. & Ong, D.E. (1994) Purification and partial characterization of a retinyl ester hydrolase from the brush border of rat small intestine mucosa: probable identity with brush border phospholipase B. *Biochemistry,* **33**, 2661–2666

Risch, H.A., Jain, M., Choi, N.W., Fodor, J.G., Pfeiffer, C.J., Howe, G.R., Harrison, L.W., Craib, K.J. & Miller, A.B. (1985) Dietary factors and the incidence of cancer of the stomach. *Am. J. Epidemiol.,* **122**, 947–959

Risch, H.A., Burch, J.D., Miller, A.B., Hill, G.B., Steele, R. & Howe, G.R. (1988) Dietary factors and the incidence of cancer of the urinary bladder. *Am. J. Epidemiol.,* **127**, 1179–1191

Ritter, S.J. & Smith, J.E. (1996) Multiple retinoids alter liver bile salt-independent retinyl ester-hydrolase activity, serum vitamin A and serum retinol-binding protein of rats. *Biochim. Biophys. Acta,* **1291**, 228–236

Robbins, S.T. & Fletcher, A.B. (1993) Early vs delayed vitamin A supplementation in very-low-birth-weight infants. *J. Parenter. Enteral. Nutr.,* **17**, 220–225

Roberts, A.B., Nichols, M.D., Newton, D.L. & Sporn, M.B. (1979) *In vitro* metabolism of retinoic acid in hamster intestine and liver. *J. Biol. Chem.,* **254**, 6296-6302

Roberts, E.S., Vaz, A.D. & Coon, M.J. (1992) Role of isozymes of rabbit microsomal cytochrome P-450 in the metabolism of retinoic acid, retinol, and retinal. *Mol. Pharmacol.,* **41**, 427–433

Rocchi, P., Arfellini, G., Capucci, A., Grilli, M.P. & Prodi, G. (1983) Effect of vitamin A palmitate on mutagenesis induced by polycyclic aromatic hydrocarbons in human cells. *Carcinogenesis,* **4**, 245–247

Rockley, N.L., Rockley, M.G., Halley, B.A. & Nelson, E.C. (1986) Fourier transform infrared spectroscopy of retinoids. *Methods Enzymol.,* **123**, 92–101

Rogers, M., Berestecky, J.M., Hossain, M.Z., Guo, H.M., Kadle, R., Nicholson, B.J. & Bertram, J.S. (1990) Retinoid-enhanced gap junctional communication is achieved by increased levels of connexin 43 mRNA and protein. *Mol. Carcinog.,* **3**, 335–343

Rohan, T.E., McMichael, A.J. & Baghurst, P.A. (1988) A population-based case-control study of diet and breast cancer in Australia. *Am. J. Epidemiol.,* **128**, 478–489

Rohan, T.E., Howe, G.R., Friedenreich, C.M., Jain, M. & Miller, A.B. (1993) Dietary fiber, vitamins A, C, and E, and risk of breast cancer: a cohort study. *Cancer Causes Control,* **4**, 29–37

Rohan, T.E., Howe, G.R., Burch, J.D. & Jain, M. (1995) Dietary factors and risk of prostate cancer: a case-control study in Ontario, Canada. *Cancer Causes Control,* **6**, 145–154

Rollman, O. & Vahlquist, A. (1985) Psoriasis and vitamin A. Plasma transport and skin content of retinol, dehydroretinol and carotenoids in adult patients versus healthy controls. *Arch. Dermatol. Res.,* **278**, 17–24

Romero, J.B., Schreiber, A., Von Hochstetter, A.R., Wagenhauser, F.J., Michel, B.A. & Theiler, R. (1996) Hyperostotic and destructive osteoarthritis in a patient with vitamin A intoxication syndrome: a case report. *Bull. Hosp. Jt. Dis.,* **54**, 169–174

Romert, L., Jansson, T., Curvall, M. & Jenssen, D. (1994) Screening for agents inhibiting the mutagenicity of extracts and constituents of tobacco products. *Mutat. Res.,* **322**, 97–110

Romney, S.L., Dwyer, A., Slagle, S., Duttagupta, C., Palan, P.R., Basu, J., Calderin, S. & Kadish, A. (1985) Chemoprevention of cervix cancer: Phase I-II: A feasibility study involving the topical vaginal administration of retinyl acetate gel. *Gynecol. Oncol.,* **20**, 109–119

Rondahl, L., Busk, L., Ahlborg, U.G. & Bergman, K. (1985) Effects of vitamin A on the metabolism and mutagenicity of 2AAF *in vitro* and on the covalent binding to rat liver DNA/RNA *in vivo. Arch. Toxicol.,* **57**, 178–183

Rosa, F.W. (1993) Retinoid embryopathy in humans. In: Koren, G. (ed.), *Retinoids in Clinical Practice. The Risk-Benefit Ratio,* New York, Marcel Dekker, pp. 77–109

Rosa, F.W., Wilk, A.L. & Kelsey, F.O. (1986) Teratogen update: vitamin A congeners. *Teratology*, **33**, 355–364

Rosales, F.J. & Ross, A.C. (1996) Inflammation in human immunodeficiency virus type 1 infection as a cause of decreased plasma retinol. *J. Infect. Dis.*, **173**, 507–509

Rosengren, R.J., Sauer, J.M., Hooser, S.B. & Sipes, I.G. (1995) The interactions between retinol and five different hepatotoxicants in the Swiss Webster mouse. *Fundam. Appl. Toxicol.*, **25**, 281–292

Ross, A.C. (1998) Vitamin A and retinoids. In: Shils, M.E., Olson, J.A., Shike, M. & Ross, A.C. (eds), *Modern Nutrition in Health and Disease*, 9th edition, Baltimore, Williams & Wilkins, pp. 305–328

Ross, A.C. & Kempner, E.S. (1993) Radiation inactivation analysis of acyl-CoA:retinol acyltransferase and lecithin:retinol acyltransferase in rat liver. *J. Lipid Res.*, **34**, 1201–1207

Ross, A.C. & Hämmerling, U.G. (1994) Retinoids and the immune system. In: Sporn, M.B., Roberts, A.B. & Goodman, D.S. (eds), *The Retinoids. Biology, Chemistry, and Medicine*, 2nd edition, New York, Raven Press, pp. 521–543

Ross, R.K., Shimizu, H., Paganini Hill, A., Honda, G. & Henderson, B.E. (1987) Case-control studies of prostate cancer in blacks and whites in southern California. *J. Natl. Cancer Inst.*, **78**, 869–874

Rossant, J., Zirngibl, R., Cado, D., Shago, M. & Giguere, V. (1991) Expression of a retinoic acid response element-hsplacZ transgene defines specific domains of transcriptional activity during mouse embryogenesis. *Genes Dev.*, **5**, 1333–1344

Rossing, M.A., Vaughan, T.L. & McKnight, B. (1989) Diet and pharyngeal cancer. *Int. J. Cancer*, **44**, 593–597

Rothman, K.J., Moore, L.L., Singer, M.R., Nguyen, U.S., Mannino, S. & Milunsky, A. (1995) Teratogenicity of high vitamin A intake. *New Engl. J. Med.*, **333**, 1369–1373

Rothman, K.J., Moore, L.L., Singer, M.R. & Milunsky, A. (1996) Re. Teratogenicity of high vitamin A intake. *New Engl. J. Med.*, **334**, 1197–1197

Roy, S.K., Islam, A., Molla, A., Akramuzzaman, S.M., Jahan, F. & Fuchs, G. (1997) Impact of a single megadose of vitamin A at delivery on breastmilk of mothers and morbidity of their infants. *Eur. J. Clin. Nutr.*, **51**, 302–307

Ruberte, E., Friederich, V., Morriss Kay, G. & Chambon, P. (1992) Differential distribution patterns of CRABP I and CRABP II transcripts during mouse embryogenesis. *Development*, **115**, 973–987

Rudland, P.S., Paterson, F.C., Davies, A.C. & Warburton, M.J. (1983) Retinoid-specific induction of differentiation and reduction of the DNA synthesis rate and tumor-forming ability of a stem cell line from a rat mammary tumor. *J. Natl. Cancer Inst.*, **70**, 949–958

Rumore, M.M. (1993) Vitamin A as an immunomodulating agent. *Clin. Pharm.*, **12**, 506–514

Russell, D.H. & Haddox, M.K. (1981) Anti-proliferative effects of retinoids related to the cell cycle-specific inhibition of ornithine decarboxylase. *Ann. N. Y. Acad. Sci.*, **359**, 281–297

Rutten, A.A., Wilmer, J.W. & Beems, R.B. (1988a) Effects of all-*trans* retinol and cigarette smoke condensate on hamster tracheal epithelium in organ culture. I. A cell proliferation study. *Virchows Arch. B. Cell Pathol. Mol. Pathol.*, **55**, 167–175

Rutten, A.A., Jongen, W.M., de Haan, L.H., Hendriksen, E.G. & Koeman, J.H. (1988b) Effect of retinol and cigarette-smoke condensate on dye-coupled intercellular communication between hamster tracheal epithelial cells. *Carcinogenesis*, **9**, 315–320

Saari, J.C. (1994) Retinoids in photosensitive systems. In: Sporn, M.B., Roberts, A.B. & Goodman, D.S. (eds), *The Retinoids: Biology, Chemistry, and Medicine*, 2nd edition, New York, Raven Press, pp. 351–385

Saffiotti, U., Montesano, R., Sellakumar, A.R. & Borg, S.A. (1967) Experimental cancer of the lung. Inhibition by vitamin A of the induction of tracheobronchial squamous metaplasia and squamous cell tumors. *Cancer*, **20**, 857–864

Samet, J.M., Skipper, B.J., Humble, C.G. & Pathak, D.R. (1985) Lung cancer risk and vitamin A consumption in New Mexico. *Am. Rev. Respir. Dis.*, **131**, 198–202

Sanders, T.A., Haines, A.P., Wormald, R., Wright, L.A. & Obeid, O. (1993) Essential fatty acids, plasma cholesterol, and fat-soluble vitamins in subjects with age-related maculopathy and matched control subjects. *Am. J. Clin. Nutr.*, **57**, 428–433

Sankaranarayanan, R., Mathew, B., Varghese, C., Sudhakaran, P.R., Menon, V., Jayadeep, A., Nair, M.K., Mathews, C., Mahalingam, T.R., Balaram, P. & Nair, P.P. (1997) Chemoprevention of oral leukoplakia with vitamin A and β-carotene: an assessment. *Eur. J. Cancer,* **33**, 231–236

Sass, J.O. (1994) 3,4-Didehydroretinol may be present in human embryos/fetuses. *Reprod. Toxicol.,* **8**, 191–191

Sass, J.O., Didierjean, L., Carraux, P., Plum, C., Nau, H. & Saurat, J.H. (1996) Metabolism of topical retinaldehyde and retinol by mouse skin *in vivo*: predominant formation of retinyl esters and identification of 14-hydroxy-4,14-retro-retinol. *Exp. Dermatol.,* **5**, 267–271

Satre, M.A. & Kochhar, D.M. (1989) Elevations in the endogenous levels of the putative morphogen retinoic acid in embryonic mouse limb-buds associated with limb dysmorphogenesis. *Dev. Biol.,* **133**, 529–536

Sauberlich, H.E., Hodges, R.E., Wallace, D.L., Kolder, H., Canham, J.E., Hood, J., Raica, N., Jr & Lowry, L.K. (1974) Vitamin A metabolism and requirements in the human studied with the use of labeled retinol. In: Harris, R.S. & Thimann, K.V. (eds), *Vitamins and Hormones*, New York, Academic Press, pp. 251–275

Schardein, J.L. (1993) Foods, nutrients, and dietary factors. In: Schardein, J.L. (ed.), *Chemically Induced Birth Defects*, New York, Marcel Dekker, pp. 539–580

Schober, S.E., Comstock, G.W., Helsing, K.J., Salkeld, R.M., Morris, J.S., Rider, A.A. & Brookmeyer, R. (1987) Serologic precursors of cancer. I. Prediagnostic serum nutrients and colon cancer risk. *Am. J. Epidemiol.,* **126**, 1033–1041

Schweigert, F.J. (1988) Insensitivity of dogs to the effects of nonspecific bound vitamin A in plasma. *Int. J. Vitam. Nutr. Res.,* **58**, 23–25

Schweigert, F.J., Rosival, I., Rambeck, W.A. & Gropp, J. (1995) Plasma transport and tissue distribution of [^{14}C] β-carotene and [^{3}H]retinol administered orally to pigs. *Int. J. Vitam. Nutr. Res.,* **65**, 95–100

Scott, W.J., Jr, Walter, R., Tzimas, G., Sass, J.O., Nau, H. & Collins, M.D. (1994) Endogenous status of retinoids and their cytosolic binding proteins in limb buds of chick vs mouse embryos. *Dev. Biol.,* **165**, 397–409

Seddon, J.M., Ajani, U.A., Sperduto, R.D., Hiller, R., Blair, N., Burton, T.C., Farber, M.D., Gragoudas, E.S., Haller, J., Miller, D.T., Yannuzzi, L.A. & Willett, W. (1994) Dietary carotenoids, vitamins A, C, and E, and advanced age-related macular degeneration. Eye Disease Case-Control Study Group. *J. Am. Med. Assoc.,* **272**, 1413–1420

Seifert, W.F., Bosma, A., Hendriks, H.F., Blaner, W.S., van Leeuwen, R.E., van Thiel de Ruiter, G.C., Wilson, J.H., Knook, D.L. & Brouwer, A. (1991) Chronic administration of ethanol with high vitamin A supplementation in a liquid diet to rats does not cause liver fibrosis. 2. Biochemical observations. *J. Hepatol.,* **13**, 249–255

Seifter, E., Rettura, G., Padawer, J., Stratford, F., Goodwin, P. & Levenson, S.M. (1983) Regression of C3HBA mouse tumor due to X-ray therapy combined with supplemental β-carotene or vitamin A. *J. Natl. Cancer Inst.,* **71**, 409–417

Semba, R.D. (1994) Vitamin A, immunity, and infection. *Clin. Infect. Dis.,* **19**, 489–499

Semba, R.D. (1998) The role of vitamin A and related retinoids in immune function. *Nutr. Rev.,* **56**, S38–48

Semba, R.D., Miotti, P.G., Chiphangwi, J.D., Saah, A.J., Canner, J.K., Dallabetta, G.A. & Hoover, D.R. (1994) Maternal vitamin A deficiency and mother-to-child transmission of HIV-1. *Lancet,* **343**, 1593–1597

Senoo, H., Stang, E., Nilsson, A., Kindberg, G.M., Berg, T., Roos, N., Norum, K.R. & Blomhoff, R. (1990) Internalization of retinol-binding protein in parenchymal and stellate cells of rat liver. *J. Lipid Res.,* **31**, 1229–1239

Senoo, H., Smeland, S., Malaba, L., Bjerknes, T., Stang, E., Roos, N., Berg, T., Norum, K.R. & Blomhoff, R. (1993) Transfer of retinol-binding protein from HepG2 human hepatoma cells to cocultured rat stellate cells. *Proc. Natl. Acad. Sci. USA,* **90**, 3616–3620

Shafi, S., Brady, S.E., Bensadoun, A. & Havel, R.J. (1994) Role of hepatic lipase in the uptake and processing of chylomicron remnants in rat liver. *J. Lipid Res.,* **35**, 709–720

Shah, J.P., Strong, E.W., DeCosse, J.J., Itri, L. & Sellers, P. (1983) Effect of retinoids on oral leukoplakia. *Am. J. Surg.,* **146**, 466–470

Shankar, S. & De Luca, L.M. (1988) Retinoic acid supplementation of a vitamin A-deficient diet inhibits retinoid loss from hamster liver and serum pools. *J. Nutr.,* **118**, 675–680

Sharieff, G.Q. & Hanten, K. (1996) Pseudotumor cerebri and hypercalcemia resulting from vitamin A toxicity. *Ann. Emergency Med.,* **27**, 518–521

Sharma, S.C., Bonnar, J. & Dostalova, L. (1986) Comparison of blood levels of vitamin A, β-carotene and vitamin E in abruptio placentae with normal pregnancy. *Int. J. Vitam. Nutr. Res.,* **56**, 3–9

Shaw, G.M., Wasserman, C.R., Block, G. & Lammer, E.J. (1996) High maternal vitamin A intake and risk of anomalies of structures with a cranial neural crest cell contribution. *Lancet,* **347**, 899–900

Shekelle, R.B., Lepper, M., Liu, S., Maliza, C., Raynor, W.J., Jr, Rossof, A.H., Paul, O., Shryock, A.M. & Stamler, J. (1981) Dietary vitamin A and risk of cancer in the Western Electric study. *Lancet,* **2**, 1185–1190

Shenai, J.P. & Chytil, F. (1990) Effect of maternal vitamin-A administration on fetal lung vitamin-A stores in the perinatal rat. *Biol. Neonate,* **58**, 318–325

Shenefelt, R.E. (1972) Morphogenesis of malformations in hamsters caused by retinoic acid: relation to dose and stage at treatment. *Teratology,* **5**, 103–118

Shetty, T.K., Francis, A.R. & Bhattacharya, R.K. (1988) Modifying role of vitamins on the mutagenic action of *N*-methyl-*N'*-nitro-*N*-nitrosoguanidine. *Carcinogenesis,* **9**, 1513–1515

Shi, H.L. & Olson, J.A. (1990) Site of conversion of endogenous all-*trans*-retinoids to 11-*cis*-retinoids in the bovine eye. *Biochim. Biophys. Acta,* **1035**, 1–5

Shibagaki, T., Kitamura, H., Inayama, Y., Ogata, T. & Kanisawa, M. (1994) Effects of vitamin A on proliferation of human distal airway epithelial cells in culture. *Virchows Arch.,* **424**, 525–531

Shibata, A., Paganini-Hill, A., Ross, R.K. & Henderson, B.E. (1992) Intake of vegetables, fruits, β-carotene, vitamin C and vitamin supplements and cancer incidence among the elderly: a prospective study. *Br. J. Cancer,* **66**, 673–679

Shih, T.W. & Hill, D.L. (1991) Conversion of retinol to retinal by rat liver microsomes. *Drug Metab. Dispos.,* **19**, 332–335

Shingleton, J.L., Skinner, M.K. & Ong, D.E. (1989) Retinol esterification in Sertoli cells by lecithin-retinol acyltransferase. *Biochemistry,* **28**, 9647–9653

Shklar, G., Schwartz, J., Grau, D., Trickler, D.P. & Wallace, K.D. (1980) Inhibition of hamster buccal pouch carcinogenesis by 13-*cis*-retinoic acid. *Oral Surg. Oral Med. Oral Pathol.,* **50**, 45–52

Siegenthaler, G. (1990) Retinoic acid formation from retinol and retinal metabolism in epidermal cells. *Methods Enzymol.,* **189**, 530–536

Silverman, S., Renstrup, G. & Pindborg, J.J. (1963) Studies in oral leukoplakias. III. Effects of vitamin A comparing clinical, histopathologic, cytologic, and hematologic responses. *Acta Odontol. Scand.,* **21**, 271–292

Simon, A., Hellman, U., Wernstedt, C. & Eriksson, U. (1995) The retinal pigment epithelial-specific 11-*cis* retinol dehydrogenase belongs to the family of short chain alcohol dehydrogenases. *J. Biol. Chem.,* **270**, 1107–1112

Singh, R.B., Ghosh, S., Niaz, M.A., Singh, R., Beegum, R., Chibo, H., Shoumin, Z. & Postiglione, A. (1995) Dietary intake, plasma levels of antioxidant vitamins, and oxidative stress in relation to coronary artery disease in elderly subjects. *Am. J. Cardiol.,* **76**, 1233–1238

Sinha, S.P. & Kumari, D. (1994) Vitamin A ameliorates the genotoxicity in mice of aflatoxin B_1- containing *Aspergillus flavus* infested food. *Cytobios,* **79**, 85–95

Sirianni, S.R., Chen, H.H. & Huang, C.C. (1981) Effects of retinoids on plating efficiency, sister-chromatid exchange (SCE) and mitomycin-C-induced SCE in cultured Chinese hamster cells. *Mutat. Res.,* **90**, 175–182

Skrede, B., Olafsdottir, A.E., Blomhoff, R. & Norum, K.R. (1993) Retinol and retinyl esters in rabbit bone marrow and blood leukocytes. *Scand. J. Clin. Lab. Invest.,* **53**, 515–519

Slattery, M.L., Abbott, T.M., Overall, J.C., Jr, Robison, L.M., French, T.K., Jolles, C., Gardner, J.W. & West, D.W. (1990) Dietary vitamins A, C, and E and selenium as risk factors for cervical cancer. *Epidemiology,* **1**, 8–15

Slattery, M.L., Jacobs, D.R., Jr, Dyer, A., Benson, J., Hilner, J.E. & Caan, B.J. (1995) Dietary antioxidants and plasma lipids: the Cardia Study. *J. Am. Coll. Nutr.,* **14**, 635–642

Smith, D.M., Rogers, A.E., Herndon, B.J. & Newberne, P.M. (1975a) Vitamin A (retinyl acetate) and benzo(a)pyrene-induced respiratory tract carcinogenesis in hamsters fed a commercial diet. *Cancer Res.*, **35**, 11–16

Smith, D.M., Rogers, A.E. & Newberne, P.M. (1975b) Vitamin A and benzo(*a*)pyrene carcinogenesis in the respiratory tract of hamsters fed a semisynthetic diet. *Cancer Res.*, **35**, 1485–1488

Soffritti, M., Mobiglia, A., Pinto, C., Bortoluzzi, L., Lefemine, G. & Maltoni, C. (1996) Results of experimental bioassays on the chemopreventive effects of vitamin A and *N*-(hydroxyphenyl)-retinamide (HPR) on mammary cancer. In: Maltoni, C., Soffritti, M. & Davis, W. (eds), *The Scientific Bases of Cancer Chemoprevention*, Amsterdam, Elsevier, pp. 241–248

Sommer, A. & West, K.P. (1996) *Vitamin A Deficiency: Health, Survival, and Vision*, Oxford, Oxford University Press

Sommer, A., Hussaini, G., Muhilal, Tarwotjo, I., Susanto, D. & Saroso, J.S. (1980) History of night-blindness: a simple tool for xerophthalmia screening. *Am. J. Clin. Nutr.*, **33**, 887–891

Soprano, D.R. & Blaner, W.S. (1994) Plasma retinol-binding protein. In: Sporn, M.B., Roberts, A.B. & Goodman, D.S. (eds), *The Retinoids: Biology, Chemistry, and Medicine*, 2nd edition, New York, Raven Press, pp. 257–281

Soprano, D.R., Soprano, K.J. & Goodman, D.S. (1986) Retinol-binding protein messenger RNA levels in the liver and in extrahepatic tissues of the rat. *J. Lipid Res.*, **27**, 166–171

Soprano, D.R., Gyda, M.3, Jiang, H., Harnish, D.C., Ugen, K., Satre, M., Chen, L., Soprano, K.J. & Kochhar, D.M. (1994) A sustained elevation in retinoic acid receptor-β 2 mRNA and protein occurs during retinoic acid-induced fetal dysmorphogenesis. *Mech. Dev.*, **45**, 243–253

Sperduto, R.D., Hu, T.S., Milton, R.C., Zhao, J.L., Everett, D.F., Cheng, Q.F., Blot, W.J., Bing, L., Taylor, P.R., Li, J.Y., Dawsey, S. & Guo, W.D. (1993) The Linxian cataract studies. Two nutrition intervention trials. *Arch. Ophthalmol.*, **111**, 1246–1253

Stansfield, S.K., Pierre Louis, M., Lerebours, G. & Augustin, A. (1993) Vitamin A supplementation and increased prevalence of childhood diarrhoea and acute respiratory infections. *Lancet*, **342**, 578–582

Stark, A.A., Pagano, D.A., Glass, G., Kamin Belsky, N. & Zeiger, E. (1994) The effects of antioxidants and enzymes involved in glutathione metabolism on mutagenesis by glutathione and L-cysteine. *Mutat. Res.*, **308**, 215–222

Stearns, M.E., Wang, M. & Fudge, K. (1993) Liarozole and 13-*cis*-retinoic acid anti-prostatic tumor activity. *Cancer Res.*, **53**, 3073–3077

Stehr, P.A., Gloninger, M.F., Kuller, L.H., Marsh, G.M., Radford, E.P. & Weinberg, G.B. (1985) Dietary vitamin A deficiencies and stomach cancer. *Am. J. Epidemiol.*, **121**, 65–70

Stephensen, C.B., Alvarez, J.O., Kohatsu, J., Hardmeier, R., Kennedy, J.I., Jr. & Gammon, R.B.J. (1994) Vitamin A is excreted in the urine during acute infection. *Am. J. Clin. Nutr.*, **60**, 388–392

Stich, H.F. & Rosin, M.P. (1984) Micronuclei in exfoliated human cells as a tool for studies in cancer risk and cancer intervention. *Cancer Lett.*, **22**, 241–253

Stich, H.F. & Tsang, S.S. (1989) Promoting activity of betel quid ingredients and their inhibition by retinol. *Cancer Lett.*, **45**, 71–77

Stich, H.F., Stich, W. & Parida, B.B. (1982) Elevated frequency of micronucleated cells in the buccal mucosa of individuals at high risk for oral cancer: betel quid chewers. *Cancer Lett.*, **17**, 125–134

Stich, H.F., Rosin, M.P. & Vallejera, M.O. (1984a) Reduction with vitamin A and beta-carotene administration of proportion of micronucleated buccal mucosal cells in Asian betel nut and tobacco chewers. *Lancet*, **1**, 1204–1206

Stich, H.F., Stich, W., Rosin, M.P. & Vallejera, M.O. (1984b) Use of the micronucleus test to monitor the effect of vitamin A, beta-carotene and canthaxanthin on the buccal mucosa of betel nut/tobacco chewers. *Int. J. Cancer*, **34**, 745–750

Stich, H.F., Hornby, A.P. & Dunn, B.P. (1985) A pilot beta-carotene intervention trial with Inuits using smokeless tobacco. *Int. J. Cancer*, **36**, 321–327

Stich, H.F., Hornby, A.P., Mathew, B., Sankaranarayanan, R. & Nair, M.K. (1988a) Response of oral leukoplakias to the administration of vitamin A. *Cancer Lett.*, **40**, 93–101

Stich, H.F., Rosin, M.P., Hornby, A.P., Mathew, B., Sankaranarayanan, R. & Nair, M.K. (1988b) Remission of oral leukoplakias and micronuclei in tobacco/betel quid chewers treated with beta-carotene and with beta-carotene plus vitamin A. *Int. J. Cancer,* **42**, 195–199

Stich, H.F., Tsang, S.S. & Palcic, B. (1990) The effect of retinoids, carotenoids and phenolics on chromosomal instability of bovine papillomavirus DNA-carrying cells. *Mutat. Res.,* **241**, 387–393

Stich, H.F., Mathew, B., Sankaranarayanan, R. & Nair, M.K. (1991a) Remission of precancerous lesions in the oral cavity of tobacco chewers and maintenance of the protective effect of β-carotene or vitamin A. *Am. J. Clin. Nutr.,* **53**, 298S–304S

Stich, H.F., Mathew, B., Sankaranarayanan, R. & Nair, M.K. (1991b) Remission of oral precancerous lesions of tobacco/areca nut chewers following administration of β-carotene or vitamin A, and maintenance of the protective effect. *Cancer Detect. Prev.,* **15**, 93–98

Sucov, H.M., Dyson, E., Gumeringer, C.L., Price, J., Chien, K.R. & Evans, R.M. (1994) RXR alpha mutant mice establish a genetic basis for vitamin A signaling in heart morphogenesis. *Genes Dev.,* **8**, 1007–1018

Suhara, A., Kato, M. & Kanai, M. (1990) Ultrastructural localization of plasma retinol-binding protein in rat liver. *J. Lipid Res.,* **31**, 1669–1681

Suharno, D., West, C.E., Muhilal, Karyadi, D. & Hautvast, J.G. (1993) Supplementation with vitamin A and iron for nutritional anaemia in pregnant women in West Java, Indonesia. *Lancet,* **342**, 1325–1328

Sulik, K.K., Dehart, D.B., Rogers, J.M. & Chernoff, N. (1995) Teratogenicity of low doses of all-*trans* retinoic acid in presomite mouse embryos. *Teratology,* **51**, 398–403

Sun, G., Alexson, S.E. & Harrison, E.H. (1997) Purification and characterization of a neutral, bile salt- independent retinyl ester hydrolase from rat liver microsomes. Relationship to rat carboxylesterase ES-2. *J. Biol. Chem.,* **272**, 24488–24493

Sundaresan, P.R. (1977) Rate of metabolism of retinol and retinoic acid-maintained rats after a single dose of radioactive retinol. *J. Nutr.,* **107**, 70–78

Surwit, E.A., Graham, V., Droegemueller, W., Alberts, D., Chvapil, M., Dorr, R.T., Davis, J.R. & Meyskens, F.L.J. (1982) Evaluation of topically applied *trans*-retinoic acid in the treatment of cervical intraepithelial lesions. *Am. J. Obstet. Gynecol.,* **143**, 821–823

Suzuki, R., Goda, T. & Takase, S. (1995) Consumption of excess vitamin A, but not excess β-carotene, causes accumulation of retinol that exceeds the binding capacity of cellular retinol-binding protein, type II in rat intestine. *J. Nutr.,* **125**, 2074–2082

Szõcsik, K., González Cabello, R., Vien, C.V., Mézes, M., Szongoth, M. & Gergely, P. (1988) Effect of vitamin A treatment on immune reactivity and lipid peroxidation in patients with Sjogren's syndrome. *Clin. Rheumatol.,* **7**, 514–519

Szuts, E.Z. & Harosi, F.I. (1991) Solubility of retinoids in water. *Arch. Biochem. Biophys.,* **287**, 297–304

Takahashi, O. (1995) Haemorrhagic toxicity of a large dose of α-, β-, γ- and δ-tocopherols, ubiquinone, β-carotene, retinol acetate and L-ascorbic acid in the rat. *Food Chem. Toxicol.,* **33**, 121–128

Takahashi, Y.I., Smith, J.E., Winick, M. & Goodman, D.S. (1975) Vitamin A deficiency and fetal growth and development in the rat. *J. Nutr.,* **105**, 1299–1310

Takase, S., Ong, D.E. & Chytil, F. (1986) Transfer of retinoic acid from its complex with cellular retinoic acid-binding protein to the nucleus. *Arch. Biochem. Biophys.,* **247**, 328–334

Talamini, R., Franceschi, S., La Vecchia, C., Serraino, D., Barra, S. & Negri, E. (1992) Diet and prostatic cancer: a case-control study in northern Italy. *Nutr. Cancer,* **18**, 277–286

Tall, A. (1995) Plasma lipid transfer proteins. *Annu. Rev. Biochem.,* **64**, 235–257

Tamura, K., Ohsugi, K. & Ide, H. (1990) Distribution of retinoids in the chick limb bud: analysis with monoclonal antibody. *Dev. Biol.,* **140**, 20–26

Tang, X. & Edenharder, R. (1997) Inhibition of the mutagenicity of 2-nitrofluorene, 3-nitrofluoranthene and 1-nitropyrene by vitamins, porphyrins and related compounds, and vegetable and fruit juices and solvent extracts. *Food Chem. Toxicol.,* **35**, 373–378

Tang, G.W. & Russell, R.M. (1990) 13-*cis*-Retinoic acid is an endogenous compound in human serum. *J. Lipid Res.*, **31**, 175–182

Tang, G. & Russell, R.M. (1991) Formation of all-*trans*-retinoic acid and 13-*cis*-retinoic acid from all-*trans*-retinyl palmitate in humans. *J. Nutr. Biochem.*, **2**, 210–213

Tanumihardjo, S.A., Koellner, P.G. & Olson, J.A. (1990) The modified relative-dose-response assay as an indicator of vitamin A status in a population of well-nourished American children. *Am. J. Clin. Nutr.*, **52**, 1064–1067

Tanumihardjo, S.A., Permaesih, D., Muherdiyantiningsih, Rustan, E., Rusmil, K., Fatah, A.C., Wilbur, S., Muhilal, Karyadi, D. & Olson, J.A. (1996) Vitamin A status of Indonesian children infected with *Ascaris lumbricoides* after dosing with vitamin A supplements and albendazole. *J. Nutr.*, **126**, 451–457

Tavan, E., Maziere, S., Narbonne, J.F. & Cassand, P. (1997) Effects of vitamins A and E on methylazoxymethanol-induced mutagenesis in *Salmonella typhimurium* strain TA100. *Mutat. Res.*, **377**, 231–237

Tavani, A., Negri, E., Franceschi, S. & La Vecchia, C. (1994) Risk factors for esophageal cancer in lifelong nonsmokers. *Cancer Epidemiol. Biomarkers. Prev.*, **3**, 387–392

Tchao, R. (1980) Keratinization and the effect of vitamin A in aggregates of a squamous carcinoma cell line NBT II. *In vitro*, **16**, 407–414

Tee, E.S. (1992) Carotenoids and retinoids in human nutrition. *Crit. Rev. Food Sci. Nutr.*, **31**, 103–163

Tembe, E.A., Honeywell, R., Buss, N.E. & Renwick, A.G. (1996) All-*trans*-retinoic acid in maternal plasma and teratogenicity in rats and rabbits. *Toxicol. Appl. Pharmacol.*, **141**, 456–472

Thaller, C. & Eichele, G. (1987) Identification and spatial distribution of retinoids in the developing chick limb bud. *Nature*, **327**, 625–628

Thaller, C. & Eichele, G. (1990) Isolation of 3,4-didehydroretinoic acid, a novel morphogenetic signal in the chick wing bud. *Nature*, **345**, 815–819

Thompson, J.N., Howell, J.M. & Pitt, G.A.J. (1964) Vitamin A and reproduction in rats. *Proc. R. Soc. London, B. Biol. Sci.*, **159**, 510–535

Thompson, H.J., Meeker, L.D., Tagliaferro, A.R. & Becci, P.J. (1982) Effect of retinyl acetate on the occurrence of ovarian hormone-responsive and -nonresponsive mammary cancers in the rat. *Cancer Res.*, **42**, 903–905

Thompson, K.H., Hughes, L.B. & Zilversmit, D.B. (1983) Lack of secretion of retinyl ester by livers of normal and cholesterol-fed rabbits. *J. Nutr.*, **113**, 1995–2001

Thorne, E.G. (1992) Long-term clinical experience with a topical retinoid. *Br. J. Dermatol.*, **127 Suppl. 41**, 31–36

Thurnham, D.I. (1997) Impact of disease on markers of micronutrient status. *Proc. Nutr. Soc.*, **56**, 421–423

Thurnham, D.I. & Singkamani, R. (1991) The acute phase response and vitamin A status in malaria. *Trans. R. Soc. Trop. Med. Hyg.*, **85**, 194–199

Thurnham, D.I., Muñoz, N., Lu, J.B., Wahrendorf, J., Zheng, S.F., Hambidge, K.M. & Crespi, M. (1988) Nutritional and haematological status of Chinese farmers: the influence of 13.5 months treatment with riboflavin, retinol and zinc. *Eur. J. Clin. Nutr.*, **42**, 647–660

Thurnham, D.I., Northrop-Clewes, C.A., Paracha, P.I. & McLoon, U.J. (1997) The possible significance of parallel changes in plasma lutein and retinol in Pakistani infants during the summer season. *Br. J. Nutr.*, **78**, 775–784

Tickle, C., Summerbell, D. & Wolpert, L. (1975) Positional signalling and specification of digits in chick limb morphogenesis. *Nature*, **254**, 199–202

Tickle, C., Alberts, B., Wolpert, L. & Lee, J. (1982) Local application of retinoic acid to the limb bond mimics the action of the polarizing region. *Nature*, **296**, 564–566

Toma, S., Albanese, M. & De Lorenzi, G. (1990) β-carotene in the treatment of oral leukoplakia. *Proc. Am. Soc. Clin. Oncol.*, **9**, 179-179

Toma, S., Mangiante, P.E., Margarino, G., Nicolo, G. & Palumbo, R. (1992) Progressive 13-*cis*-retinoic acid dosage in the treatment of oral leukoplakia. *Eur. J. Cancer, B. Oral Oncol.*, **28B**, 121–123

Tomita, Y. (1983) Immunological role of vitamin A and its related substances in prevention of cancer. *Nutr. Cancer*, **5**, 187–194

Toniolo, P., Riboli, E., Protta, F., Charrel, M. & Cappa, A.P. (1989) Calorie-providing nutrients and risk of breast cancer. *J. Natl. Cancer Inst.*, **81**, 278–286

Toyoshima, K. & Leighton, J. (1975) Vitamin A inhibition of keratinization in rat urinary bladder cancer cell line Nara Bladder Tumor No. 2 in meniscus gradient culture. *Cancer Res.*, **35**, 1873–1879

Trøen, G., Nilsson, A., Norum, K.R. & Blomhoff, R. (1994) Characterization of liver stellate cell retinyl ester storage. *Biochem. J.*, **300**, 793–798

Tsutsumi, C., Okuno, M., Tannous, L., Piantedosi, R., Allan, M., Goodman, D.S. & Blaner, W.S. (1992) Retinoids and retinoid-binding protein expression in rat adipocytes. *J. Biol. Chem.*, **267**, 1805–1810

Turpin, J., Mehta, K., Blick, M., Hester, J.P. & Lopez Berestein, G. (1990) Effect of retinoids on the release and gene expression of tumor necrosis factor-α in human peripheral blood monocytes. *J. Leukoc. Biol.*, **48**, 444–450

Tuyns, A.J., Riboli, E., Doornbos, G. & Pequignot, G. (1987) Diet and esophageal cancer in Calvados (France). *Nutr. Cancer*, **9**, 81–92

Twining, S.S., Schulte, D.P., Wilson, P.M., Fish, B.L. & Moulder, J.E. (1996) Retinol is sequestered in the bone marrow of vitamin A-deficient rats. *J. Nutr.*, **126**, 1618–1626

Tzimas, G. (1996) Investigations on the metabolism and the pharmacokinetics of retinol and retinoic acid isomers toward understanding of the interspecies variation of retinoid teratogenicity and human risk assessment (Thesis), Freie Universität Berlin

Tzimas, G., Burgin, H., Collins, M.D., Hummler, H. & Nau, H. (1994) The high sensitivity of the rabbit to the teratogenic effects of 13-*cis*-retinoic acid (isotretinoin) is a consequence of prolonged exposure of the embryo to 13-*cis*-retinoic acid and 13-*cis*-4-oxo-retinoic acid, and not of isomerization to all-*trans*-retinoic acid. *Arch. Toxicol.*, **68**, 119–128

Tzimas, G., Collins, M.D. & Nau, H. (1995) Developmental stage-associated differences in the transplacental distribution of 13-*cis*- and all-*trans*-retinoic acid as well as their glucuronides in rats and mice. *Toxicol. Appl. Pharmacol.*, **133**, 91–101

Tzimas, G., Collins, M.D., Burgin, H., Hummler, H. & Nau, H. (1996a) Embryotoxic doses of vitamin A to rabbits result in low plasma but high embryonic concentrations of all-*trans*-retinoic acid: risk of vitamin A exposure in humans. *J. Nutr.*, **126**, 2159–2171

Tzimas, G., Collins, M.D. & Nau, H. (1996b) Identification of 14-hydroxy-4,14-retro-retinol as an *in vivo* metabolite of vitamin A. *Biochim. Biophys. Acta*, **1301**, 1–6

Ueda, H., Takenawa, T., Millan, J.C., Gesell, M.S. & Brandes, D. (1980) The effects of retinoids on proliferative capacities and macromolecular synthesis in human breast cancer MCF-7 cells. *Cancer*, **46**, 2203–2209

Underwood, B.A. (1986) The safe use of vitamin A by women during the reproductive years. Washington DC, IVACG Secretariat

Underwood, B.A. (1990a) Biochemical and histological methodologies for assessing vitamin A status in human populations. *Methods Enzymol.*, **190**, 242–251

Underwood, B.A. (1990b) Methods for assessment of vitamin A status. *J. Nutr.*, **120 Suppl. 11**, 1459–1463

Underwood, B.A. & Arthur, P. (1996) The contribution of vitamin A to public health. *FASEB J.*, **10**, 1040–1048

Underwood, B.A., Loerch, J.D. & Lewis, K.C. (1979) Effects of dietary vitamin A deficiency, retinoic acid and protein quantity and quality on serially obtained plasma and liver levels of vitamin A in rats. *J. Nutr.*, **109**, 796–806

Urbach, J. & Rando, R.R. (1994) Isomerization of all-*trans*-retinoic acid to 9-*cis*-retinoic acid. *Biochem. J.*, **299**, 459–465

US Food and Drug Administration (1976) Vitamin and mineral products. Labeling and composition regulations. *Fed. Reg.*, **41**, 46156–46176

Vaessen, M.J., Meijers, J.H., Bootsma, D. & Van Kessel, A.G. (1990) The cellular retinoic-acid-binding protein is expressed in tissues associated with retinoic-acid-induced malformations. *Development*, **110**, 371–378

Vahlquist, A. (1994) Role of retinoids in normal and diseased skin. In: Blomhoff, R. (ed.), *Vitamin A in Health and Disease*, New York, Marcel Dekker, pp. 365–424

Vahlquist, A., Peterson, P.A. & Wibell, L. (1973) Metabolism of the vitamin A transporting protein complex. I. Turnover studies in normal persons and in patients with chronic renal failure. *Eur. J. Clin. Invest.*, **3**, 352–362

van Pelt, A.M. & de Rooij, D.G. (1991) Retinoic acid is able to reinitiate spermatogenesis in vitamin A-deficient rats and high replicate doses support the full development of spermatogenic cells. *Endocrinology*, **128**, 697–704

Van Rooijen, L.A., Derks, H.J., Van Wijk, R. & Bisschop, A. (1984) Relation between induction of rat hepatic ornithine decarboxylase activity by tumor promoters 12-O-tetradecanoylphorbol-13-acetate and phenobarbital and levels of the polyamines putrescine, spermidine and spermine, *in vivo*; differential effects of retinyl-acetate. *Carcinogenesis*, **5**, 225–229

Van Vliet, T. (1996) Absorption of β-carotene and other carotenoids in humans and animal models. *Eur. J. Clin. Nutr.*, **50 Suppl. 3**, S32–S37

Van Vliet, T., van Vlissingen, M.F., Van Schaik, F. & van den Berg, H. (1996) β-Carotene absorption and cleavage in rats is affected by the vitamin A concentration of the diet. *J. Nutr.*, **126**, 499–508

Van Wauwe, J., Van Nyen, G., Coene, M.C., Stoppie, P., Cools, W., Goossens, J., Borghgraef, P. & Janssen, P.A. (1992) Liarozole, an inhibitor of retinoic acid metabolism, exerts retinoid-mimetic effects *in vivo*. *J. Pharmacol. Exp. Ther.*, **261**, 773–779

van Zandwijk, N., Pastorino, U., de Vries, N., van Tinteren, H., Gras, L., Kirkpatrick, A., Dalesio, O., Lubsen, H., Copper, M.P., Grandi, C., Balm, A.J.M., Lefebvre, J.L., Lunghi, F., Jerman, J., Spasova, I., Infante, M., Vanderschueren, R.G.J.R.A. & Maioli, M. (1997) EUROSCAN. *Lung Cancer*, **18**, 86–87

Velasquez Melendez, G., Okani, E.T., Kiertsman, B. & Roncada, M.J. (1995) Vitamin A status in children with pneumonia. *Eur. J. Clin. Nutr.*, **49**, 379–384

Verhoeven, D.T., Assen, N., Goldbohm, R.A., Dorant, E., Van't Veer, P., Sturmans, F., Hermus, R.J. & van den Brandt, P.A. (1997) Vitamins C and E, retinol, beta-carotene and dietary fibre in relation to breast cancer risk: a prospective cohort study. *Br. J. Cancer*, **75**, 149–155

Verma, A.K., Shapas, B.G., Rice, H.M. & Boutwell, R.K. (1979) Correlation of the inhibition by retinoids of tumor promoter-induced mouse epidermal ornithine decarboxylase activity and of skin tumor promotion. *Cancer Res.*, **39**, 419–425

Verma, A.K., Shoemaker, A., Simsiman, R., Denning, M. & Zachman, R.D. (1992) Expression of retinoic acid nuclear receptors and tissue transglutaminase is altered in various tissues of rats fed a vitamin A-deficient diet. *J. Nutr.*, **122**, 2144–2152

Verreault, R., Chu, J., Mandelson, M. & Shy, K. (1989) A case-control study of diet and invasive cervical cancer. *Int. J. Cancer*, **43**, 1050–1054

Victorin, K., Busk, L. & Ahlborg, U.G. (1987) Retinol (vitamin A) inhibits the mutagenicity of *o*- aminoazotoluene activated by liver microsomes from several species in the Ames test. *Mutat. Res.*, **179**, 41–48

Virtanen, S.M., van't Veer, P., Kok, F., Kardinaal, A.F.M. & Aro, A. (1996) Predictors of adipose tissue carotenoid and retinol levels in nine countries. *Am. J. Epidem.*, **144**, 968–979

Volz, J., van Rissenbeck, A., Blanke, M., Melchert, F., Schneider, A. & Biesalski, H.K. (1995) Changes in the vitamin A status in dysplastic epithelium of the cervix. *Zentralbl. Gynakol.*, **117**, 472–475

Wagner, M., Han, B. & Jessell, T.M. (1992) Regional differences in retinoid release from embryonic neural tissue detected by an *in vitro* reporter assay. *Development*, **116**, 55–66

Wahrendorf, J., Muñoz, N., Lu, J.B., Thurnham, D.I., Crespi, M. & Bosch, F.X. (1988) Blood, retinol and zinc riboflavin status in relation to precancerous lesions of the esophagus: findings from a vitamin intervention trial in the People's Republic of China. *Cancer Res.*, **48**, 2280–2283

Wake, K. (1980) Perisinusoidal stellate cells (fat-storing cells, interstitial cells, lipocytes), their related structure in and around the liver sinusoids, and vitamin A-storing cells in extrahepatic organs. *Int. Rev. Cytol.*, **66**, 303–353

Wake, K. (1994) Role of perisinusoidal stellate cells in vitamin A storage. In: Blomhoff, R. (ed.), *Vitamin A in Health and Disease*, New York, Marcel Dekker, pp. 73–86

Wald, N.J., Boreham, J., Hayward, J.L. & Bulbrook, R.D. (1984) Plasma retinol, β-carotene and vitamin E levels in relation to the future risk of breast cancer. *Br. J. Cancer,* **49**, 321–324

Wang, W. & Higuchi, C.M. (1995) Induction of NAD(P)H:quinone reductase by vitamins A, E and C in Colo205 colon cancer cells. *Cancer Lett.,* **98**, 63–69

Wang, X.D., Tang, G.W., Fox, J.G., Krinsky, N.I. & Russell, R.M. (1991) Enzymatic conversion of β-carotene into β-apocarotenals and retinoids by human, monkey, ferret, and rat tissues. *Arch. Biochem. Biophys.,* **285**, 8–16

Wang, X.D., Krinsky, N.I., Tang, G.W. & Russell, R.M. (1992) Retinoic acid can be produced from excentric cleavage of β-carotene in human intestinal mucosa. *Arch. Biochem. Biophys.,* **293**, 298–304

Wang, X.D., Krinsky, N.I., Benotti, P.N. & Russell, R.M. (1994) Biosynthesis of 9-*cis*-retinoic acid from 9-*cis*-β-carotene in human intestinal mucosa *in vitro. Arch. Biochem. Biophys.,* **313**, 150–155

Ward, J. (1994) Free radicals, antioxidants and preventive geriatrics. *Aust. Fam. Physician,* **23**, 1297–1305

Ward, B.J. (1996) Retinol (vitamin A) supplements in the elderly. *Drugs Aging,* **9**, 48–59

Waters, M.D., Brady, A.L., Stack, H.F. & Brockman, H.E. (1990) Antimutagenicity profiles for some model compounds. *Mutat. Res.,* **238**, 57–85

Waters, M.D., Stack, H.F., Jackson, M.A., Brockman, H.E. & De Flora, S. (1996a) Activity profiles of antimutagens: *in vitro* and *in vivo* data. *Mutat. Res.,* **350**, 109–129

Waters, M.D., Stack, H.F., Jackson, M.A. & Brockman, H.E. (1996b) Interpretation of short-term test data: implications for assessment of chemopreventive activity. In: Stewart, B.W., McGregor, D. & Kleihues, P. (eds), *Principles of Chemoprevention,* (IARC Scientific Publications No. 139), Lyon, IARC, pp. 313–332

Watkins, M., Moore, C. & Mulinare, J. (1996) Teratogenicity of high vitamin A intake. *New Engl. J. Med.,* **334**, 1196–1196

Watson, R.R. (1986) Immunological enhancement by fat-soluble vitamins, minerals, and trace metals: a factor in cancer prevention. *Cancer Detect. Prev.,* **9**, 67–77

Watson, R.R., Moriguchi, S. & Gensler, H.L. (1987) Effects of dietary retinyl palmitate and selenium on tumoricidal capacity of macrophages in mice undergoing tumor promotion. *Cancer Lett.,* **36**, 181–187

Webster, R.P., Gawde, M.D. & Bhattacharya, R.K. (1996) Effect of different vitamin A status on carcinogen-induced DNA damage and repair enzymes in rats. *In vivo,* **10**, 113–118

Wei, S., Episkopou, V., Piantedosi, R., Maeda, S., Shimada, K., Gottesman, M.E. & Blaner, W.S. (1995) Studies on the metabolism of retinol and retinol-binding protein in transthyretin-deficient mice produced by homologous recombination. *J. Biol. Chem.,* **270**, 866–870

Wei, S.H., Lai, K., Patel, S., Piantedosi, R., Shen, H., Colantuoni, V., Kraemer, F.B. & Blaner, W.S. (1997) Retinyl ester hydrolysis and retinol efflux from BFC-1β adipocytes. *J. Biol. Chem.,* **272**, 14159–14165

Weiner, F.R., Blaner, W.S., Czaja, M.J., Shah, A. & Geerts, A. (1992) Ito cell expression of a nuclear retinoic acid receptor. *Hepatology,* **15**, 336–342

Wellik, D.M. & DeLuca, H.F. (1995) Retinol in addition to retinoic acid is required for successful gestation in vitamin A-deficient rats. *Biol. Reprod.,* **53**, 1392–1397

Wellik, D.M. & DeLuca, H.F. (1996) Metabolites of all-*trans*-retinol in day 10 conceptuses of vitamin A-deficient rats. *Arch. Biochem. Biophys.,* **330**, 355–362

Wellik, D.M., Norback, D.H. & DeLuca, H.F. (1997) Retinol is specifically required during midgestation for neonatal survival. *Am. J. Physiol.,* **272**, E25–E29

Welsch, C.W., Brown, C.K., Goodrich Smith, M., Chiusano, J. & Moon, R.C. (1980) Synergistic effect of chronic prolactin suppression and retinoid treatment in the prophylaxis of *N*-methyl-*N*-nitrosourea-induced mammary tumorigenesis in female Sprague-Dawley rats. *Cancer Res.,* **40**, 3095–3098

Welsch, C.W., Goodrich Smith, M., Brown, C.K. & Crowe, N. (1981) Enhancement by retinyl acetate of hormone-induced mammary tumorigenesis in female GR/A mice. *J. Natl. Cancer Inst.,* **67**, 935–938

Werler, M.M., Lammer, E.J., Rosenberg, L. & Mitchell, A.A. (1990) Maternal vitamin A supplementation in relation to selected birth defects. *Teratology,* **42**, 497–503

Werler, M.M., Lammer, E.J. & Mitchell, A.A. (1996) Teratogenicity of high vitamin A intake. *New Engl. J. Med.,* **334**, 1195–1196

West, D.W., Slattery, M.L., Robison, L.M., Schuman, K.L., Ford, M.H., Mahoney, A.W., Lyon, J.L. & Sorensen, A.W. (1989) Dietary intake and colon cancer: sex- and anatomic site-specific associations. *Am. J. Epidemiol.,* **130**, 883–894

West, D.W., Slattery, M.L., Robison, L.M., French, T.K. & Mahoney, A.W. (1991) Adult dietary intake and prostate cancer risk in Utah: a case-control study with special emphasis on aggressive tumors. *Cancer Causes Control,* **2**, 85–94

West, S., Vitale, S., Hallfrisch, J., Munoz, B., Muller, D., Bressler, S. & Bressler, N.M. (1994) Are antioxidants or supplements protective for age-related macular degeneration? *Arch. Ophthalmol.,* **112**, 222–227

West, K.P., LeClerq, S.C., Shrestha, S.R., Wu, L.S., Pradhan, E.K., Khatry, S.K., Katz, J., Adhikari, R. & Sommer, A. (1997) Effects of vitamin A on growth of vitamin A-deficient children: field studies in Nepal. *J. Nutr.,* **127**, 1957–1965

White, W.E., Jr & Rock, S.G. (1981) Lack of comutagenicity by norharman and other compounds on revertants induced by photolabeling with 2-azido-9-fluorenone oxime. *Mutat. Res.,* **84**, 263–271

White, J.A., Beckett Jones, B., Guo, Y.D., Dilworth, F.J., Bonasoro, J., Jones, G. & Petkovich, M. (1997a) cDNA cloning of human retinoic acid-metabolizing enzyme (hP450RAI) identifies a novel family of cytochromes P450. *J. Biol. Chem.,* **272**, 18538–18541

White, E., Shannon, J.S. & Patterson, R.E. (1997b) Relationship between vitamin and calcium supplement use and colon cancer. *Cancer Epidemiol. Biomarkers. Prev.,* **6**, 769–774

WHO (1996) *Indicators for Assessing Vitamin A Deficiency and their Application in Monitoring and Evaluating Intervention Programmes,* (Micronutrient Series, WHO/NUT/96.10), Geneva

Wiencke, J.K., Kelsey, K.T., Varkonyi, A., Semey, K., Wain, J.C., Mark, E. & Christiani, D.C. (1995) Correlation of DNA adducts in blood mononuclear cells with tobacco carcinogen-induced damage in human lung. *Cancer Res.,* **55**, 4910–4914

Wijeweera, J.B., Gandolfi, A.J., Badger, D.A., Sipes, I.G. & Brendel, K. (1996) Vitamin A potentiation of vinylidene chloride hepatotoxicity in rats and precision-cut rat liver slices. *Fundam. Appl. Toxicol.,* **34**, 73–83

Willett, W.C., Stampfer, M.J., Underwood, B.A., Taylor, J.O. & Hennekens, C.H. (1983) Vitamins A, E, and carotene: effects of supplementation on their plasma levels. *Am. J. Clin. Nutr.,* **38**, 559–566

Willett, W.C., Stampfer, M.J., Underwood, B.A., Sampson, L.A., Hennekens, C.H., Wallingford, J.C., Cooper, L., Hsieh, C.C. & Speizer, F.E. (1984a) Vitamin A supplementation and plasma retinol levels: a randomized trial among women. *J. Natl. Cancer Inst.,* **73**, 1445–1448

Willett, W.C., Polk, B.F., Underwood, B.A., Stampfer, M.J., Pressel, S., Rosner, B., Taylor, J.O., Schneider, K. & Hames, C.G. (1984b) Relation of serum vitamins A and E and carotenoids to the risk of cancer. *New Engl. J. Med.,* **310**, 430–434

Willett, W.C., Sampson, L., Stampfer, M.J., Rosner, B., Bain, C., Witschi, J., Hennekens, C.H. & Speizer, F.E. (1985) Reproducibility and validity of a semiquantitative food frequency questionnaire. *Am. J. Epidemiol.,* **122**, 51–65

Willhite, C.C., Wier, P.J. & Berry, D.L. (1989) Dose response and structure-activity considerations in retinoid-induced dysmorphogenesis. *Crit. Rev. Toxicol.,* **20**, 113–135

Williams, D.L., Dawson, P.A., Newman, T.C. & Rudel, L.L. (1985) Apolipoprotein E synthesis in peripheral tissues of nonhuman primates. *J. Biol. Chem.,* **260**, 2444–2451

Willnow, T.E., Sheng, Z., Ishibashi, S. & Herz, J. (1994) Inhibition of hepatic chylomicron remnant uptake by gene transfer of a receptor antagonist. *Science,* **264**, 1471–1474

Willnow, T.E., Armstrong, S.A., Hammer, R.E. & Herz, J. (1995) Functional expression of low density lipoprotein receptor-related protein is controlled by receptor-associated protein *in vivo. Proc. Natl. Acad. Sci. USA,* **92**, 4537–4541

Wilmer, J.W. & Spit, B.J. (1986) Influence of retinoids on the mutagenicity of cigarette-smoke condensate in *Salmonella typhimurium* TA98. *Mutat. Res.,* **173**, 9–11

Wilson, J.G. (1977) Current status of teratology: general principles and mechanisms derived from animal studies. In: Wilson, J.G. & Fraser, F.C. (eds), *Handbook of Teratology*, New York, Plenum Press, pp. 47–74

Wilson, J.G., Roth, B. & Warkany, J. (1953) An analysis of the syndrome of malformations induced by maternal vitamin A deficiency. Effects of restoration of vitamin A at various times during gestation. *Am. J. Anat.*, **92**, 189–217

Wilson, D.E., Hejazi, J., Elstad, N.L., Chan, I.F., Gleeson, J.M. & Iverius, P.H. (1987) Novel aspects of vitamin A metabolism in the dog: distribution of lipoprotein retinyl esters in vitamin A-deprived and cholesterol-fed animals. *Biochim. Biophys. Acta*, **922**, 247–258

Winkelmann, R.K., Thomas, J.R.3 & Randle, H.W. (1983) Further experience with toxic vitamin A therapy in pityriasis rubra pilaris. *Cutis*, **31**, 621–632

Winston, A. & Rando, R.R. (1998) Regulation of isomerohydrolase activity in the visual cycle. *Biochemistry*, **37**, 2044–2050

Wittpenn, J.R., Tseng, S.C. & Sommer, A. (1986) Detection of early xerophthalmia by impression cytology. *Arch. Ophthalmol.*, **104**, 237–239

Wolterbeek, A.P., Roggeband, R., van Moorsel, C.J., Baan, R.A., Koeman, J.H., Feron, V.J. & Rutten, A.A. (1995) Vitamin A and β-carotene influence the level of benzo[*a*]pyrene-induced DNA adducts and DNA-repair activities in hamster tracheal epithelium in organ culture. *Cancer Lett.*, **91**, 205–214

Woutersen, R.A. & van Garderen Hoetmer, A. (1988) Inhibition of dietary fat-promoted development of (pre)neoplastic lesions in exocrine pancreas of rats and hamsters by supplemental vitamins A, C and E. *Cancer Lett.*, **41**, 179–189

Wu, R. & Wu, M.M. (1986) Effects of retinoids on human bronchial epithelial cells: differential regulation of hyaluronate synthesis and keratin protein synthesis. *J. Cell Physiol.*, **127**, 73–82

Wu, A.H., Henderson, B.E., Pike, M.C. & Yu, M.C. (1985) Smoking and other risk factors for lung cancer in women. *J. Natl. Cancer Inst.*, **74**, 747–751

Wu, R., Martin, W.R., Robinson, C.B., St. George, J.A., Plopper, C.G., Kurland, G., Last, J.A., Cross, C.E., McDonald, R.J. & Boucher, R. (1990) Expression of mucin synthesis and secretion in human tracheobronchial epithelial cells grown in culture. *Am. J. Respir. Cell Mol. Biol.*, **3**, 467–478

Xu, X.C., Ro, J.Y., Lee, J.S., Shin, D.M., Hong, W.K. & Lotan, R. (1994) Differential expression of nuclear retinoid receptors in normal, premalignant, and malignant head and neck tissues. *Cancer Res.*, **54**, 3580–3587

Xu, X.C., Sozzi, G., Lee, J.S., Lee, J.J., Pastorino, U., Pilotti, S., Kurie, J.M., Hong, W.K. & Lotan, R. (1997) Suppression of retinoic acid receptor β in non-small-cell lung cancer *in vivo*: implications for lung cancer development. *J. Natl. Cancer Inst.*, **89**, 624–629

Yamada, M., Blaner, W.S., Soprano, D.R., Dixon, J.L., Kjeldbye, H.M. & Goodman, D.S. (1987) Biochemical characteristics of isolated rat liver stellate cells. *Hepatology*, **7**, 1224–1229

Yamada, T., Kuwano, H., Matsuda, H., Sugimachi, K. & Ishinishi, N. (1995) Effect of dietary vitamin A on forestomach tumorigenesis during the total and postinitiation stages in mice treated with high- or low-dose benzo(*a*)pyrene. *Surg. Today*, **25**, 729–736

Yamamoto, Y., Inoue, I., Takasaki, T. & Takahashi, H. (1996) Inhibitory effects of selenium, vitamin A and butylated hydroxytoluene on growth of human maxillary cancer cells *in vitro*. *Auris Nasus Larynx*, **23**, 91–97

Yen, F.T., Mann, C.J., Guermani, L.M., Hannouche, N.F., Hubert, N., Hornick, C.A., Bordeau, V.N., Agnani, G. & Bihain, B.E. (1994) Identification of a lipolysis-stimulated receptor that is distinct from the LDL receptor and the LDL receptor-related protein. *Biochemistry*, **33**, 1172–1180

Yong, L.C., Brown, C.C., Schatzkin, A., Dresser, C.M., Slesinski, M.J., Cox, C.S. & Taylor, P.R. (1997) Intake of vitamins E, C, and A and risk of lung cancer. The NHANES I epidemiologic follow-up study. First National Health and Nutrition Examination Survey. *Am. J. Epidemiol.*, **146**, 231–243

You, W.C., Blot, W.J., Chang, Y.S., Ershow, A.G., Yang, Z.T., An, Q., Henderson, B., Xu, G.W., Fraumeni, J.F., Jr & Wang, T.G. (1988) Diet and high risk of stomach cancer in Shandong, China. *Cancer Res.*, **48**, 3518–3523

Yu, M.W., Zhang, Y.J., Blaner, W.S. & Santella, R.M. (1994) Influence of vitamins A, C, and E and β-carotene on aflatoxin B_1 binding to DNA in woodchuck hepatocytes. *Cancer,* **73**, 596-604

Yu, M.W., Chiang, Y.C., Lien, J.P. & Chen, C.J. (1997) Plasma antioxidant vitamins, chronic hepatitis B virus infection and urinary aflatoxin B_1-DNA adducts in healthy males. *Carcinogenesis,* **18**, 1189–1194

Yuan, J.M., Wang, Q.S., Ross, R.K., Henderson, B.E. & Yu, M.C. (1995) Diet and breast cancer in Shanghai and Tianjin, China. *Br. J. Cancer,* **71**, 1353–1358

Yumoto, S., Yumoto, K. & Yamamoto, M. (1989) Effects of retinoic acid on Ito cells (fat-storing cells) in vitamin A-deficient rats. In: Wisse, E., Knook, D.L. & Decker, K. (eds), *Cells of the Hepatic Sinusoid,* Rijswijk, The Netherlands, Kupffer Cell Foundation, pp. 33–38

Yuspa, S.H., Elgjo, K., Morse, M.A. & Wiebel, F.J. (1977) Retinyl acetate modulation of cell growth kinetics and carcinogen-cellular interaction in mouse epidermal cell cultures. *Chem. Biol. Interact.,* **16**, 251–264

Zachman, R.D., Chen, X., Verma, A.K. & Grummer, M.A. (1992) Some effects of vitamin A deficiency on the isolated rat lung alveolar type II cell. *Int. J. Vitam. Nutr. Res.,* **62**, 113–120

Zaridze, D., Lifanova, Y., Maximovitch, D., Day, N.E. & Duffy, S.W. (1991) Diet, alcohol consumption and reproductive factors in a case-control study of breast cancer in Moscow. *Int. J. Cancer,* **48**, 493–501

Zhang, L., Blot, W.J., You, W.C., Chang, Y.S., Liu, X.Q., Kneller, R.W., Zhao, L., Liu, W.D., Li, J.Y., Jin, M.L., Xu, G.W., Fraumeni, J.F., Jr & Yang, C.S. (1994) Serum micronutrients in relation to pre-cancerous gastric lesions. *Int. J. Cancer,* **56**, 650–654

Zhao, D., McCaffery, P., Ivins, K.J., Neve, R.L., Hogan, P., Chin, W.W. & Drager, U.C. (1996) Molecular identification of a major retinoic-acid-synthesizing enzyme, a retinaldehyde-specific dehydrogenase. *Eur. J. Biochem.,* **240**, 15–22

Zheng, W., Sellers, T.A., Doyle, T.J., Kushi, L.H., Potter, J.D. & Folsom, A.R. (1995) Retinol, antioxidant vitamins, and cancers of the upper digestive tract in a prospective cohort study of postmenopausal women. *Am. J. Epidemiol.,* **142**, 955–960

Zheng, Y., Kramer, P.M., Olson, G., Lubet, R.A., Steele, V.E., Kelloff, G.J. & Pereira, M.A. (1997) Prevention by retinoids of azoxymethane-induced tumors and aberrant crypt foci and their modulation of cell proliferation in the colon of rats. *Carcinogenesis,* **18**, 2119–2125

Zhu, Z.R., Parviainen, M., Mannisto, S., Pietinen, P., Eskelinen, M., Syrjänen, K. & Uusitupa, M. (1995) Vitamin A concentration in breast adipose tissue of breast cancer patients. *Anticancer Res.,* **15**, 1593–1596

Ziari, S.A., Mireles, V.L., Cantu, C.G., Cervantes, M.3, Idrisa, A., Bobsom, D., Tsin, A.T. & Glew, R.H. (1996) Serum vitamin A, vitamin E, and β-carotene levels in preeclamptic women in northern Nigeria. *Am. J. Perinatol.,* **13**, 287–291

Ziegler, R.G., Morris, L.E., Blot, W.J., Pottern, L.M., Hoover, R. & Fraumeni, J.F. (1981) Esophageal cancer among black men in Washington, D.C. II. Role of nutrition. *J. Natl. Cancer Inst.,* **67**, 1199–1206

Ziegler, R.G., Mason, T.J., Stemhagen, A., Hoover, R., Schoenberg, J.B., Gridley, G., Virgo, P.W., Altman, R. & Fraumeni, J.F., Jr (1984) Dietary carotene and vitamin A and risk of lung cancer among white men in New Jersey. *J. Natl. Cancer Inst.,* **73**, 1429–1435

Ziegler, R.G., Brinton, L.A., Hamman, R.F., Lehman, H.F., Levine, R.S., Mallin, K., Norman, S.A., Rosenthal, J.F., Trumble, A.C. & Hoover, R.N. (1990) Diet and the risk of invasive cervical cancer among white women in the United States. *Am. J. Epidemiol.,* **132**, 432–445

Ziegler, R.G., Jones, C.J., Brinton, L.A., Norman, S.A., Mallin, K., Levine, R.S., Lehman, H.F., Hamman, R.F., Trumble, A.C., Rosenthal, J.F. & Hoover, R.N. (1991) Diet and the risk of *in situ* cervical cancer among white women in the United States. *Cancer Causes Control,* **2**, 17–29

Zovich, D.C., Orologa, A., Okuno, M., Kong, L.W., Talmage, D.A., Piantedosi, R., Goodman, D.S. & Blaner, W.S. (1992) Differentiation-dependent expression of retinoid-binding proteins in BFC-adipocytes. *J. Biol. Chem.,* **267**, 13884–13889

Appendix 1

Interconversion of units for vitamin A

1 mmol retinol	=	286 mg
1 mmol retinal	=	284 mg
1 mmol retinoic acid	=	300 mg
1 mmol retinyl acetate	=	328 mg
1 mmol retinyl palmitate	=	524 mg
1 mg all-*trans*-retinol	=	3.33 International Units (IU) of retinol or retinyl esters
		3.5 nmol all-*trans*-retinol
		1 μg retinol equivalents (RE)
		6 μg all-*trans*-β-carotene
		12 μg other all-*trans* provitamin A carotenoids

Appendix 2

Three-letter test codes used in activity profiles

Code	Definition
BID	Binding (covalent) to DNA *in vitro*
BVD	Binding (covalent) to DNA, animal cells *in vivo*
BVP	Binding (covalent) to RNA or protein, animal cells *in vivo*
CBA	Chromosomal aberrations, animal bone marrow cells *in vivo*
CCC	Chromosomal aberrations, spermatocytes treated and observed *in vivo*
CIC	Chromosomal aberrations, Chinese hamster cells *in vitro*
DIA	DNA strand breaks, cross-links or related damage, animal cells *in vitro*
DVA	DNA strand breaks, cross-links or related damage, animal cells *in vivo*
GCO	Gene mutation, Chinese hamster ovary cells *in vitro*
GIH	Gene mutation, human cells *in vitro*
G9H	Gene mutation, Chinese hamster lung V-79 cells, HPRT locus
MVM	Micronucleus test, mice *in vivo*
MVR	Micronucleus test, rats *in vivo*
SAD	*Salmonella typhimurium*, differential toxicity
SA0	*Salmonella typhimurium* TA100, reverse mutation
SA2	*Salmonella typhimurium* TA102, reverse mutation
SA4	*Salmonella typhimurium* TA104, reverse mutation
SA5	*Salmonella typhimurium* TA1535, reverse mutation
SA8	*Salmonella typhimurium* TA1538, reverse mutation
SA9	*Salmonella typhimurium* TA98, reverse mutation
SCF	*Saccharomyces cerevisiae*, forward mutation
SCR	*Saccharomyces cerevisiae*, reverse mutation
SHL	Sister chromatid exchange, human lymphocytes *in vitro*
SIC	Sister chromatid exchange, Chinese hamster cells *in vitro*
SVA	Sister chromatid exchange, animal cells *in vivo*
TCM	Cell transformation, C3H 10T1/2 mouse cells
UIA	Unscheduled DNA synthesis, other animal cells *in vitro*
URP	Unscheduled DNA synthesis, rat primary hepatocytes

Appendix 3

The concept of activity profiles of antimutagens

To facilitate an analysis of data from the open literature on antimutagenicity in short-term tests, we have applied the concept of activity profiles already used successfully for mutagenicity data (Waters *et al.*, 1988, 1990) to antimutagenicity data. The activity profiles display an overview of multi-test and multi-chemical information as an aid to the interpretation of the data. They can be organized in two general ways: for mutagens that have been tested in combination with a given antimutagen or for antimutagens that have been tested in combination with a given mutagen (Waters *et al.*, 1990). The profile presented here is an example of mutagens that have been tested in combination with a single antimutagen and they are arranged alphabetically by the names of the mutagens tested. These plots permit rapid visualization of considerable data and experimental parameters, including the inhibition as well as the enhancement of mutagenic activity. A data listing, arranged in the same order as the profile, is also given to summarize the short-term test used, the doses of mutagens and antimutagens, the response induced by the antimutagens, and the relevant publications.

The antimutagenicity profile graphically shows the doses for both the mutagen and antimutagen and the test response (either inhibition or enhancement) induced by the antimutagen. The resultant profiles are actually two parallel sets of bar graphs (Figure 1). The upper graph displays the mutagen dose and the range of antimutagen doses tested. The lower graph shows either the maximum percent inhibition represented by a bar directed upwards from the origin or the maximum percent enhancement of the genotoxic response, represented by a bar directed downwards. A short bar drawn across the origin on the lower graph indicates that no significant (generally < 20%) difference in the response was detected between the mutagen tested alone or the mutagen tested in combination with the antimutagen. Codes used to represent the short-term tests in the data listings have been reported previously (Waters *et al.*, 1988), and the subset of tests represented in this paper are shown in the Appendix.

In assembling the database on antimutagens and presumptive anticarcinogens, the literature was surveyed for the availability of antimutagenicity data (Waters *et al.*, 1990), and publications were selected that presented original, quantitative data for any of the genotoxicity assays that are in the scope of the genetic activity profiles (Waters *et al.*, 1988).

The same short-term tests used to identify mutagens and potential carcinogens are being used to identify antimutagens and potential anticarcinogens. The tests are generally those for which standardized protocols have been developed and published. Many of these tests have been evaluated by the USEPA Gene-Tox Program (Waters, 1979; Green & Auletta, 1980; Waters & Auletta, 1981; Auletta *et al.*, 1991) or the National Toxicology Program (Tennant *et al.*, 1987; Ashby & Tennant, 1991) for their performance in detecting known carcinogens and noncarcinogens or known mutagens and non-mutagens (Upton *et al.*, 1984; Waters *et al.*, 1994).

It is not clear at the present time whether antimutagenicity observed in short-term tests is a reliable indicator of anticarcinogenicity since the available data are incomplete. Information on both antimutagenicity and anticarcinogenicity *in vivo* for a number of chemical classes is required before such a conclusion can be drawn. Clearly, antimutagenicity tests performed *in vitro* will not detect those compounds that act in a carcinogenicity bioassay *in vivo,* for example, to alter the activity of one or more enzyme systems not present *in vitro*. Rather, the in-vitro tests will detect only those compounds that inhibit the metabolism of the carcinogen directly, react directly with the mutagenic species to inactivate them or otherwise show an effect that is demonstrable *in vitro*. Thus, it is essential to confirm putative antimutagenic activity observed *in vitro* through the use of animal models. Indeed, the interpretation of antimutagenicity data from short-term tests must be subjected to all of the considerations that apply in the interpretation of mutagenicity test results. Moreover, the experimental variable of the antimutagens used must be considered in addition to the variables of the mutagens and short-term tests used. Obvious examples of parameters that must be considered in evaluating results from short-term tests *in vitro* are: (1) the endpoint of the test, (2) the presence or absence of an exogenous metabolic system, (3) the inducer that may have been used in conjunction with the preparation of the metabolic system, (4) the concentration of S9 or other metabolic system used and whether that concentration has been optimized for the mutagen under test, (5) the relative time and order of presentation of the mutagen and the antimutagen to the test system, (6) the concentration ratio of the mutagen relative to the antimutagen, (7) the duration of the treatment period, and (8) the outcome of the test, i.e. inhibition or enhancement of mutagenicity. Similar considerations apply to the evaluation of in-vivo tests for antimutagenicity.

References

Ashby, J. & Tennant, R.W. (1991) Definitive relationships among chemical structure, carcinogenicity and mutagenicity for 301 chemicals tested by the US NTP. *Mutat. Res.*, **257**, 229–306

Auletta, A.E., Brown, M., Wassom, J.S. & Cimino, M.C. (1991) Current status of the Gene-Tox program. *Environ. Health Perspectives*, **96**, 33–36

Green, S. & Auletta, A. (1980) Editorial introduction to the reports of 'The Gene-Tox Program': An evaluation of bioassays in *Genetic Toxicology. Mutat. Res.*, **76**, 165–168

Tennant, R.W., Margolin, B.H., Shelby, M.D., Zeiger, E., Haseman, J.K., Spalding, J., Caspary, W., Resnick, M., Stasiewicz, S., Anderson, B. & Minor, R. (1987) Prediction of chemical carcinogenicity in rodents from in vitro genetic toxicity assays. *Science*, **236**, 933–941

Upton, A.C., Clayson, D.B., Jansen, J.D., Rosenkranz, H.S. & Williams, G.M. (1984) Report of ICPEMC Task Group 5 on the differentiation between genotoxic and non-genotoxic carcinogens. *Mutat. Res.*, **133**, 1–49

Waters, M.D. (1979) Gene-Tox Program. In: Hsie, A.W., O'Neill, J.P. & McElheny, V.K., eds, *Mammalian Cell Mutagenesis: The Maturation of Test Systems* (Banbury Report 2), Cold Spring Harbor, NY, CSH Press, pp 451–466

Waters, M.D. & Auleta, A. (1981) The GENE-TOX program: Genetic activty evaluation. *J. chem. Inf. Computer Sci.*, **21**, 35–38

Waters, M.D., Stack, H.F., Brady, A.L., Lohman, P.H.M., Haroun, L. & Vainio, H. (1988) Use of computerized data listings and activity profiles of genetic and related effects in the review of 195 compounds. *Mutat. Res.*, **205**, 295–312

Waters, M.D., Brady, A.L., Stack, H.E. & Brockman, H.E. (1990) Antimutagenicity profiles for some model compounds. *Mutat. Res.*, **238**, 57–85

Waters, M.D., Stack, H.F., Jackson, M.A., Bridges, B.A. & Adler, I.-D. (1994) The performance of short-test tests in identifying potential germ cell mutagens: A qualitative and quantitative analysis. *Mutat. Res.*, **341**, 109–131

Figure 1. Schematic diagram of an antimutagenicity profile. Profiles are organized to display either the antimutagenic activity of various antimutagens in combination with a single mutagen or the activity of a single antimutagen with various mutagens. The upper bar graph displays the mutagen concentration and the range of antimutagen concentrations tested. The lower graph shows either the maximum percent inhibition, represented by a bar directed upwards from the origin, or the maximum percent enhancement of the genotoxic response, represented by a bar directed downwards. As illustrated in the lower graph, a bar across the origin indicates that no significant (< 20%) effect was detected (designated as 'negative data' in the text). Test codes are defined in Appendix 2.

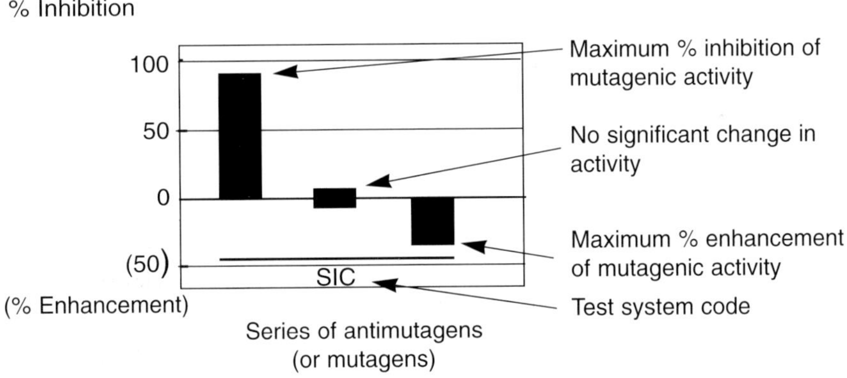

Appendix 4

Activity profiles for genetic and related effects

Methods

The *x*-axis of the activity profile (Waters *et al.*, 1987, 1988) represents the bioassays in phylogenetic sequence by end-point, and the values on the *y*-axis represent the logarithmically transformed lowest effective doses (LED) and highest ineffective doses (HID) tested. The term 'dose', as used in this report, does not take into consideration length of treatment or exposure and may therefore be considered synonymous with concentration. In practice, the concentrations used in all the in-vitro tests were converted to μg/mL, and those for in-vivo tests were expressed as mg/kg bw. Because dose units are plotted on a log scale, differences in the relative molecular masses of compounds do not, in most cases, greatly influence comparisons of their activity profiles. Conventions for dose conversions are given below.

Profile-line height (the magnitude of each bar) is a function of the LED or HID, which is associated with the characteristics of each individual test system — such as population size, cell-cycle kinetics and metabolic competence. Thus, the detection limit of each test system is different, and, across a given activity profile, responses will vary substantially. No attempt is made to adjust or relate responses in one test system to those of another.

Line heights are derived as follows: for negative test results, the highest dose tested without appreciable toxicity is defined as the HID. If there was evidence of extreme toxicity, the next highest dose is used. A single dose tested with a negative result is considered to be equivalent to the HID. Similarly, for positive results, the LED is recorded. If the original data were analysed statistically by the author, the dose recorded is that at which the response was significant ($p < 0.05$). If the available data were not analysed statistically, the dose required to produce an effect is estimated as follows: when a dose-related positive response is observed with two or more doses, the lower of the doses is taken as the LED; a single dose resulting in a positive response is considered to be equivalent to the LED.

In order to accommodate both the wide range of doses encountered and positive and negative responses on a continuous scale, doses are transformed logarithmically, so that effective (LED) and ineffective (HID) doses are represented by positive and negative numbers, respectively. The response, or logarithmic dose unit (LDU_{ij}), for a given test system *i* and chemical *j* is represented by the expressions

$LDU_{ij} = -\log_{10}$ (dose), for HID values; $LDU \leq 0$

and

$LDU_{ij} = -\log_{10}$ (dose $\times$ 10^{-5}), for LED values; $LDU \geq 0$.

These simple relationships define a dose range of 0 to –5 logarithmic units for ineffective doses (1–100 000 μg/mL or mg/kg bw) and 0 to +8 logarithmic units for effective doses (100 000–0.001 mg/mL or mg/kg bw). A scale illustrating the LDU values is shown in Figure 1. Negative responses at doses less than 1 mg/mL (mg/kg bw) are set equal to 1. Effectively, an LED value ≥ 100 000 or an HID value ≤ 1 produces an LDU = 0; no quantitative information is gained from such extreme values. The dotted lines at the levels of log dose units 1 and –1 define a 'zone of uncertainty' in which positive results are reported at such high doses (between 10 000 and 100 000 mg/mL or mg/kg bw) or negative results are reported at such low doses (1 to 10 mg/ml or mg/kg bw) as to call into question the adequacy of the test.

Figure 1. Scale of log dose units used on the y-axis of activity profiles

Positive units (µg/mL or mg/kg bw)	Negative (mg/mL or mg/kg bw)	Log dose	
0.001		8	----
0.01		7	--
0.1		6	--
1.0		5	--
10		4	--
100		3	--
1000		2	--
10 000		1	--
100 000	1	0	----
	10	−1	--
	100	−2	--
	1000	−3	--
	10 000	−4	--
	100 000	−5	----

In practice, an activity profile is computer generated. A data entry programme is used to store abstracted data from published reports. A sequential file (in ASCII) is created for each compound, and a record within that file consists of the name and Chemical Abstracts Service number of the compound, a three-letter code for the test system (see below), the qualitative test result (with and without an exogenous metabolic system), dose (LED or HID), citation number and additional source information. An abbreviated citation for each publication is stored in a segment of a record accessing both the test data file and the citation file. During processing of the data file, an average of the logarithmic values of the data sub-set is calculated, and the length of the profile line represents this average value. All dose values are plotted for each profile line, regardless of whether results are positive or negative. Results obtained in the absence of an exogenous metabolic system are indicated by a bar (–), and results obtained in the presence of an exogenous metabolic system are indicated by an upward-directed arrow (↑). When all results for a given assay are either positive or negative, the mean of the LDU values is plotted as a solid line; when conflicting data are reported for the same assay (i.e. both positive and negative results), the majority data are shown by a solid line and the minority data by a dashed line (drawn to the extreme conflicting response). In the few cases in which the numbers of positive and negative results are equal, the solid line is drawn in the positive direction and the maximal negative response is indicated with a dashed line. Profile lines are identified by three-letter code words representing the commonly used tests. Code words for most of the test systems in current use in genetic toxicology were defined for the US Environmental Protection Agency's GENE-TOX Program (Waters, 1979; Waters & Auletta, 1981). For *IARC Monographs* Supplement 6, Volume 44 and subsequent volumes, as well as the present series, codes were redefined in a manner that should facilitate inclusion of additional tests. Naming conventions are described below.

Data listings are presented in the text and include end-point and test codes, a short test code definition, results, either with (M) or without (NM) an exogenous activation system, the associated LED or HID value and a short citation. Test codes are organized phylogenetically and by end-point from left to right across each activity profile and from top to bottom of the corresponding data listing. End-points are defined as follows: A, aneuploidy; C, chromosomal aberrations; D, DNA damage; F, assays of body fluids; G, gene mutation; H, host-mediated assays; I, inhibition of intercellular communication; M, micronuclei; P, sperm morphology; R, mitotic recombination or gene conversion; S, sister chromatid exchange; and T, cell transformation.

Dose conversions for activity profiles

Doses are converted to mg/mL for in-vitro tests and to mg/kg bw per day for in-vivo experiments.

1. In-vitro test systems

(*a*) Weight/volume converts directly to mg/mL.

(*b*) Molar (M) concentration × molecular weight = mg/mL = 103 mg/mL; mM concentration × molecular weight = mg/mL.

(*c*) Soluble solids expressed as % concentration are assumed to be in units of mass per volume (i.e. 1% = 0.01 g/mL = 10 000 µg/mL; also, 1 ppm = 1 mg/mL).

(*d*) Liquids and gases expressed as % concentration are assumed to be given in units of volume per volume. Liquids are converted to weight per volume using the density (D) of the solution (D = g/mL). Gases are con verted from volume to mass using the ideal gas law, $PV = nRT$. For exposure at 20–37 °C at standard atmospheric pressure, 1% (v/v) = 0.4 mg/mL × molecular weight of the gas. Also, 1 ppm (v/v) = 4 × 10^5 mg/mL × molecular weight.

(*e*) In microbial plate tests, it is usual for the doses to be reported as weight/plate, whereas concentrations are required to enter data on the activity profile chart. While remaining cognisant of the errors involved in the process, it is assumed that a 2-mL volume of top agar is delivered to each plate and that the test substance remains in solution within it; concentrations are derived from the reported weight/plate values by dividing by this arbitrary volume. For spot tests, a 1-mL volume is used in the calculation.

(f) Conversion of particulate concentrations given in mg/cm^2 is based on the area (A) of the dish and the volume of medium per dish; i.e. for a 100-mm dish: $A = \pi R^2 = \pi \times (5\ cm)^2 = 78.5\ cm^2$. If the volume of medium is 10 mL, then 78.5 cm^2 = 10 mL and 1 cm^2 = 0.13 mL.

2. In-vitro systems using in-vivo activation

For the body fluid-urine (BF-) test, the concentration used is the dose (in mg/kg bw) of the compound administered to test animals or patients.

3. In-vivo test systems

(*a*) Doses are converted to mg/kg bw per day of exposure, assuming 100% absorption. Standard values are used for each sex and species of rodent, including body weight and average intake per day, as reported by Gold *et al.* (1984). For example, in a test using male mice fed 50 ppm of the agent in the diet, the standard food intake per day is 12% of body weight, and the conversion is dose = 50 ppm × 12% = 6 mg/kg bw per day. Standard values used for humans are: weight—males, 70 kg; females, 55 kg; surface area, 1.7 m^2; inhalation rate, 20 L/min for light work, 30 L/min for mild exercise.

(*b*) When reported, the dose at the target site is used. For example, doses given in studies of lymphocytes of humans exposed *in vivo* are the measured blood concentrations in mg/mL.

Codes for test systems

For specific nonmammalian test systems, the first two letters of the three-symbol code word define the test organism (e.g. SA- for *Salmonella typhimurium*, EC- for *Escherichia coli*). If the species is not known, the convention used is -S-. The third symbol may be used to define the tester strain (e.g. SA8 for *S. typhimurium* TA1538, ECW for *E. coli* WP2uvrA). When strain designation is not indicated, the third letter is used to define the specific genetic end-point under investigation (e.g. --D for differential toxicity, --F for forward mutation, --G for gene conversion or genetic crossing-over, --N for aneuploidy, --R for reverse mutation, --U for unscheduled DNA synthesis). The third letter may also be used to define the general end-point under investigation when a more complete definition is not possible or relevant (e.g. --M for mutation, --C for chromosomal aberration). For mammalian test systems, the first letter of the three-letter code word defines the genetic end-point under investigation: A-- for aneuploidy, B-- for binding, C-- for chromosomal aberration, D-- for DNA strand breaks, G-- for gene mutation, I-- for inhibition of intercellular communication, M-- for micronucleus formation, R-- for DNA repair, S-- for sister chromatid exchange, T-- for cell transformation and U-- for unscheduled DNA synthesis.

For animal (i.e. non-human) test systems *in vitro*, when the cell type is not specified, the code letters -IA are used. For such assays *in vivo*, when the animal species is not specified, the code letters -VA are used. Commonly used animal species are identified by the third letter (e.g. --C for Chinese hamster, --M for mouse, --R for rat, --S for Syrian hamster).

For test systems using human cells *in vitro*, when the cell type is not specified, the code letters -IH are used. For assays on humans *in vivo*, when the cell type is not specified, the code letters -VH are used. Otherwise, the second letter specifies the cell type under investigation (e.g. -BH for bone marrow, -LH for lymphocytes).

Some other specific coding conventions used for mammalian systems are as follows: BF- for body fluids, HM- for host-mediated, --L for leukocytes or lymphocytes *in vitro* (-AL, animals; -HL, humans), -L- for leukocytes *in vivo* (-LA, animals; -LH, humans),--T for transformed cells.

Note that these are examples of major conventions used to define the assay code words. The alphabetized listing of codes must be examined to confirm a specific code word. As might be expected from the limitation to three symbols, some codes do not fit the naming conventions precisely. In a few cases, test systems are defined by first-letter code words, for example: MST, mouse spot test; SLP, mouse specific locus mutation, postspermatogonia; SLO, mouse specific locus mutation, other stages; DLM, dominant lethal mutation in mice; DLR, dominant lethal mutation in rats; MHT, mouse heritable translocation.

The genetic activity profiles and listings were prepared in collaboration with Environmental Health Research and Testing Inc. (EHRT) under contract to the United States Environmental Protection Agency; EHRT also determined the doses used. The references cited in each genetic activity profile listing can be found in the list of references in the appropriate volume.

References

Garrett, N.E., Stack, H.F., Gross, M.R. & Waters, M.D. (1984) An analysis of the spectra of genetic activity produced by known or suspected human carcinogens. *Mutat. Res.*, **134**, 89–111

Gold, L.S., Sawyer, C.B., Magaw, R., Backman, G.M., de Veciana, M., Levinson, R., Hooper, N.K., Havender, W.R., Bernstein, L., Peto, R., Pike, M.C. & Ames, B.N. (1984) A carcinogenic potency database of the standardized results of animal bioassays. *Environ. Health Perspect.*, **58**, 9–319

Waters, M.D. (1979) *The GENE-TOX program*. In: Hsie, A.W., O'Neill, J.P. & McElheny, V.K., eds, Mammalian Cell Mutagenesis: *The Maturation of Test Systems* (Banbury Report 2), Cold Spring Harbor, NY, CSH Press, pp. 449–467

Waters, M.D. & Auletta, A. (1981) The GENE-TOX program: genetic activity evaluation. *J. chem. Inf. comput. Sci.*, 21, 35–38

Waters, M.D., Stack, H.F., Brady, A.L., Lohman, P.H.M., Haroun, L. & Vainio, H. (1987) Appendix 1: Activity profiles for genetic and related tests. In: *IARC Monographs on the Evaluation of the Carcinogenic Risk of Chemicals to Humans,* Suppl. 6, *Genetic and Related Effects: An Updating of Selected* IARC Monographs *from Volumes 1 to 42*, Lyon, IARC, pp. 687–696

Waters, M.D., Stack, H.F., Brady, A.L., Lohman, P.H.M., Haroun, L. & Vainio, H. (1988) Use of computerized data listings and activity profiles of genetic and related effects in the review of 195 compounds. *Mutat. Res.*, **205**, 295–312

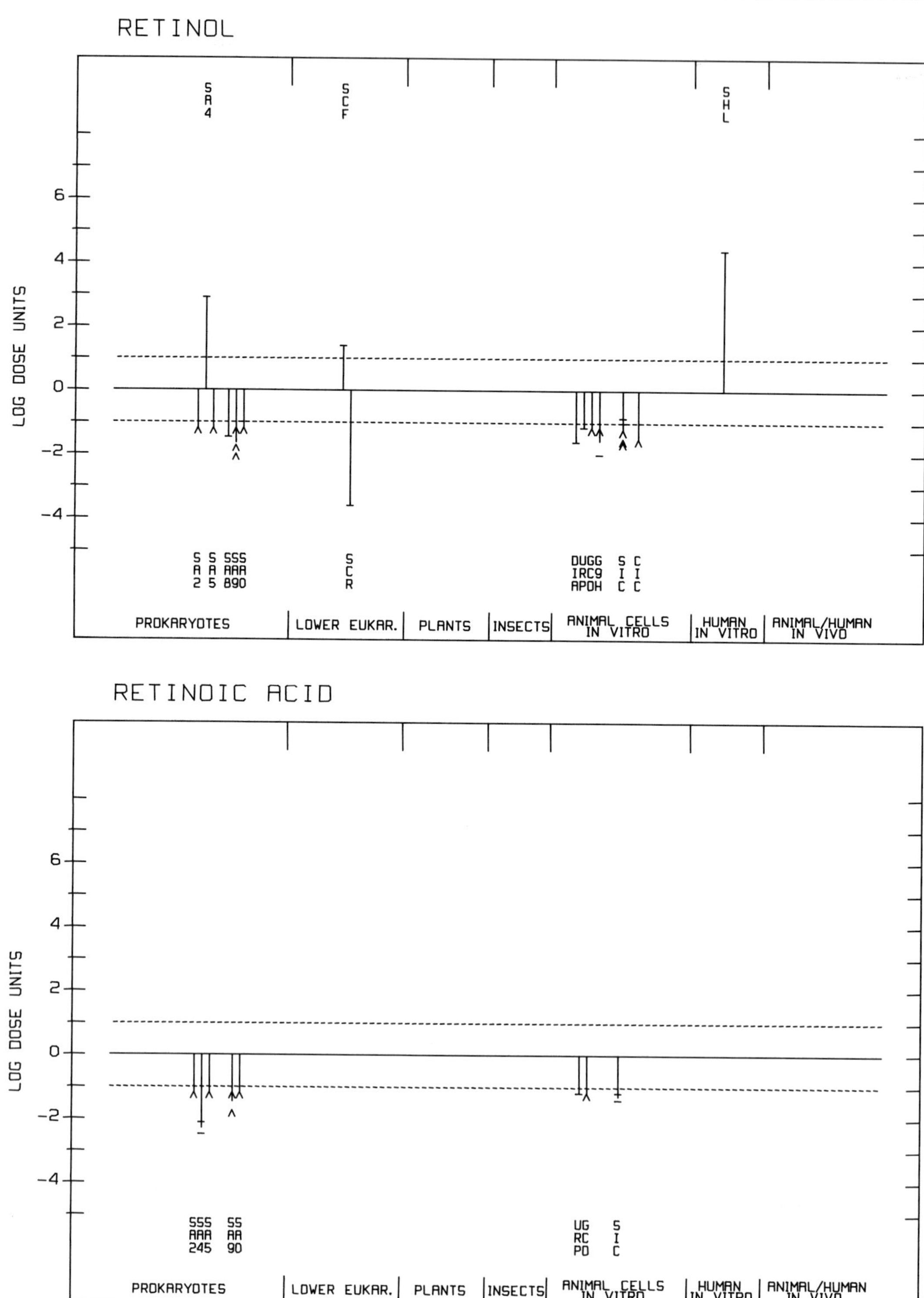

RETINOL
LOG DOSE UNITS
6
4
2
0
-2
-4
S A 4
S C F
S H L
S S SSS
A A AAA
2 5 890
S C R
DUGG S C
IRC9 I I
APOH C C
PROKARYOTES
LOWER EUKAR.
PLANTS
INSECTS
ANIMAL CELLS IN VITRO
HUMAN IN VITRO
ANIMAL/HUMAN IN VIVO
RETINOIC ACID
LOG DOSE UNITS
6
4
2
0
-2
-4
SSS SS
AAA AA
245 90
UG S
RC I
PD C
PROKARYOTES
LOWER EUKAR.
PLANTS
INSECTS
ANIMAL CELLS IN VITRO
HUMAN IN VITRO
ANIMAL/HUMAN IN VIVO

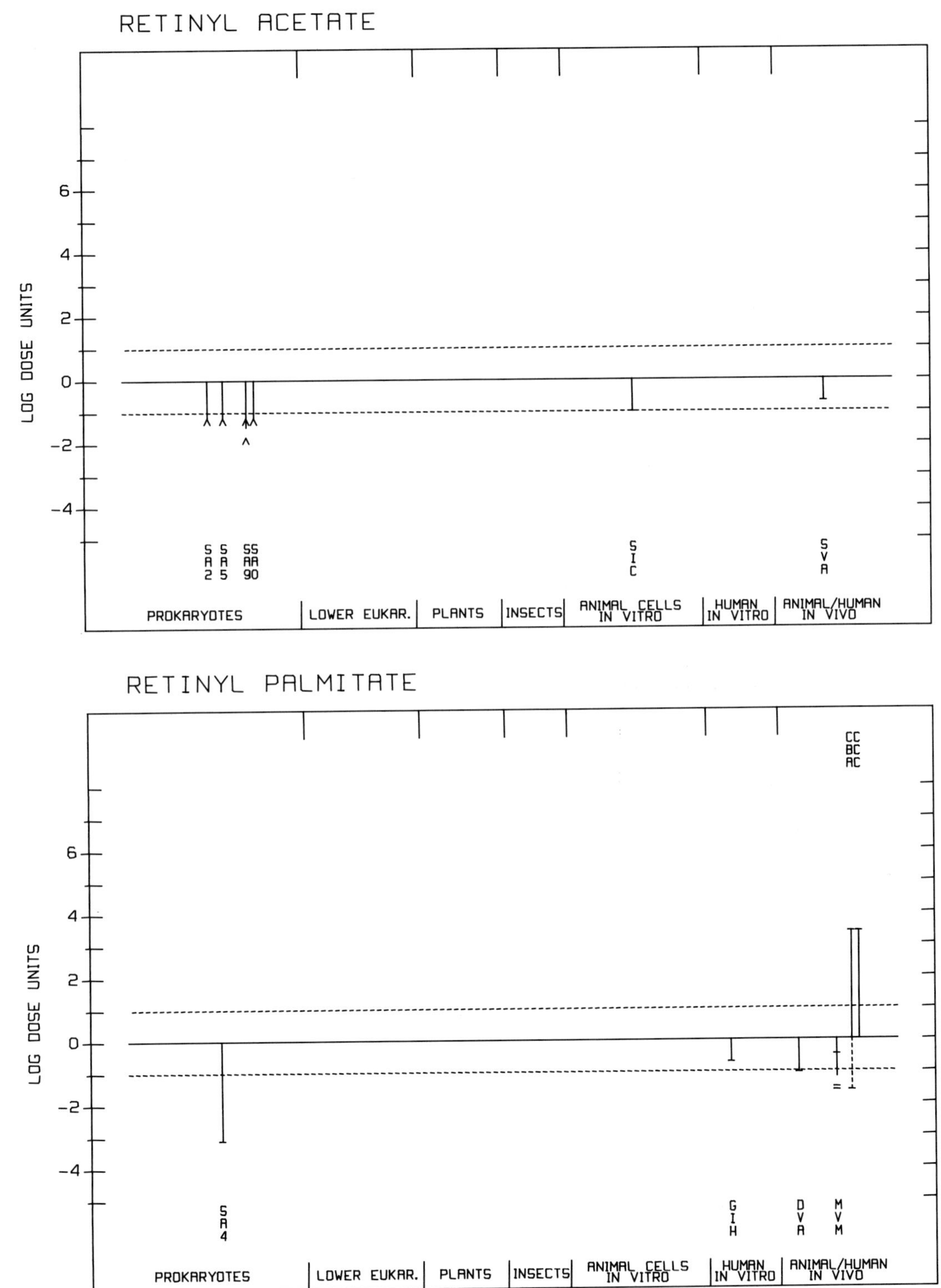
RETINYL ACETATE
LOG DOSE UNITS
6
4
2
0
-2
-4
S A 2
S A 5
SS AA 90
S I C
S V A
PROKARYOTES
LOWER EUKAR.
PLANTS
INSECTS
ANIMAL CELLS IN VITRO
HUMAN IN VITRO
ANIMAL/HUMAN IN VIVO
RETINYL PALMITATE
LOG DOSE UNITS
6
4
2
0
-2
-4
S A 4
G I H
D V A
M V M
CC BC AC
PROKARYOTES
LOWER EUKAR.
PLANTS
INSECTS
ANIMAL CELLS IN VITRO
HUMAN IN VITRO
ANIMAL/HUMAN IN VIVO

IARC Monographs on the Evaluation of Carcinogenic Risks to Humans

ISSN 0250 9555

*Volume 1**
Some Inorganic Substances, Chlorinated Hydrocarbons, Aromatic Amines, N-Nitroso Compounds, and Natural Products
1972; 184 pages; ISBN 92 832 1201 0

*Volume 2**
Some Inorganic and Organometallic Compounds
1973; 181 pages; ISBN 92 832 1202 9

*Volume 3**
Certain Polycyclic Aromatic Hydrocarbons and Heterocyclic Compounds
1973; 271 pages; ISBN 92 832 1203 7

Volume 4
Some Aromatic Amines, Hydrazine and Related Substances, *N*-Nitroso Compounds and Miscellaneous Alkylating Agents
1974; 286 pages; ISBN 92 832 1204 5

*Volume 5**
Some Organochlorine Pesticides
1974; 241 pages; ISBN 92 832 1205 3

*Volume 6**
Sex Hormones
1974; 243 pages; ISBN 92 832 1206 1

*Volume 7**
Some Anti-Thyroid and Related Substances, Nitrofurans and Industrial Chemicals
1974; 326 pages; ISBN 92 832 1207 X

Volume 8
Some Aromatic Azo Compounds
1975; 357 pages; ISBN 92 832 1208 8

Volume 9
Some Aziridines, *N*-, *S*- and *O*-Mustards and Selenium
1975; 268 pages; ISBN 92 832 1209 6

*Volume 10**
Some Naturally Occurring Substances
1976; 353 pages; ISBN 92 832 1210 X

*Volume 11**
Cadmium, Nickel, Some Epoxides, Miscellaneous Industrial Chemicals and General Considerations on Volatile Anaesthetics
1976; 306 pages; ISBN 92 832 1211 8

*Volume 12**
Some Carbamates, Thiocarbamates and Carbazides
1976; 282 pages; ISBN 92 832 1212 6

Volume 13
Some Miscellaneous Pharmaceuticals
1977; 255 pages; ISBN 92 832 1213 4

*Volume 14**
Asbestos
1977; 106 pages; ISBN 92 832 1214 2

*Volume 15**
Some Fumigants, the Herbicides 2,4-D and 2,4,5-T, Chlorinated Dibenzodioxins and Miscellaneous Industrial Chemicals
1977; 354 pages; ISBN 92 832 1215 0

Volume 16
Some Aromatic Amines and Related Nitro Compounds – Hair Dyes, Colouring Agents and Miscellaneous Industrial Chemicals
1978; 400 pages; ISBN 92 832 1216 9

Volume 17
Some N-Nitroso Compounds
1978; 365 pages; ISBN 92 832 1217 7

*Volume 18**
Polychlorinated Biphenyls and Polybrominated Biphenyls
1978; 140 pages; ISBN 92 832 1218 5

*Volume 19**
Some Monomers, Plastics and Synthetic Elastomers, and Acrolein
1979; 513 pages; ISBN 92 832 1219 3

*Volume 20**
Some Halogenated Hydrocarbons
1979; 609 pages; ISBN 92 832 1220 7

Volume 21
Sex Hormones (II)
1979; 583 pages; ISBN 92 832 1521 4

Volume 22
Some Non-Nutritive Sweetening Agents
1980; 208 pages; ISBN 92 832 1522 2

*Volume 23**
Some Metals and Metallic Compounds
1980; 438 pages; ISBN 92 832 1523 0

Volume 24
Some Pharmaceutical Drugs
1980; 337 pages; ISBN 92 832 1524 9

Volume 25
Wood, Leather and Some Associated Industries
1981; 412 pages; ISBN 92 832 1525 7

Volume 26
Some Antineoplastic and Immunosuppressive Agents
1981; 411 pages; ISBN 92 832 1526 5

Volume 27
Some Aromatic Amines, Anthraquinones and Nitroso Compounds, and Inorganic Fluorides Used in Drinking Water and Dental Preparations
1982; 341 pages; ISBN 92 832 1527 3

Volume 28
The Rubber Industry
1982; 486 pages; ISBN 92 832 1528 1

Volume 29
Some Industrial Chemicals and Dyestuffs
1982; 416 pages; ISBN 92 832 1529 X

Volume 30
Miscellaneous Pesticides
1983; 424 pages; ISBN 92 832 1530 3

*Volume 31**
Some Food Additives, Feed Additives and Naturally Occurring Substances
1983; 314 pages; ISBN 92 832 1531 1

*Volume 32**
Polynuclear Aromatic Compounds, Part 1: Chemical, Environmental and Experimental Data
1983; 477 pages; ISBN 92 832 1532 X

*Volume 33**
Polynuclear Aromatic Compounds, Part 2: Carbon Blacks, Mineral Oils and Some Nitroarenes
1984; 245 pages; ISBN 92 832 1533 8

Volume 34
Polynuclear Aromatic Compounds, Part 3: Industrial Exposures in Aluminium Production, Coal Gasification, Coke Production, and Iron and Steel Founding
1984; 219 pages; ISBN 92 832 1534 6

Volume 35
Polynuclear Aromatic Compounds: Part 4: Bitumens, Coal-Tars and Derived Products, Shale-Oils and Soots
1985; 271 pages; ISBN 92 832 1535 4

*Out-of-print

Volume 36
Allyl Compounds, Aldehydes, Epoxides and Peroxides
1985; 369 pages; ISBN 92 832 1536 2

Volume 37
Tobacco Habits Other than Smoking; Betel-Quid and Areca-Nut Chewing; and Some Related Nitrosamines
1985; 291 pages; ISBN 92 832 1537 0

Volume 38
Tobacco Smoking
1986; 421 pages; ISBN 92 832 1538 9

Volume 39
Some Chemicals Used in Plastics and Elastomers
1986; 403 pages; ISBN 92 832 1239 8

Volume 40
Some Naturally Occurring and Synthetic Food Components, Furocoumarins and Ultraviolet Radiation
1986; 444 pages; ISBN 92 832 1240 1

Volume 41
Some Halogenated Hydrocarbons and Pesticide Exposures
1986; 434 pages; ISBN 92 832 1241 X

Volume 42
Silica and Some Silicates
1987; 289 pages; ISBN 92 832 1242 8

Volume 43
Man-Made Mineral Fibres and Radon
1988; 300 pages; ISBN 92 832 1243 6

Volume 44
Alcohol Drinking
1988; 416 pages; ISBN 92 832 1244 4

Volume 45
Occupational Exposures in Petroleum Refining; Crude Oil and Major Petroleum Fuels
1989; 322 pages; ISBN 92 832 1245 2

Volume 46
Diesel and Gasoline Engine Exhausts and Some Nitroarenes
1989; 458 pages; ISBN 92 832 1246 0

Volume 47
Some Organic Solvents, Resin Monomers and Related Compounds, Pigments and Occupational Exposures in Paint Manufacture and Painting
1989; 535 pages; ISBN 92 832 1247 9

Volume 48
Some Flame Retardants and Textile Chemicals, and Exposures in the Textile Manufacturing Industry
1990; 345 pages; ISBN: 92 832 1248 7

Volume 49
Chromium, Nickel and Welding
1990; 677 pages; ISBN: 92 832 1249 5

Volume 50
Some Pharmaceutical Drugs
1990; 415 pages; ISBN: 92 832 1259 9

Volume 51
Coffee, Tea, Mate, Methylxanthines and Methylglyoxal
1991; 513 pages; ISBN: 92 832 1251 7

Volume 52
Chlorinated Drinking-Water; Chlorination By-products; Some other Halogenated Compounds; Cobalt and Cobalt Compounds
1991; 544 pages; ISBN: 92 832 1252 5

Volume 53
Occupational Exposures in Insecticide Application, and Some Pesticides
1991; 612 pages; ISBN 92 832 1253 3

Volume 54
Occupational Exposures to Mists and Vapours from Strong Inorganic Acids; and other Industrial Chemicals
1992; 336 pages; ISBN 92 832 1254 1

Volume 55
Solar and Ultraviolet Radiation
1992; 316 pages; ISBN 92 832 1255 X

Volume 56
Some Naturally Occurring Substances: Food Items and Constituents, Heterocyclic Aromatic Amines and Mycotoxins
1993; 600 pages; ISBN 92 832 1256 8

Volume 57
Occupational Exposures of Hairdressers and Barbers and Personal Use of Hair Colourants; Some Hair Dyes, Cosmetic Colourants, Industrial Dyestuffs and Aromatic Amines
1993; 428 pages; ISBN 92 832 1257 6

Volume 58
Beryllium, Cadmium, Mercury and Exposures in the Glass Manufacturing Industry
1994; 444 pages; ISBN 92 832 1258 4

Volume 59
Hepatitis Viruses
1994; 286 pages; ISBN 92 832 1259 2

Volume 60
Some Industrial Chemicals
1994; 560 pages; ISBN 92 832 1260 6

Volume 61
Schistosomes, Liver Flukes and *Helicobacter pylori*
1994; 280 pages; ISBN 92 832 1261 4

Volume 62
Wood Dusts and Formaldehyde
1995; 405 pages; ISBN 92 832 1262 2

Volume 63
Dry cleaning, Some Chlorinated Solvents and Other Industrial Chemicals
1995; 558 pages; ISBN 92 832 1263 0

Volume 64
Human Papillomaviruses
1995; 409 pages; ISBN 92 832 1264 9

Volume 65
Printing Processes and Printing Inks, Carbon Black and Some Nitro Compounds
1996; 578 pages; ISBN 92 832 1265 7

Volume 66
Some Pharmaceutical Drugs
1996; 514 pages; ISBN 92 832 1266 5

Volume 67
Human Immunodeficiency Viruses and Human T-cell Lymphotropic Viruses
1996; 424 pages; ISBN 92 832 1267 3

Volume 68
Silica, Some Silicates, Coal Dust and *para*-Aramid Fibrils
1997; 506 pages; ISBN 92 832 1268 1

Volume 69
Polychlorinated Dibenzo-para-dioxins and Polychlorinated Dibenzofurans
1997; 666 pages; ISBN 92 832 1269 X

Volume 70
Epstein-Barr Virus and Kaposi's Sarcoma Herpesvirus/Human Herpesvirus 8
1998; 524 pages; ISBN 92 832 1270 3

Supplements to Monographs

*Supplement No.1**
Chemicals and Industrial Processes Associated with Cancer in Humans (Volumes 1 to 20)
1979; 71 pages; ISBN 92 832 1404 8

Supplement No. 2
Long-Term and Short-Term Screening Assays for Carcinogens: A Critical Appraisal
1980; 426 pages; ISBN 92 832 1404 8

*Supplement No. 3**
Cross Index of Synonyms and Trade Names in Volumes 1 to 26
1982; 199 pages; ISBN 92 832 1405 6

*Supplement No.4**
Chemicals, Industrial Processes and Industries Associated with Cancer in Humans (Volumes 1 to 29)
1982; 292 pages; ISBN 92 832 1407 2

*Supplement No. 5**
Cross Index of Synonyms and Trade Names in Volumes 1 to 36
1985; 259 pages; ISBN 92 832 1408 0

Supplement No. 6
Genetic and Related Effects: An Updating of Selected IARC Monographs from Volumes 1 to 42
1987; 729 pages; ISBN 92 832 1409 9

Supplement No. 7
Overall Evaluations of Carcinogenicity: An Updating of IARC Monographs Volumes 1 to 42
1987; 440 pages; ISBN 92 832 1411 0

*Supplement No. 8**
Cross Index of Synonyms and Trade Names in Volumes 1 to 46
1989; 346 pages; ISBN 92 832 1417 X

IARC Scientific Publications
ISSN 0300 5085

*No. 1**
Liver Cancer
1971; 176 pages; ISBN 0 19 723000 8

No. 2
Oncogenesis and Herpesviruses
Edited by P.M. Biggs, G. de Thé and L.N. Payne
1972; 515 pages; ISBN 0 19 723001 6

*No. 3**
***N*-Nitroso Compounds: Analysis and Formation**
Edited by P. Bogovski, R. Preussman and E.A. Walker
1972; 140 pages; ISBN 0 19 723002 4

*No. 4**
Transplacental Carcinogenesis
Edited by L. Tomatis and U. Mohr
1973; 181 pages; ISBN 0 19 723003 2

No. 5/6
Pathology of Tumours in Laboratory Animals. Volume 1: Tumours of the Rat
Edited by V.S. Turusov
1973/1976; 533 pages; ISBN 92 832 1410 2

*No. 7**
Host Environment Interactions in the Etiology of Cancer in Man
Edited by R. Doll and I. Vodopija
1973; 464 pages; ISBN 0 19 723006 7

*No. 8**
Biological Effects of Asbestos
Edited by P. Bogovski, J.C. Gilson, V. Timbrell and J.C. Wagner
1973; 346 pages; ISBN 0 19 723007 5

No. 9
N-Nitroso Compounds in the Environment
Edited by P. Bogovski and E.A. Walker
1974; 243 pages; ISBN 0 19 723008 3

*No. 10**
Chemical Carcinogenesis Essays
Edited by R. Montesano and L. Tomatis
1974; 230 pages; ISBN 0 19 723009 1

*No. 11**
Oncogenesis and Herpes-viruses II
Edited by G. de-Thé, M.A. Epstein and H. zur Hausen
1975; Two volumes, 511 pages and 403 pages; ISBN 0 19 723010 5

No. 12
Screening Tests in Chemical Carcinogenesis
Edited by R. Montesano, H. Bartsch and L. Tomatis
1976; 666 pages; ISBN 0 19 723051 2

*No. 13**
Environmental Pollution and Carcinogenic Risks
Edited by C. Rosenfeld and W. Davis
1975; 441 pages; ISBN 0 19 723012 1

No. 14
Environmental N-Nitroso Compounds. Analysis and Formation
Edited by E.A. Walker, P. Bogovski and L. Griciute
1976; 512 pages; ISBN 0 19 723013 X

*No. 15**
Cancer Incidence in Five Continents, Volume III
Edited by J.A.H. Waterhouse, C. Muir, P. Correa and J. Powell
1976; 584 pages; ISBN 0 19 723014 8

*No. 16**
Air Pollution and Cancer in Man
Edited by U. Mohr, D. Schmähl and L. Tomatis
1977; 328 pages; ISBN 0 19 723015 6

*No. 17**
Directory of On-Going Research in Cancer Epidemiology 1977
Edited by C.S. Muir and G. Wagner
1977; 599 pages; ISBN 92 832 1117 0

*No. 18**
Environmental Carcinogens. Selected Methods of Analysis. Volume 1: Analysis of Volatile Nitrosamines in Food
Editor-in-Chief: H. Egan
1978; 212 pages; ISBN 92 932 1118 9

*No. 19**
Environmental Aspects of N-Nitroso Compounds
Edited by E.A. Walker, M. Castegnaro, L. Griciute and R.E. Lyle
1978; 561 pages; ISBN 0 19 723018 0

*No. 20**
Nasopharyngeal Carcinoma: Etiology and Control
Edited by G. de Thé and Y. Ito
1978; 606 pages; ISBN 0 19 723019 9

*No. 21**
Cancer Registration and its Techniques
Edited by R. MacLennan, C. Muir, R. Steinitz and A. Winkler
1978; 235 pages; ISBN 0 19 723020 2

*out-of-print

No. 22
Environmental Carcinogens: Selected Methods of Analysis. Volume 2: Methods for the Measurement of Vinyl Chloride in Poly(vinyl chloride), Air, Water and Foodstuffs
Editor-in-Chief: H. Egan
1978; 142 pages; ISBN 92 832 1122 7

*No. 23**
Pathology of Tumours in Laboratory Animals. Volume II: Tumours of the Mouse
Editor-in-Chief: V.S. Turusov
1979; 669 pages; ISBN 0 19 723022 9

*No. 24**
Oncogenesis and Herpesviruses III
Edited by G. de-Thé, W. Henle and F. Rapp
1978; Part I: 580 pages, Part II: 512 pages; ISBN 0 19 723023 7

No. 25
Carcinogenic Risk: Strategies for Intervention
Edited by W. Davis and C. Rosenfeld
1979; 280 pages; ISBN 0 19 723025 3

*No. 26**
Directory of On-going Research in Cancer Epidemiology 1978
Edited by C.S. Muir and G. Wagner
1978; 550 pages; ISBN 0 19 723026 1

No. 27
Molecular and Cellular Aspects of Carcinogen Screening Tests
Edited by R. Montesano, H. Bartsch and L. Tomatis
1980; 372 pages; ISBN 0 19 723027 X

*No. 28**
Directory of On-going Research in Cancer Epidemiology 1979
Edited by C.S. Muir and G. Wagner
1979; 672 pages; ISBN 92 832 1128 6

*No. 29**
Environmental Carcinogens. Selected Methods of Analysis. Volume 3: Analysis of Polycyclic Aromatic Hydrocarbons in Environmental Samples
Editor-in-Chief: H. Egan
1979; 240 pages; ISBN 0 92 932 1129 4

*No. 30**
Biological Effects of Mineral Fibres
Editor-in-Chief: J.C. Wagner
1980; Two volumes, 494 pages & 513 pages; ISBN 0 19 723030 X

No. 31
***N*-Nitroso Compounds: Analysis, Formation and Occurrence**
Edited by E.A. Walker, L. Griciute, M. Castegnaro and M. Börzsönyi
1980; 835 pages; ISBN 0 19 723031 8

No. 32
Statistical Methods in Cancer Research. Volume 1: The Analysis of Case-control Studies
By N.E. Breslow and N.E. Day
1980; 338 pages; ISBN 92 832 0132 9

*No. 33**
Handling Chemical Carcinogens in the Laboratory
Edited by R. Montesano, H. Bartsch, E. Boyland, G. Della Porta, L. Fishbein, R.A. Griesemer, A.B. Swan and L. Tomatis
1979; 32 pages; ISBN 0 19 723033 4

No. 34
Pathology of Tumours in Laboratory Animals. Volume III: Tumours of the Hamster
Editor-in-Chief: V.S. Turusov
1982; 461 pages; ISBN 0 19 723034 2

*No. 35**
Directory of On-going Research in Cancer Epidemiology 1980
Edited by C.S. Muir and G. Wagner
1980; 660 pages; ISBN 0 19 723035 0

No. 36
Cancer Mortality by Occupation and Social Class 1851–1971
Edited by W.P.D. Logan
1982; 253 pages; ISBN 0 19 723036 9

No. 37
Laboratory Decontamination and Destruction of Aflatoxins B_1, B_2, G_1, G_2 in Laboratory Wastes
Edited by M. Castegnaro, D.C. Hunt, E.B. Sansone, P.L. Schuller, M.G. Siriwardana, G.M. Telling, H.P. van Egmond and E.A. Walker
1980; 56 pages; ISBN 92 832 1137 5

*No. 38**
Directory of On-going Research in Cancer Epidemiology 1981
Edited by C.S. Muir and G. Wagner
1981; 696 pages; ISBN 0 19 723038 5

No. 39
Host Factors in Human Carcinogenesis
Edited by H. Bartsch and B. Armstrong
1982; 583 pages;
ISBN 0 19 723039 3

No. 40
Environmental Carcinogens: Selected Methods of Analysis. Volume 4: Some Aromatic Amines and Azo Dyes in the General and Industrial Environment
Edited by L. Fishbein, M. Castegnaro, I.K. O'Neill and H. Bartsch
1981; 347 pages; ISBN 0 92 932 1140 5

*No. 41**
***N*-Nitroso Compounds: Occurrence and Biological Effects**
Edited by H. Bartsch, I.K. O'Neill, M. Castegnaro and M. Okada
1982; 755 pages; ISBN 0 19 723041 5

*No. 42**
Cancer Incidence in Five Continents Volume IV
Edited by J. Waterhouse, C. Muir, K. Shanmugaratnam and J. Powell
1982; 811 pages; ISBN 0 19 723042 3

No. 43
Laboratory Decontamination and Destruction of Carcinogens in Laboratory Wastes: Some *N*-Nitrosamines
Edited by M. Castegnaro, G. Eisenbrand, G. Ellen, L. Keefer, D. Klein, E.B. Sansone, D. Spincer, G. Telling and K. Webb
1982; 73 pages; ISBN 92 832 1143 X

No. 44
Environmental Carcinogens: Selected Methods of Analysis.
Volume 5: Some Mycotoxins
Edited by L. Stoloff, M. Castegnaro, P. Scott, I.K. O'Neill and H. Bartsch
1983; 455 pages; ISBN 92 932 1144 8

*No. 45**
Environmental Carcinogens: Selected Methods of Analysis. Volume 6: *N*-Nitroso Compounds
Edited by R. Preussmann, I.K. O'Neill, G. Eisenbrand, B. Spiegelhalder and H. Bartsch
1983; 508 pages; ISBN 92 832 1145 6

*No. 46**
Directory of On-going Research in Cancer Epidemiology 1982
Edited by C.S. Muir and G. Wagner
1982; 722 pages; ISBN 0 19 723046 6

*No. 47**
Cancer Incidence in Singapore 1968–1977
Edited by K. Shanmugaratnam, H.P. Lee and N.E. Day
1983; 171 pages; ISBN 0 19 723047 4

*No. 48**
Cancer Incidence in the USSR (2nd Revised Edition)
Edited by N.P. Napalkov, G.F. Tserkovny, V.M. Merabishvili, D.M. Parkin, M. Smans and C.S. Muir
1983; 75 pages; ISBN 0 19 723048 2

*Out-of-print

No. 49
Laboratory Decontamination and Destruction of Carcinogens in Laboratory Wastes: Some Polycyclic Aromatic Hydrocarbons
Edited by M. Castegnaro, G. Grimmer, O. Hutzinger, W. Karcher, H. Kunte, M. Lafontaine, H.C. Van der Plas, E.B. Sansone and S.P. Tucker
1983; 87 pages; ISBN 92 832 1149 9

*No. 50**
Directory of On-going Research in Cancer Epidemiology 1983
Edited by C.S. Muir and G. Wagner
1983; 731 pages; ISBN 0 19 723050 4

No. 51
Modulators of Experimental Carcinogenesis
Edited by V. Turusov and R. Montesano
1983; 307 pages; ISBN 0 19 723060 1

No. 52
Second Cancers in Relation to Radiation Treatment for Cervical Cancer: Results of a Cancer Registry Collaboration
Edited by N.E. Day and J.C. Boice, Jr
1984; 207 pages; ISBN 0 19 723052 0

No. 53
Nickel in the Human Environment
Editor-in-Chief: F.W. Sunderman, Jr
1984; 529 pages; ISBN 0 19 723059 8

No. 54
Laboratory Decontamination and Destruction of Carcinogens in Laboratory Wastes: Some Hydrazines
Edited by M. Castegnaro, G. Ellen, M. Lafontaine, H.C. van der Plas, E.B. Sansone and S.P. Tucker
1983; 87 pages; ISBN 92 832 11545

No. 55
Laboratory Decontamination and Destruction of Carcinogens in Laboratory Wastes: Some *N*-Nitrosamides
Edited by M. Castegnaro, M. Bernard, L.W. van Broekhoven, D. Fine, R. Massey, E.B. Sansone, P.L.R. Smith, B. Spiegelhalder, A. Stacchini, G. Telling and J.J. Vallon
1984; 66 pages; ISBN 92 832 1155 3

No. 56
Models, Mechanisms and Etiology of Tumour Promotion
Edited by M. Börzsönyi, N.E. Day, K. Lapis and H. Yamasaki
1984; 532 pages; ISBN 92 832 1156 1

*No. 57**
N-Nitroso Compounds: Occurrence, Biological Effects and Relevance to Human Cancer
Edited by I.K. O'Neill, R.C. von Borstel, C.T. Miller, J. Long and H. Bartsch
1984; 1013 pages; ISBN 92 832 1157 X

No 58
Age-related Factors in Carcinogenesis
Edited by A. Likhachev, V. Anisimov and R. Montesano
1985; 288 pages; ISBN 92 832 1158 8

No. 59
Monitoring Human Exposure to Carcinogenic and Mutagenic Agents
Edited by A. Berlin, M. Draper, K. Hemminki and H. Vainio
1984; 457 pages; ISBN 0 19 723056 3

No. 60
Burkitt's Lymphoma: A Human Cancer Model
Edited by G. Lenoir, G. O'Conor and C.L.M. Olweny
1985; 484 pages; ISBN 0 19 723057 1

No. 61
Laboratory Decontamination and Destruction of Carcinogens in Laboratory Wastes: Some Haloethers
Edited by M. Castegnaro, M. Alvarez, M. Iovu, E.B. Sansone, G.M. Telling and D.T. Williams
1985; 55 pages; ISBN 92 832 11618

*No. 62**
Directory of On-going Research in Cancer Epidemiology 1984
Edited by C.S. Muir and G. Wagner
1984; 717 pages; ISBN 0 19 723062 8

No. 63
Virus-associated Cancers in Africa
Edited by A.O. Williams, G.T. O'Conor, G.B. de Thé and C.A. Johnson
1984; 773 pages; ISBN 0 19 723063 6

No. 64
Laboratory Decontamination and Destruction of Carcinogens in Laboratory Wastes: Some Aromatic Amines and 4-Nitrobiphenyl
Edited by M. Castegnaro, J. Barek, J. Dennis, G. Ellen, M. Klibanov, M. Lafontaine, R. Mitchum, P. van Roosmalen, E.B. Sansone, L.A. Sternson and M. Vahl
1985; 84 pages; ISBN: 92 832 1164 2

No. 65
Interpretation of Negative Epidemiological Evidence for Carcinogenicity
Edited by N.J. Wald and R. Doll
1985; 232 pages; ISBN 92 832 1165 0

No. 66
The Role of the Registry in Cancer Control
Edited by D.M. Parkin, G. Wagner and C.S. Muir
1985; 152 pages; ISBN 92 832 0166 3

No. 67
Transformation Assay of Established Cell Lines: Mechanisms and Application
Edited by T. Kakunaga and H. Yamasaki
1985; 225 pages; ISBN 92 832 1167 7

*No. 68**
Environmental Carcinogens: Selected Methods of Analysis. Volume 7: Some Volatile Halogenated Hydrocarbons
Edited by L. Fishbein and I.K. O'Neill
1985; 479 pages; ISBN 92 832 1168 5

*No. 69**
Directory of On-going Research in Cancer Epidemiology 1985
Edited by C.S. Muir and G. Wagner
1985; 745 pages; ISBN 92 823 1169 3

No. 70
The Role of Cyclic Nucleic Acid Adducts in Carcinogenesis and Mutagenesis
Edited by B. Singer and H. Bartsch
1986; 467 pages; ISBN 92 832 1170 7

No. 71
Environmental Carcinogens: Selected Methods of Analysis. Volume 8: Some Metals: As, Be, Cd, Cr, Ni, Pb, Se, Zn
Edited by I.K. O'Neill, P. Schuller and L. Fishbein
1986; 485 pages; ISBN 92 832 1171 5

No. 72
Atlas of Cancer in Scotland, 1975–1980: Incidence and Epidemiological Perspective
Edited by I. Kemp, P. Boyle, M. Smans and C.S. Muir
1985; 285 pages; ISBN 92 832 1172 3

No. 73
Laboratory Decontamination and Destruction of Carcinogens in Laboratory Wastes: Some Antineoplastic Agents
Edited by M. Castegnaro, J. Adams, M.A. Armour, J. Barek, J. Benvenuto, C. Confalonieri, U. Goff, G. Telling
1985; 163 pages; ISBN 92 832 1173 1

No. 74
Tobacco: A Major International Health Hazard
Edited by D. Zaridze and R. Peto
1986; 324 pages; ISBN 92 832 1174 X

*Out-of-print

No. 75
Cancer Occurrence in Developing Countries
Edited by D.M. Parkin
1986; 339 pages; ISBN 92 832 1175 8

No. 76
Screening for Cancer of the Uterine Cervix
Edited by M. Hakama, A.B. Miller and N.E. Day
1986; 315 pages; ISBN 92 832 1176 6

No. 77
Hexachlorobenzene: Proceedings of an International Symposium
Edited by C.R. Morris and J.R.P. Cabral
1986; 668 pages; ISBN 92 832 1177 4

No. 78
Carcinogenicity of Alkylating Cytostatic Drugs
Edited by D. Schmähl and J.M. Kaldor
1986; 337 pages; ISBN 92 832 1178 2

No. 79
Statistical Methods in Cancer Research. Volume III: The Design and Analysis of Long-term Animal Experiments
By J.J. Gart, D. Krewski, P.N. Lee, R.E. Tarone and J. Wahrendorf
1986; 213 pages; ISBN 92 832 1179 0

*No. 80**
Directory of On-going Research in Cancer Epidemiology 1986
Edited by C.S. Muir and G. Wagner
1986; 805 pages; ISBN 92 832 1180 4

No. 81
Environmental Carcinogens: Methods of Analysis and Exposure Measure-ment. Volume 9: Passive Smoking
Edited by I.K. O'Neill, K.D. Brunnemann, B. Dodet and D. Hoffmann
1987; 383 pages; ISBN 92 832 1181 2

No. 82
Statistical Methods in Cancer Research. Volume II: The Design and Analysis of Cohort Studies
By N.E. Breslow and N.E. Day
1987; 404 pages; ISBN 92 832 0182 5

No. 83
Long-term and Short-term Assays for Carcinogens: A Critical Appraisal
Edited by R. Montesano, H. Bartsch, H. Vainio, J. Wilbourn and H. Yamasaki
1986; 575 pages; ISBN 92 832 1183 9

No. 84
The Relevance of *N*-Nitroso Compounds to Human Cancer: Exposure and Mechanisms
Edited by H. Bartsch, I.K. O'Neill and R. Schulte-Hermann
1987; 671 pages; ISBN 92 832 1184 7

No. 85
Environmental Carcinogens: Methods of Analysis and Exposure Measurement. Volume 10: Benzene and Alkylated Benzenes
Edited by L. Fishbein and I.K. O'Neill
1988; 327 pages; ISBN 92 832 1185 5

*No. 86**
Directory of On-going Research in Cancer Epidemiology 1987
Edited by D.M. Parkin and J. Wahrendorf
1987; 685 pages; ISBN: 92 832 1186 3

*No. 87**
International Incidence of Childhood Cancer
Edited by D.M. Parkin, C.A. Stiller, C.A. Bieber, G.J. Draper. B. Terracini and J.L. Young
1988; 401 page; ISBN 92 832 1187 1

*No. 88**
Cancer Incidence in Five Continents, Volume V
Edited by C. Muir, J. Waterhouse, T. Mack, J. Powell and S. Whelan
1987; 1004 pages; ISBN 92 832 1188 X

*No. 89**
Methods for Detecting DNA Damaging Agents in Humans: Applications in Cancer Epidemiology and Prevention
Edited by H. Bartsch, K. Hemminki and I.K. O'Neill
1988; 518 pages; ISBN 92 832 1189 8

No. 90
Non-occupational Exposure to Mineral Fibres
Edited by J. Bignon, J. Peto and R. Saracci
1989; 500 pages; ISBN 92 832 1190 1

No. 91
Trends in Cancer Incidence in Singapore 1968–1982
Edited by H.P. Lee, N.E. Day and K. Shanmugaratnam
1988; 160 pages; ISBN 92 832 1191 X

No. 92
Cell Differentiation, Genes and Cancer
Edited by T. Kakunaga, T. Sugimura, L. Tomatis and H. Yamasaki
1988; 204 pages; ISBN 92 832 1192 8

*No. 93**
Directory of On-going Research in Cancer Epidemiology 1988
Edited by M. Coleman and J. Wahrendorf
1988; 662 pages; ISBN 92 832 1193 6

No. 94
Human Papillomavirus and Cervical Cancer
Edited by N. Muñoz, F.X. Bosch and O.M. Jensen
1989; 154 pages; ISBN 92 832 1194 4

No. 95
Cancer Registration: Principles and Methods
Edited by O.M. Jensen, D.M. Parkin, R. MacLennan, C.S. Muir and R. Skeet
1991; 296 pages; ISBN 92 832 1195 2

Registros de cancer: Principios y Métodos
Edited by O.M. Jensen, D.M. Parkin, R. MacLennan, C.S. Muir and R. Skeet
1995; 286 pages; ISBN 92 832 0403 4

Enregistrement des Cancers: Principes et Methodes
Edited by O.M. Jensen, D.M. Parkin, R. MacLennan, C.S. Muir and R. Skeet
1996; 211 pages; ISBN 92 832 0404 2

No. 96
Perinatal and Multigeneration Carcinogenesis
Edited by N.P. Napalkov, J.M. Rice, L. Tomatis and H. Yamasaki
1989; 436 pages; ISBN 92 832 1196 0

No. 97
Occupational Exposure to Silica and Cancer Risk
Edited by L. Simonato, A.C. Fletcher, R. Saracci and T. Thomas
1990; 124 pages; ISBN 92 832 1197 9

No. 98
Cancer Incidence in Jewish Migrants to Israel, 1961-1981
Edited by R. Steinitz, D.M. Parkin, J.L. Young, C.A. Bieber and L. Katz
1989; 320 pages; ISBN 92 832 1198 7

No. 99
Pathology of Tumours in Laboratory Animals, Second Edition, Volume 1, Tumours of the Rat
Edited by V.S. Turusov and U. Mohr
1990; 740 pages; ISBN 92 832 1199 5

*Out-of-print

No. 100
Cancer: Causes, Occurrence and Control
Editor-in-Chief: L. Tomatis
1990; 352 pages; ISBN 92 832 0110 8

*No. 101**
Directory of On-going Research in Cancer Epidemiology 1989/90
Edited by M. Coleman and J. Wahrendorf
1989; 828 pages; ISBN 92 832 2101 X

No. 102
Patterns of Cancer in Five Continents
Edited by S.L. Whelan, D.M. Parkin and E. Masuyer
1990; 160 pages; ISBN 92 832 2102 8

*No. 103**
Evaluating Effectiveness of Primary Prevention of Cancer
Edited by M. Hakama, V. Beral, J.W. Cullen and D.M. Parkin
1990; 206 pages; ISBN 92 832 2103 6

No. 104
Complex Mixtures and Cancer Risk
Edited by H. Vainio, M. Sorsa and A.J. McMichael
1990; 441 pages; ISBN 92 832 2104 4

No. 105
Relevance to Human Cancer of *N*-Nitroso Compounds, Tobacco Smoke and Mycotoxins
Edited by I.K. O'Neill, J. Chen and H. Bartsch
1991; 614 pages; ISBN 92 832 2105 2

No. 106
Atlas of Cancer Incidence in the Former German Democratic Republic
Edited by W.H. Mehnert, M. Smans, C.S. Muir, M. Möhner and D. Schön
1992; 384 pages; ISBN 92 832 2106 0

No. 107
Atlas of Cancer Mortality in the European Economic Community
Edited by M. Smans, C. Muir and P. Boyle
1992; 213 pages + 44 coloured maps; ISBN 92 832 2107 9

No. 108
Environmental Carcinogens: Methods of Analysis and Exposure Measurement. Volume 11: Polychlorinated Dioxins and Dibenzofurans
Edited by C. Rappe, H.R. Buser, B. Dodet and I.K. O'Neill
1991; 400 pages; ISBN 92 832 2108 7

No. 109
Environmental Carcinogens: Methods of Analysis and Exposure Measurement. Volume 12: Indoor Air
Edited by B. Seifert, H. van de Wiel, B. Dodet and I.K. O'Neill
1993; 385 pages; ISBN 92 832 2109 5

*No. 110**
Directory of On-going Research in Cancer Epidemiology 1991
Edited by M.P. Coleman and J. Wahrendorf
1991; 753 pages; ISBN 92 832 2110 9

No. 111
Pathology of Tumours in Laboratory Animals, Second Edition. Volume 2: Tumours of the Mouse
Edited by V. Turusov and U. Mohr
1994; 800 pages; ISBN 92 832 2111 1

No. 112
Autopsy in Epidemiology and Medical Research
Edited by E. Riboli and M. Delendi
1991; 288 pages; ISBN 92 832 2112 5

No. 113
Laboratory Decontamination and Destruction of Carcinogens in Laboratory Wastes: Some Mycotoxins
Edited by M. Castegnaro, J. Barek, J.M. Frémy, M. Lafontaine, M. Miraglia, E.B. Sansone and G.M. Telling
1991; 63 pages; ISBN 92 832 2113 3

No. 114
Laboratory Decontamination and Destruction of Carcinogens in Laboratory Wastes: Some Polycyclic Heterocyclic Hydrocarbons
Edited by M. Castegnaro, J. Barek, J. Jacob, U. Kirso, M. Lafontaine, E.B. Sansone, G.M. Telling and T. Vu Duc
1991; 50 pages; ISBN 92 832 2114 1

No. 115
Mycotoxins, Endemic Nephropathy and Urinary Tract Tumours
Edited by M. Castegnaro, R. Plestina, G. Dirheimer, I.N. Chernozemsky and H. Bartsch
1991; 340 pages; ISBN 92 832 2115 X

No. 116
Mechanisms of Carcinogenesis in Risk Identification
Edited by H. Vainio, P. Magee, D. McGregor and A.J. McMichael
1992; 615 pages; ISBN 92 832 2116 8

*No. 117**
Directory of On-going Research in Cancer Epidemiology 1992
Edited by M. Coleman, E. Demaret and J. Wahrendorf
1992; 773 pages; ISBN 92 832 2117 6

No. 118
Cadmium in the Human Environment: Toxicity and Carcinogenicity
Edited by G.F. Nordberg, R.F.M. Herber and L. Alessio
1992; 470 pages; ISBN 92 832 2118 4

*No. 119**
The Epidemiology of Cervical Cancer and Human Papillomavirus
Edited by N. Muñoz, F.X. Bosch, K.V. Shah and A. Meheus
1992; 288 pages; ISBN 92 832 2119 2

*No. 120**
Cancer Incidence in Five Continents, Vol. VI
Edited by D.M. Parkin, C.S. Muir, S.L. Whelan, Y.T. Gao, J. Ferlay and J. Powell
1992; 1020 pages; ISBN 92 832 2120 6

No. 121
Time Trends in Cancer Incidence and Mortality
By M. Coleman, J. Estéve, P. Damiecki, A. Arslan and H. Renard
1993; 820 pages; ISBN 92 832 2121 4

No. 122
International Classification of Rodent Tumours. Part I. The Rat
Editor-in-Chief: U. Mohr

Respiratory System
1992; 57 pages; ISBN 92 832 0121 3

Soft Tissue and Muscoskeletal System
1992; 62 pages: ISBN 92 832 01221

Urinary System
1993; 27 pages; ISBN 92 832 0123 X

Haematopoietic System
1992; 46 pages; ISBN 92 832 0124

Integumentary System
1993; 45 pages; ISBN 92 832 0125 6

Endocrine System
1994; 75 pages; ISBN 92 832 0126 4

Central Nervous System: Heart; Eye, Mesothelium
1994; 80 pages; ISBN 92 832 0127 2
Male Genital System
1997; 52 pages; ISBN 92 832 0128 0

*Out-of-print

Female Genital System
1997; 83 pages; ISBN 92 832 0129 9

Digestive System
1997; 109 pages; ISBN 92 832 0130 2

No. 123
Cancer in Italian Migrant Populations
Edited by M. Geddes, D.M. Parkin, M. Khlat, D. Balzi and E. Buiatti
1993; 292 pages; ISBN 92 832 2123 0

No. 124
Postlabelling Methods for the Detection of DNA Damage
Edited by D.H. Phillips, M. Castegnaro and H. Bartsch
1993; 392 pages; ISBN 92 832 2124 9

No. 125
DNA Adducts: Identification and Biological Significance
Edited by K. Hemminki, A. Dipple, D.E.G. Shuker, F.F. Kadlubar, D. Segerbäck and H. Bartsch
1994; 478 pages; ISBN 92 832 2125 7

No. 126
Pathology of Tumours in Laboratory Animals, Second Edition. Volume 3: Tumours of the Hamster
Edited by U. Mohr and V. Turosov
1996; 464 pages; ISBN 92 832 2126 5

No. 127
Butadiene and Styrene: Assessment of Health Hazards
Edited by M. Sorsa, K. Peltonen, H. Vainio and K. Hemminki
1993; 412 pages; ISBN 92 832 2127 3

No. 128
Statistical Methods in Cancer Research. Volume IV. Descriptive Epidemiology
By J. Estève, E. Benhamou and L. Raymond
1994; 302 pages; ISBN 92 832 2128 1

No. 129
Occupational Cancer in Developing Countries
Edited by N. Pearce, E. Matos, H. Vainio, P. Boffetta and M. Kogevinas
1994; 191 pages; ISBN 92 832 2129 X

*No. 130**
Directory of On-going Research in Cancer Epidemiology 1994
Edited by R. Sankaranarayanan, J. Wahrendorf and E. Démaret
1994; 800 pages; ISBN 92 832 2130 3

No. 132
Survival of Cancer Patients in Europe: The EUROCARE Study
Edited by F. Berrino, M. Sant, A. Verdecchia, R. Capocaccia, T. Hakulinen and J. Estève
1995; 463 pages; ISBN 92 832 2132 X

No. 134
Atlas of Cancer Mortality in Central Europe
W. Zatonski, J. Estéve, M. Smans, J. Tyczynski and P. Boyle
1996; 175 pages plus 40 coloured maps; ISBN 92 832 2134 6

No. 135
Methods for Investigating Localized Clustering of Disease
Edited by F.E. Alexander and P. Boyle
1996; 235 pages; ISBN 92 832 2135 4

No. 136
Chemoprevention in Cancer Control
Edited by M. Hakama, V. Beral, E. Buiatti, J. Faivre and D.M. Parkin
1996; 160 pages; ISBN 92 832 2136 2

No. 137
Directory of On-going Research in Cancer Epidemiology 1996
Edited by R. Sankaranarayan, J. Warendorf and E. Démaret
1996; 810 pages; ISBN 92 832 2137 0

No. 138
Social Inequalities and Cancer
Edited by M. Kogevinas, N. Pearce, M. Susser and P. Boffetta
1997; 412 pages; ISBN 92 832 8138 9

No. 139
Principles of Chemoprevention
Edited by B.W. Stewart, D. McGregor and P. Kleihues
1996; 358 pages; ISBN 92 832 2139 7

No. 140
Mechanisms of Fibre Carcinogenesis
Edited by A.B. Kane, R. Saracci, P. Boffetta and J.D. Wilbourn
1996; 135 pages; ISBN 92 832 2140 0

No. 142
Application of Biomarkers in Cancer Epidemiology
Edited by P. Toniolo, P. Boffetta, D.E.G. Shuker, N. Rothman, B. Hulka and N. Pearce
1997; 318 pages; ISBN 92 832 2142 7

No. 143
Cancer Incidence in Five Continentss Vol VII.
Edited by D.M. Parkin, S.L. Whelan, J. Ferlay, L. Raymond and J. Young
1997; 1240 pages; ISBN 92 832 2143 5

No. 144
International Incidence of Childhood Cancer, Vol. II
Edited by D.M. Parkin, E. Kramárová, C.A. Stiller, J.G.J. Draper, E. Masuyer, J. Michaelis, J. Neglia and S. Qureshi
Publication due November 1998; c. 500 pages; ISBN 92 832 2144 3

No. 145
Cancer Survival in Developing Countries
Edited by R. Sankaranarayanan, R.J. Black and D.M. Parkin
Publication due November 1998; c. 250 pages; ISBN 92 832 2145 1

No. 146
Short- and Medium-term Carcinogenicity Tests, Mutation Analysis, and Multistage Models in Risk Identification
Publication due November 1998
c. 320 pages; ISBN 92 832 2146 X

IARC Technical Reports

No. 1
Cancer in Costa Rica
Edited by R. Sierra, R. Barrantes, G. Muñoz Leiva, D.M. Parkin, C.A. Bieber and N. Muñoz Calero
1988; 124 pages;
ISBN 92 832 1412 9

*No. 2**
SEARCH: A Computer Package to Assist the Statistical Analysis of Case-Control Studies
Edited by G.J. Macfarlane, P. Boyle and P. Maisonneuve
1991; 80 pages; ISBN 92 832 1413 7

No. 3
Cancer Registration in the European Economic Community
Edited by M.P. Coleman and E. Démaret
1988; 188 pages; ISBN 92 832 1414 5

*No. 4**
Diet, Hormones and Cancer: Methodological Issues for Prospective Studies
Edited by E. Riboli and R. Saracci
1988; 156 pages; ISBN 92 832 1415 3

*No. 5**
Cancer in the Philippines
Edited by A.V. Laudico, D. Esteban and D.M. Parkin
1989; 186 pages; ISBN 92 832 1416 1

No. 6
La genèse du Centre international de recherche sur le cancer
By R. Sohier and A.G.B. Sutherland
1990, 102 pages; ISBN 92 832 1418 8

No. 7
Epidémiologie du cancer dans les pays de langue latine
1990, 292 pages; ISBN 92 832 1419 6

No. 8
Comparative Study of Anti-smoking Legislation in Countries of the European Economic Community
By A. J. Sasco, P. Dalla-Vorgia and P. Van Der Elst
1992; 82 pages; ISBN: 92 832 1421 8

Etude comparative des Législations de Contrôle du Tabagisme dans les Pays de la Communauté économique européenne
By A. J. Sasco, P. Dalla-Vorgia and P. Van Der Elst
1995; 82 pages; ISBN 92 832 2402 7

*No. 9**
Epidémiologie du cancer dans les pays de langue latine
1991; 346 pages; ISBN 92 832 1423 4

No. 10
Manual for Cancer Registry Personnel
Edited by D. Esteban, S. Whelan, A. Laudico and D.M. Parkin
1995; 400 pages; ISBN 92 832 1424 2

No. 11
Nitroso Compounds: Biological Mechanisms, Exposures and Cancer Etiology
Edited by I. O'Neill and H. Bartsch
1992; 150 pages; ISBN 92 832 1425 0

*No. 12**
Epidémiologie du cancer dans les pays de langue latine
1992; 375 pages; ISBN 92 832 1426 9

No. 13
Health, Solar UV Radiation and Environmental Change
By A. Kricker, B.K. Armstrong, M.E. Jones and R.C. Burton
1993; 213 pages; ISBN 92 832 1427 7

*No. 14**
Epidémiologie du cancer dans les pays de langue latine
1993; 400 pages; ISBN 92 832 1428 5

No. 15
Cancer in the African Population of Bulawayo, Zimbabwe, 1963–1977
By M.E.G. Skinner, D.M. Parkin, A.P. Vizcaino and A. Ndhlovu
1993; 120 pages; ISBN 92 832 1429 3

No. 16
Cancer in Thailand 1984–1991
By V. Vatanasapt, N. Martin, H. Sriplung, K. Chindavijak, S. Sontipong, S. Sriamporn, D.M. Parkin and J. Ferlay
1993; 164 pages; ISBN 92 832 1430 7

No. 18
Intervention Trials for Cancer Prevention
By E. Buiatti
1994; reprinted 1996, 52 pages; ISBN 92 832 1432 3

No. 19
Comparability and Quality Control in Cancer Registration
By D.M. Parkin, V.W. Chen, J. Ferlay, J. Galceran, H.H. Storm and S.L. Whelan
1994; revised 1996, 110 pages plus diskette;
ISBN 92 832 1433 1

Comparabilidad y Control de Calidad en los Registros de Cancer
By D.M. Parkin, V.W. Chen, J. Ferlay, J. Galceran, H.H. Storm and S.L. Whelan
1995; 125 pages + diskette
ISBN 92 832 0402 6

Comparabilité et Contrôle de Qualité dans 'Enriegistrement des Cancers
By D.M. Parkin, V.W. Chen, J. Ferlay, J. Galceran, H.H. Storm and S.L. Whelan
1996; 123 pages + diskette
ISBN 92 832 0403 5

No. 20
Epidémiologie du cancer dans les pays de langue latine
1994; 346 pages; ISBN 92 832 1434 X

*No. 21**
ICD Conversion Programs for Cancer
By J. Ferlay
1994; 24 pages plus diskette;
ISBN 92 832 1435 8

*No. 22**
Cancer in Tianjin
By Q.S. Wang, P. Boffetta, M. Kogevinas and D.M. Parkin
1994; 96 pages; ISBN 92 832 1437 4

*No. 23**
An Evaluation Programme for Cancer Preventive Agents
By Bernard W. Stewart
1995; 40 pages; ISBN 92 832 1438 2

No. 24
Peroxisome Proliferation and its Role in Carcinogenesis
1995; 85 pages; ISBN 92 832 1439 0

No. 25
Combined Analysis of Cancer Mortality in Nuclear Workers in Canada, the United Kingdom and the United States of America
By E. Cardis *et al.* 1995; 160 pages;
ISBN 92 832 1440 4

No. 26
Mortalité par Cancer des Immigrés en France, 1979-1985
By C. Bouchardy, M. Khlat, P. Wanner and D.M. Parkin
1998; 150 pages; ISBN 92 832 2404 3

No. 27
The Risk of Cancer in Three Generations of Young Israelis
By J. Iscovich and D.M. Parkin
1998; 92 pages; ISBN 92 832 1441 2

No. 28
Survey of Cancer Registries in the European Union
By H. Storm, I. Clemmensen and R. Black
1998; c. 64 pages; ISBN 92 832 1442 0

No. 29
International Classification of Childhood Cancer 1996
By E. Kramárová, C.A. Stiller, J. Ferlay, D.M. Parkin, G.J. Draper, J. Michaelis, J. Neglia and S. Qureshi
1997; 48 pages + diskette; ISBN 92 832 1443 9

No. 30
Cancer Risk from Occupational Exposure to Wood Dust:
By P. Demers and P. Boffetta
1998; 95 pages; ISBN 92 832 1444 7

No. 31
Histological Groups for Comparative Studies
By D.M. Parkin, K. Shanmugaratnam, L. Sobin, J. Ferlay and S. Whelan
1998; 67 pages + diskette; ISBN 92 832 1145

No. 32
Automated Data Collection in Cancer Registration
By R.J. Black, L. Simonato and H. Storm
1998; 52 pages; ISBN 92 832 1146 3 US$ 26

No. 33
European Multicentre Case-Control Study of Lung Cancer in Non-smokers
By P. Boffetta et al. 1998; 340 pages; ISBN 92 832 2405 1

IARC CancerBases
ISSN 1027 5614

No. 1
EUCAN90: Cancer in the European Union (Electronic Database with Graphic Display)
By J. Ferlay, R.J. Black, P. Pisani, M.T. Valdivieso and D.M. Parkin
1996; Computer software on 3.5" IBM diskette + user's guide (50 pages); ISBN 92 832 1450 1

No. 2
CIVII: Electronic Database of Cancer Incidence in Five Continents Vol. VII
By J. Ferlay
1997; Computer software on 3.5" IBM diskettes + user's guide (63 pages); ISBN 92 832 1449 8

No. 3
Globocan 1: Cancer Incidence and Mortality Worldwide
By J. Ferlay, D.M. Parkin & P. Pisani
1998; CD Rom

IARC Handbooks of Cancer Prevention
ISSN 1027 5622

Volume 1
Non-Steroidal Anti-Inflammatory Drugs
1997; 202 pages
ISBN 92 832 3001 9

Volume 2
Carotenoids
1998; 326 pages
ISBN 92 832 3002 7

Volume 3
Vitamin A
1998; c. 260 pages
ISBN 92 832 3003 5

IARC Non-Serial Publications

Alcool et Cancer
By A. Tuyns
1978; 48 pages

Cancer Morbidity and Causes of Death among Danish Brewery Workers
By O.M. Jensen
1980; 143 pages;1SBN 92 832 1403 X

Directory of Computer Systems Used in Cancer Registries*
By H.R. Menck and D.M. Parkin
1986; 236 pages

Facts and Figures of Cancer in the European Community
By J. Estève, A. Kricker, J. Ferlay and D.M. Parkin
1993; 52 pages; ISBN 92 832 1427

Cancer Epidemiology: Principles and Methods
By I. dos Santos Silva
Publications due November 1998, c. 400 pages; ISBN 92 832 0405 0
Also to be published in Spanish and French

Pathology and Genetics of Tumours of the Nervous System
Edited by P. Kleihues and W.K. Cavanee
1997; 255 pages; ISBN 92 832 1148 X US$ 85

All IARC Publications are available directly from
IARCPress, 150 Cours Albert Thomas, F-69372 Lyon cedex 08, France (Fax: +33 4 72 73 83 02; E-mail:press@iarc.fr).

IARC Monographs and Technical Reports are also available from the
World Health Organization Distribution and Sales, CH-1211 Geneva 27 (Fax: +41 22 791 4857) and from WHO Sales Agents worldwide.

IARC Scientific Publications, IARC Handbooks and IARC CancerBases are also available from
Oxford University Press, Walton Street, Oxford, UK OX2 6DP (Fax: +44 1865 267782).